MEASURING HEALTH

Second Edition

MEASURING HEALTH

A REVIEW OF
QUALITY OF LIFE
MEASUREMENT
SCALES

Second Edition

Ann Bowling

Open University Press
Buckingham · Philadelphia

Open University Press
Celtic Court
22 Ballmoor
Buckingham
MK18 1XW

email: enquiries@openup.co.uk
world wide web: http://www.openup.co.uk

and
325 Chestnut Street
Philadelphia, PA 19106, USA

First published 1991
Reprinted 1992, 1993, 1994, 1995
First published in this second edition 1997
Reprinted in this second edition 1998, 1999

ISBN 0-335-19754 X (pbk)   0-335-19755 8 (hbk)

Library of Congress Cataloging-in-Publication Data

Bowling, Ann.
    Measuring health : a review of quality of life
measurement scales / Ann Bowling. – 2nd ed.
        p.   cm.
    Includes bibliographical references and index.
    ISBN 0-335-19754-X (pb). – ISBN 0-335-19755-8 (hb)
    1. Health status indicators.   2. Quality of
life.   I. Title. [DNLM: 1. Health Status
Indicators.   2. Quality of Life.   3. Relative
Value Scales.   WA 900.1 8787m 1997]
RA407.B69   1997
613'.028'7—dc21
DNLM/DLC
for Library of Congress   96-50373
                                            CIP

Typeset by Type Study, Scarborough
Printed in Great Britain by St Edmundsbury Press,
Bury St Edmunds, Suffolk

CONTENTS

6 MEASURING SOCIAL NETWORKS AND SOCIAL SUPPORT

7 MEASURES OF LIFE SATISFACTION AND MORALE

PREFACE TO
REVISED EDITION

Since the first edition of *Measuring Health* was published in 1991, the emphasis on patient-based evaluation of health care has increased, and there have been several rapid developments in relation to the measurement of health status and health-related quality of life. The most well known of these is the international testing and use of the Short Form-36 (SF-36). A review of this scale has been included in this new edition of *Measuring Health*, along with the recently developed shorter version (the SF-12) and several other new inclusions (such as the Dartmouth COOP Function Charts, Sense of Coherence Scale, the second version of the Arthritis Impact Measurement Scales, the Social Support Scale (from the Rand Medical Outcomes Study), the Network Assessment Instrument, and the Rand Depression Screener). In addition, previous reviews have been updated in cases where relevant literature has been published. Overlap with the author's *Measuring Disease, A Review of Disease Specific Quality of Life Measurement Scales* (1995a) has been kept to a minimum, but is inevitable for a few scales which have both a widespread disease specific and generic or domain specific use.

While this volume includes a wide selection of popularly used generic and domain specific measurement scales, there are inevitable omissions. For example, scales of stress and coping ability have been omitted (some adjustment and coping scales were reviewed in *Measuring Disease*). This is a complex area and interested readers are referred to Kasl and Cooper (1987) and Maes *et al.* (1987).

Copyright permission was sought to reproduce the items from the scales reproduced in this volume, and the author is grateful to the scale developers and distributors for their consent. Some scales are too long to reproduce in full here, and others are strictly copyrighted and only available commercially (which prevents reproduction of full scales). It was, as before, decided to aim for consistency and only reproduce a selection of scale items as examples. Potential users are advised to consult the authors of scales (where a contact address has been given) before use in order to avoid copyright infringement. Informed use also assists authors of scale to compile bibliographies of users and results, and handbooks or user guides may be available. A selection of useful addresses has been incorporated at the end of this revised volume in order to assist readers. Where a contact address has not been given for a particular scale, it is usually because there is no current contact for that scale, and readers should consult the references to the scale for further details. Where no address has been given for a scale, the scale has usually been reproduced in full in one of the key publications listed in the references (e.g. many of the social support scales have been reproduced in this way). The current addresses of scale developers and distributors are not always easy to trace, and I would like to repeat a plea made by Wilkin *et al.* (1992), and emphasized in the preface to *Measuring Disease*, that authors should be encouraged to publish their scales in full in key journal publications or, where copyright, length or commercial reasons prevent this, to, at minimum, publish the address of the scale distributor. Finally, as before, section summaries recommending a 'best buy' have not been included as each scale has its strengths and weaknesses, most scales are being continually developed or tested, and ultimately the choice of which scale to use is dependent on the aims of the study, its population type and the judgement of the investigators. While a number of the scales have not been subjected to full or adequate psychometric testing, their developers are still to be commended for their efforts, given that such testing can be expensive and take many years. Investigators are encouraged to include routine tests for reliability and validity in order to develop the knowledge bases of the scales they have selected.

ACKNOWLEDGEMENTS

I would like to thank Dr Robert Edelmann for his valuable advice and comments, and Jenny Stanley and Lesley Marriott for their help in collating the references.

LIST OF
ABBREVIATIONS

ABS	Affect–Balance Scale	ICD	International Classification of Diseases
ADL	Activities of Daily Living		
AIMS	Arthritis Impact Measurement Scales	ISEL	Interpersonal Support Evaluation List
AMTS	Abbreviated Mental Test Score		
APA	American Psychiatric Association	ISSB	Inventory of Socially Supportive Behaviours
ASSIS	Arizona Social Support Interview Schedule		
		ISSI	Interview Schedule for Social Interaction
BDI	Beck Depression Inventory		
CAPE	Clifton Assessment Procedures for the Elderly	LASA	Linear Analogue Self Assessment
		LSIA	Life Satisfaction Index A
CMI	Cornell Medical Index	LSIB	Life Satisfaction Index B
CRBRS	Crichton Royal Behaviour Rating Scale	LSIZ	Life Satisfaction Index Z
		MHIQ	McMaster Health Index Questionnaire
D–TFS	Delighted–Terrible Faces Scale		
DSM	Diagnostic and Statistical Manual	MOS	Medical Outcomes Study (Rand)
FAI	Functional Assessment Inventory	MPQ	McGill Pain Questionnaire
FIM+FAM	Functional Independence Measure and Functional Assessment	MSQ	Mental Status Questionnaire
		NHP	Nottingham Health Profile
FLP	Functional Limitations Profile	OARS	Older Americans' Resources and Services Schedule
FRI	Family Relationship Index		
GHQ	General Health Questionnaire	QL	(Spitzer) Quality of Life Index
GMS	Geriatric Mental State	QWBS	Quality of Well-Being Scale
GWBS	(Psychological) General Well-Being Schedule	SAD	Symptoms of Anxiety and Depression Scale
		SEIQOL	Schedule for the Evaluation of Individual Quality of Life
HAD	Hospital Anxiety and Depression Scale		
HAQ	(Stanford Arthritis Center) Health Assessment Questionnaire	SF–36	Short Form-36
		SF–12	Short Form-12
HIS	Health Insurance Study (Rand)	SIP	Sickness Impact Profile
HSQ-12	Health Status Questionnaire-12	SNS	Social Network Scale
IADL	Instrumental Activities of Daily Living	SOC	Sense of Coherence Scale
		SS-A	Social Support Appraisals Scale

SS-B	Social Support Behaviours Scale	WHOQOL	World Health Organization Quality of Life Group
VAS	Visual Analogue Scale	WONCA	World Organization of Family Doctors
WHO	World Health Organization		

1

THE CONCEPTUALIZATION OF FUNCTIONING, HEALTH AND QUALITY OF LIFE

Clinicians and researchers interested in health care are increasingly focusing their attention on the measurement of health outcomes, or consequences, of care. The conceptualization and measurement of outcomes are controversial. There is now recognition that meaningful measures of health-related quality of life should be used to evaluate health-care interventions. Most existing indicators reflect a 'disease' model. The 'disease' model is a medical conception of pathological abnormality which is indicated by signs and symptoms. A person's 'ill health' is indicated by feelings of pain and discomfort or perceptions of change in usual functioning and feeling. Illnesses can be the result of pathological abnormality, but not necessarily so. A person can feel ill without medical science being able to detect disease. Measures of health status need to take both concepts into account. What matters in the 20th century is how the patient feels, rather than how doctors think they ought to feel on the basis of clinical measurements. Symptom response or survival rates are no longer enough; and, particularly where people are treated for chronic or life-threatening conditions, the therapy has to be evaluated in terms of whether it is more or less likely to lead to an outcome of a life worth living in social and psychological, as well as physical, terms.

MEASURING HEALTH OUTCOME

In order to measure health outcome a measure of health status is required which in turn must be based on a concept of health. The limitations of the widely used negative definition of health as the absence of disease and the World Health Organization's (WHO) 1946 definition of health as total social, psychological and physical well-being have long been recognized (WHO 1958). In the absence of satisfactory definitions of this basic concept how should health outcome be defined? Typical indices of health status in current use in the Western world focus on disease, illness and negative concepts. They include mortality rates and biochemical data (e.g. haemoglobin levels); routinely collected statistics on health-service use; subjective indicators: self- or other-reported morbidity, disability and behavioural data (e.g. smoking, alcohol use, etc.).

Mortality and morbidity indicators used by clinicians

Clinicians ultimately tend to judge the value of a therapy in terms of the five-year-survival period. In the developed world mortality rates are routinely collected; on the other hand, mortality statistics are subject to error and also ignore the living – many health-care programmes and interventions will have little or no impact on mortality rates. Survival time needs to be interpreted more broadly in terms of the impact and consequences of treatment.

The major outcome measures in most clinical trials are mortality and morbidity. Measures of morbidity used by clinicians in assessing outcome commonly focus on results of biochemical tests, observed symptom rates or role performance (e.g. number of days off work, bed disability days). Wilson Barnett (1981) has reviewed research attempting to measure outcome among post-operative cardiac patients. She reported that the most frequently used measures related to mortality rates (length of survival), morbidity (serious complication), physical condition (e.g. exercise testing, cardiac function, angiography), patency of grafts, symptoms (pain, dyspnoea) and return to work. Return to work is one of the most commonly used non-biological indicators of health status. This is of limited value as it is influenced by economic and social opportunities and age.

Service utilization

Another source of data to which there is relatively easy access in the USA and the UK in particular is service-use information. The USA relies heavily on health insurance data for information about service use, the UK relies on routinely collected information from the National Health Service about deaths and discharges from hospital by condition, age and sex. Some information is also available from periodic morbidity surveys in general medical practice. Much of Europe has little tradition of data collection of this type. All routinely collected data about usage is subject to problems of inaccuracy. Also, while hospital readmission rates, length of hospital stay and other indices of service use are frequently used as outcome and morbidity measures, they often reflect the policies of individual clinicians and service provision, and provide no information about the impact of the treatment on the patient's life. Service-use rates also reflect people's illness behaviour – the extent to which they perceive, react to and act upon symptoms of ill health.

Subjective health indicators

More detailed information about health and illness can be collected using surveys. These take the form of either community-based population surveys, which collect data about individuals' self-reports of illness and disability, or studies of clinic populations based on patient-, and sometimes physician-assessed, morbidity.

An example of a physician-assessed morbidity-rating scale is the Olsson Health Scale which was developed using New York Heart Association gradings which range from 'dead' to 'alive' with various complications, to 'alive' with I to IV grades of activity limitation (Olsson *et al.* 1986). The classifications give no indication of the effects of the condition on specific areas of physical, economic, psychological, social and domestic functioning. This also provides an example of how, in relation to the assessment of morbidity, health is generally conceptualized as being at one extreme of a continuum, generally defined negatively as the absence of symptoms, and with death at the other. There are differing views as to the gradations that may exist between 'perfect health' and 'death'. For example, Dorn (1955) represents the health spectrum as perfect health at one end, passing through conditions predisposing to disease (e.g. obesity), latent or incipient disease, early apparent disease, far advanced disease and then to death. The problem with such frameworks is that each stage is blurred as a disease may or may not manifest itself for a period of time and may or may not be recognized by the individual or presented to, and diagnosed by, a doctor. Moreover, in passing along the continuum, the point at which a state of health no longer exists is unknown.

A more positive model is a scale of feeling, or well-being. Merrell and Reed (1949) proposed a graded scale of health from positive to negative health:

> On such a scale people would be classified from those who are in top-notch condition with abundant energy, through to people who are well, to fairly well, down to people who are feeling rather poorly, and finally to the definitely ill. The word health rather than illness is chosen deliberately to emphasise the positive side of this scale, for in the past we have focussed our attention thoroughly on the disease side.

The authors criticize scales which range from 'no reported illness' to 'hospitalization' or 'confinement to bed' as they do not break down the title 'no reported illness' into different degrees of positive health and well-being. Classifications along continuums, whether negative or positive in orientation, appear relatively crude. They are reflective of the underdeveloped state of measures of health outcome.

Routine information about illness, obtained from individuals responding to large community samples, has been collected annually by government interview surveys in the USA since 1956, in Britain since 1971, and in Finland since 1964. There is also an increasing number of *ad hoc* surveys carried out by research organizations, university and health departments.

Routine government health surveys typically report on the incidence of acute illness and injuries requiring either medical attention or restriction of daily activity; number of days of restricted activity and activity limitation resulting from various diseases and conditions; absence from work or school; self-reported chronic diseases and impairments; and discharges from hospital. Some also include symptom check-lists. Early methodologies concentrated on the collection of morbidity data, reflecting a disease model. More recent studies also reflect this model but are also more likely to encompass a behavioural approach – e.g. the annual British General Household Survey often includes questions on behaviour such as alcohol and tobacco use.

There are multiple influences upon patient outcome, and these require a broad model of health. The non-biological factors which can affect recovery and outcome include patient psychology, motivation and adherence to therapy-coping strategies, socioeconomic status, availability of health care, social support networks and individual and cultural beliefs and behaviours. Outcome should thus also be measured more comprehensively in relation to people's value systems. More recently developed 'subjective health indicators' reflect these non-biological inputs. They are also recognized in research on health behaviour, for example the health-belief model refers to people's perceptions of the severity of an illness, their susceptibility to it, and the costs and benefits incurred in following a particular course of action (Becker 1974).

Health has been operationalized in most survey and broader clinical outcomes research in terms of self-reported health status and, perhaps most commonly, by functional ability. The following sections examine the concepts of functional ability and status, followed by the broader concepts of positive health, social health, and quality of life.

THE CONCEPT OF FUNCTIONAL ABILITY

One of the most common methods of assessing outcome of care in a broader sense is in terms of people's ability to perform tasks of daily living. Disability measures are more meaningful to people's lives than objective biochemical measures or measures of timed walking or grip strength.

The terms 'impairment', 'disability' and 'handicap' are often erroneously used interchangeably. The increasing use of the concept of functional dependency has recently added to the confusion. The distinctions between these concepts first requires clarification. The World Health Organization's (1980) *International Classification of Impairments, Disabilities and Handicaps* provides a consistent terminology and a classification system. This defines the terms 'impairment', 'disability' and 'handicap' and links them together conceptually:

Disease or Disorder $\rightarrow$ Impairment $\rightarrow$ Disability $\rightarrow$ Handicap

e.g.:

Blindness	$\rightarrow$ Vision	$\rightarrow$ Seeing	$\rightarrow$ Orientation
Rheumatism	$\rightarrow$ Skeletal	$\rightarrow$ Walking	$\rightarrow$ Mobility

Impairment is defined as: 'In the context of health experience, an impairment is any loss or abnormality of psychological, physiological or anatomical structure or function.' It represents deviation from some norm in the individual's biomedical status. While impairment is concerned with biological function, disability is concerned with activities expected of the person or the body.

Disability is defined as 'In the context of health experience, a disability is any restriction or lack (resulting from an impairment) of ability to perform an activity in the manner or within the range considered normal for a human being.'

Functional handicap represents the social consequences of impairments or disabilities. It is thus a social phenomenon and a relative concept. The attitudes and values of the non-handicapped play a major part in defining a handicap. It is defined as:

In the context of health experience, a handicap is a disadvantage for a given individual, resulting from an impairment or a disability, that limits or prevents the fulfilment of a role that is normal (depending on age, sex and social and cultural factors) for that individual.

These constitute working definitions of impairment, disability and handicap. A working definition, as distinct from an operational definition, must be precise enough to suggest the content of the indicators but must not be so precise that it cannot be generalized to a variety of contexts. Operational definitions, in contrast, are usually specific to a particular measurement instrument and even to a particular type of study. They define the specific behaviours and the ways in which they are to be classified.

These concepts lead to the concept of dependency on other people or service providers. Impairment and disability may or may not lead to dependency in the same way they lead to handicap. As with the concept of handicap, functional 'dependency' is a social consequence – societal attitudes decide on its definition and existence. Wilkin (1987) defined dependency as 'A state in which an individual is reliant upon other(s) for assistance in meeting recognized needs.'

In summary, impairment and disability may lead to dependency in the same way they lead to handicap. However, they cannot be equated with dependency, nor is there a necessary relationship.

Working definitions are limited to specific contexts which, in the case of dependency, means that they tend to deal with particular types of dependency, for example, the type of help necessary for survival that has to be obtained from others.

Operational definitions, on the whole, concentrate upon activities of daily living, often subdivided into domestic and self-care activities. Thus the operational definition of dependency is failure to perform certain specified activities independently to a pre-defined standard.

Functional status

On the basis of the previous definitions, functional status can be defined as the degree to which an individual is able to perform socially allocated roles free of physically (or mentally in the case of mental illness) related limitations.

There is a clear distinction from general health status. Functional status is directly related to the ability to perform social roles, which a measure of general health need not take into account. Functional status is just one component of health – it is a measure of the effects of disease rather than the disease itself.

THE CONCEPT OF POSITIVE HEALTH

Health is usually referred to negatively as the absence of disease, illness and sickness. All measures of health status take health as a baseline and then measure deviations away from this. They are really measuring ill health. It is easier to measure departures from health rather than to find indices of health itself. When studying severely ill populations, the best strategy may be to employ measures of negative health status. However, only approximately 15 per cent of a general population in a Western society will have chronic physical limitations, and some 10–20 per cent will have substantial psychiatric impairment (Stewart *et al.* 1978; Ware *et al.* 1979). Thus reliance on a negative definition of health provides little information about the health of the remaining 80–90 per cent of general populations. A positive conception of health is difficult to measure because of the lack of agreement over its definition. Clinical judgements focus upon the absence of disease; lay people may hold a variety of concepts such as the ability to carry out normal everyday tasks, feeling strong, good, fit and so on. Without an operational definition it is not possible to determine if and when a state of health has been achieved by a population.

The WHO has recommended the development of measures of positive health (Scottish Health Education Group 1984). In its 1946 constitution (WHO 1958), the WHO specified that 'Health is a state of complete physical, mental and social well-being and not merely the absence of disease and infirmity.' No conceptual or operational definitions were provided. Despite the controversy provoked by this utopian definition, it has generated a new focus on a broader, more positive concept of health, rather than a narrow, negative (disease-based) focus (Seedhouse 1986). The World

Health Organization's (1985) ideal of *Health for all by the Year 2000* and the *Ottawa Charter for Health Promotion* (1986) with its emphasis on assisting the individual to increase control over and improve health, both employ broader definitions of health than those traditionally employed. They highlight the inadequacy of existing negative concepts of health (Thuriaux 1988).

There is now broad agreement that the concept of positive health is more than the mere absence of disease or disability and implies 'completeness' and 'full functioning' or 'efficiency' of mind and body and social adjustment. Beyond this there is no one accepted definition. Positive health could be described as the ability to cope with stressful situations, the maintenance of a strong social-support system, integration in the community, high morale and life satisfaction, psychological well-being, and even levels of physical fitness as well as physical health (Lamb *et al.* 1988). It is composed of distinct components that must be measured and interpreted separately.

Partly confusing conceptual issues further are the other related multi-faceted concepts such as 'social well-being' or 'social health' and 'quality of life', which are components of a broad concept of positive health.

THE CONCEPT OF SOCIAL HEALTH

Donald *et al.* (1978) have called a broader view of health than the reporting of symptoms, illness and functional ability 'social health'. Social health was viewed as a dimension of individual well-being distinct from both physical and mental health. They conceptualized social health both as a component of health-status outcomes (as a dependent variable) and, following Caplan (1974) and Cassel (1976):

in terms of social support systems that might intervene and modify the effect of the environment and life stress events on physical and mental health (as an intervening variable). Measurement of social health focuses on the individual and is defined in terms of interpersonal interactions (e.g. visits with friends) and social participation (e.g.

membership in clubs). Both objective and subjective constructs (e.g. number of friends and a rating of how well one is getting along, respectively) are included in this definition.

(Donald *et al.* 1978)

The authors attempted to measure social health, or social well-being as they also sometimes called it, in the Rand Health Insurance Study.

Other authors have also conceptualized social health as a separate component of health status, defining it in terms of the degree to which people function adequately as members of the community (Renne 1974; Greenblatt 1975). Lerner (1973) noted that health status may be a function of non-health factors external to the individual, such as the environment, the community and significant social groups. He recommended that social well-being measures focus on constructs such as role-related coping, family health and social participation. He hypothesized that socially healthy persons would be more able to cope successfully with day-to-day challenges arising from performance of major social roles; would live in families that are more stable, integrated and cohesive; would be more likely to participate in community activities; and would be more likely to conform to societal norms. In relation to psychiatric illness, Leighton (1959) has described how individual personalities can be influenced by the quality and quantity of interpersonal relationships. Lack of social integration may produce psychological stress and decrease the individual's resources for dealing with it, possibly resulting in psychiatric disorders. Lack of social support has also been implicated in poor outcome of depressive illness (George *et al.* 1989).

Social support can thus be regarded as a key concept in theory and research on 'social health'. Kaplan (1975) outlined several areas of social support, including work achievements and position in the hierarchy; family support, social activity and friendships; financial adequacy; personal life (e.g. existence of a confidante); personal achievements and philosophy and sexual satisfaction. In sum, studies of social health tend to focus on the individual, rather than on the community and the concept is used as a dimension of another imprecisely defined term: 'quality of life'.

THE CONCEPT OF QUALITY OF LIFE

In general terms quality can be defined as a grade of 'goodness'. Quality of life in relation to health is a broader concept than personal health status and also takes social well-being, as described above, into account. There is no consensus over a definition of quality of life. The literature covers a range of components: functional ability including role functioning (e.g. domestic, return to work), the degree and quality of social and community interaction, psychological well-being, somatic sensation (e.g. pain) and life satisfaction. It is becoming fashionable to equate all non-clinical data with 'quality of life' which is likely to be a source of conceptual confusion. Health and functional status are just two dimensions of health-related quality of life.

There is little empirical research attempting to define those qualities which make life and survival valuable. Mendola and Pelligrini (1979) have defined quality of life as 'the individual's achievement of a satisfactory social situation within the limits of perceived physical capacity'. This is a fairly limited definition and no more easy to operationalize than more complex definitions. Shin and Johnson (1978) have suggested that quality of life consists of 'the possession of resources necessary to the satisfaction of individual needs, wants and desires, participation in activities enabling personal development and self actualization and satisfactory comparison between oneself and others', all of which are dependent on previous experience and knowledge. Patterson (1975) approached this differently by identifying certain characteristics deemed essential to any evaluation of quality of life. These included general health, performance status, general comfort, emotional status and economic status, all of which are contributory to the proposition made by Shin and Johnson. Basically, quality of life is recognized as a concept representing individual responses to the physical, mental and social effects of illness on daily living which influence the extent to which personal satisfaction with life circumstances can be achieved. It encompasses more than adequate physical well-being, it includes perceptions of well-being, a basic level of satisfaction and a general sense of self-worth. The wide range of definitions of quality of life, and their inconsistent structures, has been reviewed by Farquhar (1995a),

and the diverse contributions of sociology (functionalism) and psychology (subjective well-being) to the theoretical foundation of the conceptualization of quality of life have been described by Patrick and Erickson (1993).

There is increasing re-recognition of the importance of another sociological approach – phenomenology – to the study of quality of life (the evaluation of quality of life is dependent on the individual who experiences it) (Ziller 1974; Benner 1985) and attempts are being made to compromise by taking greater account of human meanings within conventional measurement scales (O'Boyle *et al*. 1989; Rosenberg 1995). These approaches were described in the author's *Measuring Disease*. In this vein, the WHOQOL Group (1993), at the World Health Organization, has included in their definition of quality of life, the individual's perception of their position in life in the context of the culture and value systems in which they live and in relation to their goals. Bowling (1995b) carried out a national survey asking people open questions about important areas of life. Respondents prioritized relationships with family/relatives, their health, the health of close others, their finances, followed by social life/leisure activities. Farquhar (1995b) asked a sample of 70 people aged 65+ and 85+ about the quality of their lives, and, confirming Bowling's (1995b) results, respondents freely defined it in relation to relationships, their health, material circumstances and activities. However, in Bowling's study, different areas were subsequently prioritized by respondents in relation to the most important effects of illness on their lives, demonstrating the complexity of the concept, and its measurement. It is an abstract and complex concept comprising diverse areas, all of which contribute to the whole, personal satisfaction and self-esteem.

Studies of quality of life after various therapies have been reviewed by several authors. They have consistently reached the same conclusion that most studies of quality of life are hampered by poor design and inadequate assessment methods. Earlier reviews of clinical trials of treatment also reported that elements of quality of life were mentioned in between 3–50 per cent of studies and measured in fewer than 2–7 per cent (Bardelli and Saracci 1978; McPeek and McPeek 1984; O'Young and McPeek 1987).

Wilson Barnett (1981) in her review of studies of

recovery after cardiac surgery reported that measures purporting to tap quality of life in a social and psychological sense were rarely used. Rarely used measures included activity levels (other than work), compliance with medical advice, social activities (hobbies), financial status, sexual activity and patient satisfaction with the operation. Exceptionally, evaluation criteria used to assess outcome included psychological status (affect, adjustment, self-esteem, perception of health status), resumption of normal life, 'minor' physical problems, patient satisfaction with advice and guidance, and patient understanding of treatment. She concluded that the implication is that more social and psychological measures are needed. Since these reviews, the use of broader outcome measures of health status has escalated, in recognition of the need to assess patients' views of the impact of treatments on their everyday lives. In addition, the design and use of disease specific indicators of quality of life is increasing (see the author's *Measuring Disease*), as well as broader scales which aim to capture the essence of quality of life and health–related quality of life (e.g. Evans and Cope 1994; WHOQOL Group 1995).

QUALITY OF LIFE AS AN OUTCOME MEASURE: WHOSE ASSESSMENT?

Existing global measurement scales of health outcome, aiming to encompass the measurement of 'quality of life' are based on either physicians' or individuals' own assessments.

The question arises about who should measure quality of life. McNeil *et al.*'s (1978; 1981) research shows that doctors, nurses, medical students, volunteers and patients disagreed over treatment of choice for lung cancer and cancer of the larynx. Research indicates wide discrepancies between patients' and doctors' ratings of outcome after specific therapies (Orth-Gomer *et al.* 1979; Thomas and Lyttle 1980; Jachuck *et al.* 1982). There are also studies reporting wide discrepancies between patients and doctors in relation to preferences for treatments (Liddle *et al.* 1993; Schneiderman *et al.* 1993).

Slevin *et al.* (1988) attempted to determine whether assessments of quality of life of cancer patients by health professionals are meaningful and reliable by analysing the associations between professionals' and patients' assessments. The instruments used were the Karnofsky Performance Index, the Spitzer Quality of Life Index, the Hospital Anxiety and Depression Scale and a series of linear analogue self-assessment scales. The wide discrepancies between doctors' and patients' assessments led the authors to conclude that doctors could not adequately measure the patients' quality of life. The implication is that measures of outcome should take account of individuals' self-assessments. While a number of self-rating scales exist and will be reviewed in the following chapters, few indicators attempt to measure patients' perceptions of improvement or satisfaction with level of performance; yet it is this element which is largely responsible for predicting whether individuals seek care, accept treatment and consider themselves to be well and 'recovered'.

MEASURES OF HEALTH STATUS IN RELATION TO QUALITY OF LIFE

Developments in measures of health status have been largely confined to the USA and the UK. An evaluation of the 32 European member states of the WHO (Thuriaux 1988) reported that attempts at quantitative measurement of health status were only mentioned in two countries; and data on the measurement of freedom from disability such as independence in activities of daily living, the proportion of disabled people in employment or measures of temporary or long-term disability, were provided by only five member states. Information generally available was largely limited to indicators such as overall tobacco and cigarette consumption from trade sources, and proportions of low-birthweight babies. This situation is rapidly changing with the development of international, collaborative research groups who aim to test health-status measures for international application, e.g. the International Quality of Life Assessment Project (Aaronson *et al.* 1992) and the Short Form-36 collaborative project (Ware *et al.* 1993).

Whilst a plethora of quantitative tools exist which operationalize and attempt to measure aspects of quality of life which are regarded as pertinent to health status, such as life satisfaction, well-being and morale, functional ability, social interaction, stress and psychiatric disturbance, attempts to combine them into a single tool have been less successful. Most of these attempts have been made in the USA, generally producing diverse, unwieldy and time-consuming scales of measurement. Moreover, the conceptual confusion which surrounds definitions of health in relation to quality of life is reflected in these measurement tools.

During the 1980s, as a result of the increasing focus on health promotion, the search for indicators of positive health had intensified and has again been stimulated by the WHO (Abelin *et al.* 1986; Anderson *et al.* 1989). The WHO's concept of health in social, psychological and physical terms has become accepted to the extent that a measure of health status that fails to incorporate one of these dimensions is subject to negative evaluation (Kaplan 1985). Attempts have been made to measure well-being. One example is the McMaster Health Index Questionnaire (Chambers 1982) which includes questions on general well-being. An index of psychological well-being was developed by Bradburn (1969) and a similar one by Dupuy (1984). These types of scales are gradually being incorporated into studies of health-related quality of life. However, there have been few attempts to encompass perceptions of physical fitness in health-status scales, as opposed to feelings of illness. Progress is sometimes slow due to the differences of opinion between researchers and policy makers with regard to the definition and measurement of health. Researchers are increasingly inclining towards self-ratings of present health; personal evaluation of physical condition; feelings of anxiety, nerves, depression; feelings of general positive affect; and future expectations about health. On the other hand, policy makers may prefer more explicit indicators in their formation of health policy: limitations in activities of daily living; confinement to bed due to ill health; ratings of intensity, duration and frequency of pain (Noack and McQueen 1988).

Whatever perspective is adopted, the reliability and validity of existing measures are still questionable, especially as most were derived from professional conceptions of well-being. Two measures which were derived from interviews with lay people are the Sickness Impact Profile and the Nottingham Health Profile, but these both limited respondents to assessing the effects of illness on behaviour, rather than global conceptualizations of health-related quality of life. The range of available health indicators consists of *ad hoc* measures that may or may not focus on functioning and health-related behaviours, morbidity and perceived health. Many of these measures have serious limitations in terms of reliability, validity and techniques of analysis, although attempts are continuing to refine and develop the most popular scales. The regular publication of bibliographies of health-related quality of life research (e.g. Spilker *et al.* 1990; 1992a; 1992b; Mulder and Sluijs 1993; World Health Organization 1994; Berzon *et al.* 1995) has facilitated easier access to information about the psychometric properties of popular scales.

2

THEORY OF MEASUREMENT

CHOICE OF HEALTH INDICATOR

When deciding on which measure to use, the investigator should assess whether a disease-specific or broad-ranging instrument is required; the type of scoring that the instrument is based on (whether scores can be easily analysed in relation to other variables); the reliability, validity and sensitivity of the scale; the appropriateness of the instrument for the study population; and the acceptability of the instrument to the group under study (Hunt *et al.* 1986). It is also important to decide whether the study requires measurement on a nominal-, ordinal-, interval- or ratio-scale level; these terms are explained below.

MEASUREMENT THEORY

Descriptions can be placed on a nominal or an ordinal, interval or ratio scale. The requisite level of measurement depends on the intended applications of the indicator and on the question the researcher is attempting to answer.

With a *nominal* scale, numbers or other symbols are used simply to classify a characteristic or item. This is measurement at its weakest level. For example, functional disability states and perceived health are defined by descriptions and thus a nominal or classification scale is constructed. For the purpose of the comparative evaluation of the outcome of intervention A in comparison with the outcome of intervention B a nominal scale may be sufficient (for example, 'died' or 'survived').

Hypotheses can be tested regarding the distribution of cases among categories by using the nonparametric test, x^2, and also Fisher's exact probability test. The most common measure of association (correlation) for nominal data is the contingency coefficient.

An *ordinal* (or ranking) scale is applicable where objects in one category of a scale are not simply different from objects in other categories of that scale, but they stand in some kind of relation to them. For example, typical relations may be higher than, more preferred, more difficult (in effect, greater than). This is an ordinal scale. Many disability and health-status measures are strictly of this type.

The most appropriate statistic for describing the central tendency of scores in an ordinal scale is the median, since the median is not affected by changes of any scores above or below it as long as the number of scores above and below remain the same. Hypotheses can be tested using nonparametric statistics such as correlation coefficients based on rankings (e.g. Spearman r or the Kendall r). An ordinal scale is sufficient only for answering basic questions such as 'How does X compare with Y?'

An *interval* scale is obtained when a scale has all the characteristics of an ordinal scale, and when in addition the distances between any two numbers on the scale are of known size. Measurement considerably stronger than ordinality has thus been achieved. An interval scale is characterized by a common and constant unit of measurement which assigns a real number, but the zero point and unit of measurement are arbitrary (e.g. temperature – two scales are commonly used as the zero point differs on each and is arbitrary).

The interval scale is a truly quantitative scale and all the common parametric statistics (means, standard deviations, Pearson correlations, etc.) are applicable as are the common statistical tests of significance (t test, F test, etc.). Parametric tests should be used as nonparametric methods would not usually take advantage of all information contained in the research data. Interval scales are appropriate if the question is 'How different is X to Y?'

The *ratio* scale exists when a scale has all the characteristics of an interval scale and in addition has a true zero point as its origin. The ratio of any two scale points is independent of the unit of measurement. Weight is one example. Any statistical test is usable when ratio measurement has been achieved. Ratio scales are needed if the question is: 'Proportionately how different is X to Y?'

The most rigorous methods of data analysis require quantitative data. Whenever possible, measures which yield interval or ratio data should be used, although this is often difficult in social science. Measures of functional disability and health status never strictly reach a ratio- or interval-scale of measurement. However, methods of data transformation do exist which permit even nominal data to be made quantitative for purposes of analysis.

MEASUREMENT PROBLEMS

Measurement problems are rife when attempting to measure health outcomes. Indicators may work well or badly and are usually assessed by tests of validity and reliability.

Authors of the various measures often make claims for reliability and validity based on achieved coefficients without any reference to acceptable levels. Suggestions for acceptable levels for reliability and validity range from 0.85 to 0.94, although often 0.50 is regarded as acceptable for correlation coefficients (Ware *et al*. 1980). A full discussion of the problems of achieving reliability and validity can be found in Streiner and Norman (1989).

Validity

Validity is concerned with whether the indicator actually does measure the underlying attribute or not. One of the most problematic aspects of assessing validity is the varying terminology. Textbooks have tended to focus on content validity, criterion validity and construct validity. More recently, more different types of validity have emerged. Construct validity has been differentiated into various dimensions such as discriminant validity and convergent validity. However, all types of validity are addressing the same issue of the degree of confidence that can be placed on the inferences drawn from scale scores. These issues have been addressed more fully by Messick (1980) and Streiner and Norman (1989).

The assessment of validity involves assessment against a standard criterion. Because there is no 'gold standard' of health against which health-status indices can be compared, the validation methods commonly used in the behavioural sciences are the assessment of content and construct validity (American Psychological Association 1974). The criteria of validity which should be met in general are:

Content validity

Do the components of the scale/item cover *all* aspects of the attribute to be measured? Does the content of the variable match the name which it has been given? Each item should fall into at least one of the content areas being tapped. If it does not, then the item is not relevant to the scale's objectives, or the list of scale objectives is not comprehensive. The number of items in each area should also reflect its importance to the attribute.

Face validity

This is one form of content validity. Is the indicator, on the face of it, a reasonable one – do the items appear to be measuring the variables they claim to measure? Is the meaning and relevance of the indicator self-evident?

Criterion validity

Can the variable be measured with accuracy? The traditional definition of criterion validity is the correlation of a scale with some other measure of the trait under study, ideally a 'gold standard'. Criterion validity is usually divided into two types: concurrent and predictive validity:

Concurrent validity

This refers to a scale's substitutability and involves the correlation of the new scale with the criterion measure; both scales are administered to subjects at the same time. It is most often used when attempting to develop a replacement scale which is simpler or less expensive to administer than an existing scale.

Predictive validity

Does the measure predict future differences? With predictive validity, the criterion will be unavailable until some future end point.

Construct validity

This type of validity is relevant in more abstract areas such as psychology and sociology where the variable of interest cannot be directly observed. Underlying psychological or sociological factors are referred to as hypothetical constructs. These are the theories which attempt to explain behaviours and attitudes. There is no one single study that can satisfy the criteria for establishing construct validity (or testing constructs), it is an ongoing process. There are many predictions that could be made from one construct. Unlike other types of validity testing, testing for construct validity involves assessing both theory and method simultaneously. The problem is that, if the predictions made on the basis of theory are not confirmed, then the problem could be with the validity of the measure or the validity of the theory. This type of validity is generally divided into convergent and discriminant validity:

Convergent-Discriminant validity

This involves assessing the extent to which the new scale is related to other variables and measures of the same construct to which it should be related. For example, if the theory states that depressed subjects will perceive their level of social support to be lower than non-depressed people, then the scores from scales measuring these two dimensions should be correlated. The interpretation is sometimes problematic with the measurement of similar concepts, as scale scores that correlate too highly may be measuring the same dimension. Convergent validity also requires that a new scale should correlate with other measures of this construct. Thus, while convergent validity requires correlation with related variables, discriminant validity requires that the construct should not correlate with dissimilar variables.

Factor analysis is an increasingly used technique for the assessment of the number of dimensions that underlie a set of variables. If items relate to a single dimension, then the combination of items into a single measure is supported. If the items relate to a number of different dimensions, then refinement of the scale or sub-scale analyses are more appropriate in recognition of this (Harman 1976).

Reliability

An instrument will also require testing for reliability. A measure is judged to be reliable when it consistently produces the same results, particularly when applied to the same subjects at different time periods when there is no evidence of change. The methods of testing for reliability include multiple form, basic tests of internal consistency (for example split-half, item-item correlations and item-total correlations), test-retest, intra-rater and inter-rater agreement, and sensitivity to change. In addition, tests of internal consistency based on statistical models, for example using factor analysis are becoming more widespread (Harman 1976).

Multiple form reliability

This is used where two instruments, which have been developed in parallel, and which measure the same attribute, are administered and the scores on each correlated. A high correlation indicates a reliable test. This overlaps with validity, and results are usually presented in the context of testing for validity.

Internal consistency

Internal consistency involves testing for homogeneity. Correlations between the items in the scale, or within each scale domain, or between the two halves of the scale where the scale can be divided into two equivalent parts (split-half reliability), and correlations between the items and the total score are performed. Cronbach's alpha should be calculated (Cronbach 1951), which is based on the average correlation among the items and the number of items in the instrument (values range from 0 to 1). A low coefficient alpha (e.g. below 0.50) indicates that the item does not come from the same conceptual domain. More detailed information on the appropriate statistical methods to employ, and minimum acceptable values, are given in the author's *Measuring Disease*.

As questions that deliberately tap different dimensions within a scale cannot be expected to necessarily have high item-item or item-total correlations, factor analysis should be used to identify the separate factors (e.g. domains) within the scale. Each item within a factor is judged to be worthy of retention in a scale if its eigenvalue (a measure of its power to explain variation between subjects) exceeds a certain value (usually 1.5).

Test-retest reliability

The test is administered to the same population on two occasions and the results are compared, usually by correlation. The main problem with this is that the first administration may affect responses on the second. There can be problems with interpretation of observed change, given the potential for observer errors with any scale, and the potential for genuine individual change between administration which affects the estimate of reliability.

Intra-rater and Inter-rater agreements

Intra-rater agreement is the reliability of the same rater's scores, of the same subjects, on different occasions. Inter-rater agreement is the concordance of scores achieved by different raters on the same occasion.

Sensitivity to change

Finally, if the study aims to assess outcome or change, then the instrument's responsiveness to change will need to be measured. This involves correlating its scores with other measures which reflect any anticipated changes (e.g. in the case of a depression scale, it will need to be correlated with a structured psychiatric interview and any indicated changes in psychological status between the two methods of assessment compared).

The achievement of standards of validity and reliability requires time and effort. It is a powerful reason for using existing scales.

TYPES OF INSTRUMENTS

Most instruments used in social science rely on self-reporting of feelings, attitudes and behaviour by people in an interview situation or in response to a self-administered questionnaire. Other measurement approaches include the use of records and the observation of behaviour. Each approach has its strengths and limitations. The optimal measurement strategy is to measure the same phenomenon using several different approaches (Webb *et al.* 1966).

SELF-REPORT MEASURES

Self-report measures are essential for much research because of the need to obtain subjective assessments of experiences (e.g. feelings about recovery, level of health and well-being). They have a broad appeal as they are often quick to administer and involve little interpretation by the investigator. Self-report measures may take a variety of forms:

Single-item measures
These are self-report questions which use a single question, rating or item to measure the concept of interest.

Battery
A series of self-report questions, ratings or items used to measure a concept. The responses are not summed or weighted. A battery is like a series of single-item measures, all tapping the same concept.

Scale
A series of self-report questions, ratings or items used to measure a concept. The response categories

of the items are all in the same format, are summed and may be weighted.

Sometimes researchers do not wish to use a long scale, because their questionnaires are already fairly lengthy, and prefer single-item questions. Generally, where questionnaire length permits, scales are preferred because they contain a larger number of items and are suitable for statistical calculations using summed and weighted scores. Single-item measures are least preferable because it is doubtful that one question can effectively tap a given phenomenon and it is also difficult to assess the adequacy of a single-item instrument.

SCALING ITEM RESPONSES

There is a wide variety of scaling methods for item responses. The finer the distinctions that can be made between subjects' responses, the greater the precision of the measure. For example, rather than asking a person to simply agree or disagree with a statement (which yields only two-response (nominal) categories), it is preferable to ask respondents to indicate their opinions along a continuum of agreement: e.g. 'strongly disagree, disagree, no opinion, agree or strongly agree' (Likert 1952). Attitudinal and behavioural issues are not easily dichotomized; they often lie on a continuum. A question about any difficulty in washing oneself can elicit a range of responses from 'no difficulty', to 'slight', 'moderate' or 'severe' difficulty, to 'cannot do this at all'. Offering a wide range of choices is likely to reduce the potential for error due to confusion, although the continuum should not be too great, or meaningless responses will be elicited.

If the aim of the research is to elicit continuous rather than categorical responses, there are several techniques available. One approach is to ask respondents to indicate their replies on a visual analogue scale – for example, a line of 100 mm, with descriptions such as 'very depressed' to 'not at all depressed' at each end. Respondents are asked to place a mark on the line corresponding to their state. There is little evidence that different methods (e.g. categorical response choices or a visual analogue scale) produce different responses and the choice of method is ultimately the investigator's preference.

A common method for developing scales is Thurstone's method. This involves asking respondents to rank statements relating to the variable of interest, which are typed on to cards, into hierarchical order, from the most to the least desirable. The details and scoring systems of this technique are described by Streiner and Norman (1989) and in most psychology and methodology textbooks.

In relation to functional status, many methods exist of scoring or assessing 'function' by scaling, whereby a set of items can be put in a hierarchy of severity. The notion is that patients who can perform a particular task will be able to perform all tasks more easily. Conversely, if they cannot perform a particular task, they will be unable to perform tasks rated as higher. Guttman's (1944) scaling of disability was one of the earliest attempts in this field. He ranked degrees of patient disability in respect of a number of activities, such as feeding, continence, ambulation, dressing and bathing. This method assumes that disabilities can be ordered. Provided that disability progressed steadily from one activity to another (i.e. patients first have difficulty in bathing, then in bathing and dressing, and so on until they are disabled in respect of all five activities), this method of scaling yields a single rating from 1 (no disability) to 6 (disabled on all five). For example, four disabilities always score worse than three, and a score of 6 would assume that all disability items 2–5 had been affirmed. Examples of well-known measures using this scaling method are the Index of Activities of Daily Living (ADL) and the Arthritis Impact Measurement Scales (AIMS). A more recent Guttman scaling instrument has been developed by Williams et al. (1976). The activities which make up the scale are not comprehensive in terms of describing activities of daily living. The instrument has the advantage of having two scales, one for men and one for women. Work on developing and refining the scale is continuing. Guttman scaling, although popular, has been criticized for its method of attributing equal weights to item responses. For example, with responses per item ranging from 1 to 6, the higher the score the greater the debility; it cannot be assumed that 6 is six times as bad as 1 (Skinner and Yett 1972).

WEIGHTING SCALE ITEMS

Many scales simply involve summing the item scores, each of which has been given an equal weight. This is the easiest solution to the scale scoring. There is a fundamental problem with this method: some items may be more important to the construct underlying the scale than others and should therefore contribute more to the total score. Summing also erroneously converts what is at best ordinal data into interval levels of measurement when applying statistical techniques. Statistical caution is required.

The problem with many scoring methods, particularly when equal weight for each item is applied, is that a given score can be arrived at in different ways. A person who is cheerful and lucid but unable to walk due to arthritis may achieve the same scale score as someone who is physically mobile but disoriented and withdrawn. While this may be useful for assessments of staff workload, it is not useful in assessing patient outcome in any detail. Scoring may exacerbate the instrument's distortion of the experiences of individuals. The problem may be avoided by treating all aspects of disability and health status as equal contributors to overall severity, and expressing the results for each item separately. The disadvantage of this method is that multiple disabilities are not then evident and this type of breakdown can be cumbersome in analysis. The alternative is to assign different values (weights) to different scale items for scoring purposes. The Normative Scale relies on the classification of items into major or minor categories, e.g. with disability items, 'being able to feed oneself' is given twice the weight of 'being able to dress oneself'. Principal Component Scaling relies on the internal evidence of the data being scaled, thus calculating the relative weights to be given to each item to construct a linear additive index. Numerous health-index questionnaires fall into these categories. The main methods of weighting have been clearly and fully described by Streiner and Norman (1989). The most common is to use a different number of items to measure the various aspects of the trait, proportional to its importance within the construct. The total for any sub-scale would be the number of items with a response of interest divided by the total number of items within the sub-scale. The sub-scale scores can be added together for the scale total. Thus, each sub-scale contributes equally to the scale's total score, even though each may consist of a different number of items.

In practice, however, it is frequently found that weighting items makes little difference to subjects' relative scores, despite the inherent logic of this technique. This is because people who score high on one scale variant often score high on others. Examples of this have been given by Streiner and Norman (1989). On the other hand, weighting items can increase the predictive ability of an index (Perloff and Persons 1988). Streiner and Norman (1989) conclude that when the scale contains at least 40 items, or when the items are fairly homogeneous, then differential weighting contributes little (except complexity in scoring).

UTILITY RATING SCALES

Finally, economists have devised a series of econometric scaling techniques in an attempt to assign a numerical value to a health state. These are known as utility ratings, the most well-known application of these being the quality-adjusted life year (Chiange 1965; Rosser and Watts 1971; Kaplan and Bush 1982). A QALY is a year of full life quality. Poor health may reduce the quality of a year. In QALYs, improvements in the length and quality of life are combined into one single index. Each life year is quality-adjusted with a utility value, where 1 = full health. QALYs are not measures of quality of life but measures of units of benefit from a medical intervention, aiming to reflect the change in survival with a weighting factor for quality of life.

Different types of medical interventions are then compared by calculations of costs per gained QALY (Williams 1985). QALYs can be derived by several different methods (e.g. the Rosser Index of Disability (Rosser and Watts 1972), standard gamble, trade-off and rating scale techniques (Torrance et al. 1972, 1982; Torrance 1986, 1987). These will be only briefly referred to here; interested readers should consult specialist texts for their evaluation (e.g. Torrance 1986; Teeling Smith 1988).

The rating scale

The rating scale is suitable for measuring preferences for chronic or temporary health states. A typical rating scale consists of a line drawn on a page with clearly defined end points such as 'death/least desirable' at one end and 'healthy/most desirable' at the other. The remaining health states are then located on the line between these two in order of their preference, such that the intervals between them correspond to the differences in preference between the health states, as perceived by the respondent. This is the interval-scaling technique. The scale is measured from 0 assigned to the worst health state of the group and 1 assigned to the best. The person is asked to select the best and worst health states from the group and then locate the other states on the scale relative to each other, according to the interval-scaling principle.

The standard gamble

With this technique, people are asked to choose between a gamble, with a desirable outcome, with risk P, and a less desirable outcome, with risk 1-P, and a certain option of intermediate desirability. The person is asked what probability of getting the desirable or less desirable outcome will make him indifferent between the gamble and the certainty.

An example of the standard gamble is to take a person faced with the choice of remaining in a poor state of health versus taking a gamble on treatment that could fully restore health or result in death (e.g. surgery for angina). If the probability of restoring full health is varied there will be a point where the person is indifferent between her current poor state of health and taking the gamble of surgery. If the person perceives her poor health state as particularly undesirable, she will be more likely to accept a greater probability of death in order to escape it.

Equivalence

A similar technique is the 'equivalence technique' whereby respondents are asked to identify their point of indifference between keeping alive a group of people in a state of fairly good health and a larger group, whose size is determined by the respondent, of less well people.

Time trade-off

With this method, the technique is to vary the length of time in each health state with treatment choice. For example, the respondent is presented with two alternatives and asked to select the more preferred. Alternative 1 offers the respondent a particular health outcome for a specified length of time fol-

lowed by death, and alternative 2 offers a different outcome for a different length of time. The time is varied until the respondent is indifferent between the two alternatives.

This technique then requires people to judge how long a period in one state of health could be 'traded' for a different period in another state of health. The assumption underlying this concept is that the better their state of health, the shorter period of life people would accept as a 'trade-off' for longer survival in a less desirable state.

All utility scales achieve interval scales. Research has found that people find the trade-off techniques the easiest of the utility measures, the standard gamble has been found to be more difficult for people, and the rating scale the most difficult. One main criticism of these techniques is that disease sufferers probably assign more positive utilities to states of ill health than normal people in hypothetical disease states. Very elderly persons may feel that a frail and painful existence is just as valuable to them as someone else's apparently healthier state.

Such models suffer from several limitations. They have not been adequately tested for validity and reliability, and they rarely ask sufferers themselves to make ratings (Carr-Hill 1989; Carr-Hill and Morris 1991). Judgements are usually made by 'experts' (e.g. doctors, nurses and medical students). They assume that people are rational when assessing quality of life, and that individual value judgements are not interfering with their ratings. It is also difficult to quantify quality of life, which is a multi-dimensional concept, in terms of one figure.

The following chapters present relatively concise reviews of generic health-status measures, and measures of specific domains of broader health-related quality of life. A generic scale is useful when the investigator aims to make comparisons between conditions or diseases; a domain specific scale should be used when the area is of particular interest to the investigator. Some domain specific scales overlap with disease specific scales (e.g. scales of physical functioning and psychological well-being). Disease specific scales are useful when the attributes of particular diseases or conditions require assessment, as they will usually be more relevant to the condition and more sensitive. Disease specific scales were reviewed in the author's *Measuring Disease*.

3

THE MEASUREMENT OF
FUNCTIONAL ABILITY

There are a number of methodological techniques available for measuring function: direct physical tests of function, direct observation of behaviour and interviews with the person concerned or a third party. Each method has its limitations, as has been indicated. Direct observation is rarely used because it is so time consuming. Direct tests of functioning, such as range-of-limb movement, grip strength, walking time or standards such as joint swelling, pain scores, morning stiffness, erythrocyte sedimentation rate and joint counts, while objective, may not necessarily give an accurate indication of ability or performance. Grip strength will tell you how much a patient can and will squeeze a bag on a particular day. Patients may be more concerned with subjective feelings and reductions in activities associated with daily living.

Most measures of functional disability are self-report methods. Respondents are asked to report limitations on their activities. Sometimes researchers do not wish to use a long scale to measure functional status, usually because their questionnaires are already fairly lengthy, and they therefore prefer single-item questions. One well-known example is the British government's annual General Household Survey which limits its measure of functional status to questions such as

Do you have any longstanding illness, disability or infirmity? By longstanding I mean anything that has troubled you over a period of time or that is likely to affect you over a period of time?

(IF YES):

(a) What is the matter with you?
(b) Does this illness or disability limit your activities in any way?
   (Office of Population Censuses and Surveys 1987)

The main criticism of this type of measure is: how limited does a person have to be to answer 'yes'? Subjectivity is involved: people who are short sighted might reply 'yes' or they might not define their condition as a 'longstanding illness, disability or infirmity' or as limiting. Also, people who are used to their conditions and the restrictions they impose may no longer define them as limiting. However, if a measure of perceived health status is required, rather than objective morbidity indicators, then this inherent subjectivity is the strength of the measure.

There are many measures of functional ability. Some measures focus simply on basic functioning (e.g. mobility) but, more commonly, they include items of instrumental, or extended, activities of daily living, which encompass the activities that are required for the maintenance of independence, as well as optimum levels of functioning (e.g. doing laundry, housework, preparing meals).

Only those which are either most well tested for validity and reliability, of current topical interest, are frequently used or are potentially applicable in Europe as well as in the USA, are presented in detail. Other scales which are less well tested, but which are popular or are frequently used, are also presented but in less detail (e.g. the Katz Index of Activities of Daily Living, Barthel Index and the Karnofsky Scale).

There are also several available measures of broader health status which incorporate measures of functional ability. These are discussed in Chapter 4 along with other broad health status measures.

Measures of functional ability – e.g. self-care (e.g. eating, bathing, dressing), mobility and physical activities – are frequently used measures because they are socially relevant and interpretable. However, self-care limitations are rare in a general population – less than 0.5 per cent report limitations in eating, dressing, bathing or using the toilet due to poor health. Thus in studies of the general population these items should be selected sparingly in contrast to studies of the severely ill or very elderly where self-care measures may be more appropriate. Broad measures of function are also likely to miss specific effects of disease and generic measures should be supplemented with highly focused measures of disease impact.

Most measures narrowly focus on a range of mobility, domestic and self-care tasks, often, however, ignoring financial, emotional and social needs which may be equally or more important. Measures of physical functioning and activity limitations do not always provide assessments of functioning in everyday social roles, mental functioning, sexual functioning, pain and comfort. More meaningful aspects of household roles are also largely ignored: for example, the effect of the condition on the time taken to perform chores such as cleaning, cooking, shopping, errands, child-care and other caring roles. Assessments of patients' satisfaction and choice with regard to level of functioning are seldom made. People may prefer to have a strip wash rather than to risk slipping while getting into the bath. On scales of function it is generally assumed that respondents achieving a low score due to immobility necessarily have a poorer quality of life than a patient with a higher score. Thus someone who is wheelchair bound might have a low ADL score, despite the fact s/he may be receiving good-quality social support.

Moreover, most scales have been developed on the basis of professionals' (e.g. doctors') judgements about essential abilities for daily living. Berg *et al.* (1976) asked 150 health workers to assign weight from 0 to 10 for 50 listed abilities or functions; open-ended questions to elicit functions not listed were also used. Serious problems were documented in finding simple and meaningful terms to describe functional loss to many respondents. Respondents assigned the largest average values to ability to use one's mental abilities, to see, to think clearly, to love and be loved, to make decisions for oneself, to live at home, to walk, to maintain contact with family and friends, and to talk. Although the sample was limited to health workers, the results indicate a need to consider lay person's judgements of essential functions and to include these in measures of health outcomes.

The problem of measuring functional disability is compounded by conceptual difficulties and interactive factors. One of the major problems with using a functional index is that different people may react differently to apparently similar levels of physical impairment, depending on their expectations, priorities, goals, social-support networks and so on. Functional disability, like dependency, is a multi-dimensional concept which may relate to physical, mental, cognitive, social, economic or environmental factors (Wilkin 1987). Thus it is an interactive concept – it is not a necessary consequence of impairment but perhaps, for example, of the siting of bathrooms, toilets and other facilities and the necessity for negotiating stairs. In terms of dependency, severity might be a function of the existence of aids or the frequency and timing of help. Perceptions of severity with both disability and dependency will also be influenced by previous history and expectations for the future. Meaning apart, most scales are not sensitive enough as they simply ask respondents whether they have no or some difficulty with a task, or whether they are unable to perform it at all. The problem emerges of how limited does one have to be to answer in the affirmative? More sensitive scales with greater response choices based on degrees of severity require development.

Also there are often differing viewpoints of how people ought to be performing, for instance, on the part of surgeon and patients. The patient may want to walk without aids or limp, whilst the surgeon may regard 'walking with aids and limp' as indicative of a satisfactory outcome.

Finally, caution is needed when deciding on which measures to use. Measures tend to be developed, administered and validated on one of two types of samples – people living in the community or in institutions. The measures are not necessarily interchangeable between samples. The measures must be appropriate for the population type. Many measures have been developed to be optimally suitable for a particular age group and may be inappropriate for use with other age groups.

THE OLDER AMERICANS' RESOURCES AND SERVICES SCHEDULE (OARS): MULTI-DIMENSIONAL FUNCTIONAL ASSESSMENT QUESTIONNAIRE

The OARS Multi-dimensional Functional Assessment Questionnaire was developed in order to measure the level of functioning and need for services of older people. It was developed at Duke University Center for the Study of Ageing and Human Development (Fillenbaum 1978; 1988; Fillenbaum and Smyer 1981). The measure was developed for use with adults aged 55 and over and should be restricted to this age group. Gatz *et al.* (1987) tested OARS on a sample of over 1,000 people aged 26–86 and reported that the global test scores can be misleading when applied to different age groups. It can be used with community or institutional samples. When used with institutionalized samples some questions are omitted, and institution-relevant items are added.

OARS measures five dimensions of personal functioning, including mental impairment. Despite its popularity, little work has been done on the measurement properties of the mental-health scale.

The numerous applications of the OARS during its construction are described in the OARS handbook (Fillenbaum 1978). One of the most well-known studies using the OARS questionnaire was the survey of social support in relation to mortality carried out in Durham, North Carolina (Blazer 1982). This was based on 331 people aged 65 years and over, taken from a wider community sample survey of 997 people. This sub-sample was followed up 30 months after baseline interview which assessed functional status, social support, depressive symptoms, physical-health status and cognitive

functioning, stressful life events and cigarette smoking. Increased mortality risk was found for those with impaired social support and social interaction. The OARS questionnaire has been widely used throughout the USA and has also been used in Australia. Two Spanish translations are available for use with Spanish-speaking people in America.

Administration time is on average 45 minutes but probably takes an hour generally to administer. The main limitation of OARS is its length. A shorter version of OARS is available, known as the Functional Assessment Inventory (FAI), although this still takes approximately 35 minutes to administer. The FAI contains the functional assessment items, but not the detailed service-use items. Interviewer training, which takes two days, is recommended. Its administration is also explained in a manual which can be purchased from the authors. As with most scales, OARS is strictly copyrighted and permission for its use must be obtained from the authors.

Content

The questionnaire consists of two independent sections. Part A assesses functional status in relation to social, economic, mental and physical health, and activities of daily living. Interviewers also make ratings of ability. The responses to the items in each area are summarized on a six-point scale (e.g. level of functioning: 1 = excellent to 6 = totally impaired). These five ratings yield a profile showing concomitant functioning across the five areas. Part B is a services assessment that directs enquiry into 24 generically defined services, determining for each the current use, the extent of use in the past six months, the type of service provider and perceived need. There is also a demographic section. Information is sought from the respondent, proxy interviews are permitted. If sub-questions are included, the total number of items asked is 120. Examples of the items are:

Can you get to places out of walking distance?

2 Without help (can travel alone on buses, taxis, or drive your own car).
1 With some help (need someone to help you or go with you when travelling).

0 Or are you unable to travel unless emergency arrangements are made for a specialized vehicle like an ambulance?
— Not answered.

Can you go shopping for groceries or clothes (assuming subject has transportation)?

2 Without help (taking care of all shopping needs yourself, assuming you had transportation).
1 With some help (need someone to go with you on all shopping trips).
0 Or are you completely unable to go shopping?
— Not answered.

Can you prepare your own meals?

2 Without help (plan and cook full meals yourself).
1 With some help (can prepare some things but unable to cook full meals yourself).
0 Or are you completely unable to prepare any meals?
— Not answered.

Can you do your own housework?

2 Without help (can scrub floors, etc.).
1 With some help (can do light housework but need help with heavy work).
0 Or are you completely unable to do any housework?
— Not answered.

Scoring

There are various methods of aggregation. The 1–6 ratings on each of the five scales may be summed (5: excellent functioning in each area to 30: total overall impairment), although summing is problematic as was indicated earlier. Alternatively, the number of areas of functioning that are impaired can be counted. To do this, it is necessary first to establish which level of functioning indicates impairment. Ratings of 1 and 2 may be combined and compared with ratings of 3–6 (i.e. non-impaired versus impaired) or the contrast may be between ratings of 1–3 and 4–6. Summed over areas, this yields a 6-class system (0 areas of functioning impaired to 5 areas impaired). A more complex classification based on a trichotomized scale (1 + 2/3 + 4/5 + 6) which takes account of both number of areas of impairment and severity of impairment has also been developed; full details are contained in the handbook. It is also possible to examine the responses to each individual question and treat the items as separate units. For clinical purposes it might be important to maintain the distinctions but not for population purposes.

However, a classification based on summed information assumes that areas are equivalent; at present the validity of this assumption has not been established. Consequently a classification system that maintains distinctions between areas may be preferred.

Validity

OARS and the shorter FAI were extensively tested for validity at the various stages of its development (Fillenbaum 1978; Cairl et al. 1983). Both instruments appear to have face and content validity, although discriminant and predictive validity have not yet been adequately tested.

Criterion validity was tested on 33 patients from a family medical practice. Spearman correlation between separate criterion ratings and the economic items was 0.68, 0.67 for mental health, 0.82 for physical health, and 0.89 for self-care ability. On another study of 82 community residents, the Spearmen correlation between independent psychiatrists' ratings and the mental-health items was 0.62, and between physician assistants' ratings and the physical-health items was 0.70. Detailed results for reliability and validity of OARS can be found in Fillenbaum (1978) and Fillenbaum and Smyer (1981), and results for the FAI can be found in Cairl et al. (1983).

Reliability

OARS and the FAI has been extensively tested for reliability. Tests of agreement of the raters' assessments have been carried out involving 11 raters who assessed 30 patients. Intraclass correlations ranged from 0.66 for physical health to 0.87 for self-care. Raters were in complete agreement for 74 per cent of the ratings (Fillenbaum 1978). Reliability ratings of the Community Service Questionnaire gave inter-rater Kendall coefficients of concordance between 0.70 and 0.93. Test-retest reliability, conducted 12–18 months apart, gave correlations of between 0.47 and 1.00. Five-week test-retest correlations based on ratings of 30 elderly people gave results of 0.82 for the physical Activities of Daily Living (ADL) questions, such as personal care, 0.71 for the Instrumental Activities of Daily Living (IADL) questions, such as housework, and 0.79 for the economic resources items. For social resources the correlation was 0.71 and for subjective questions it was 0.53. Coefficients for life satisfaction and mental health were lower: 0.42 and 0.32 respectively.

Although much of the data on reliability and validity refers to previous versions of the instrument, the OARS appears to be a superior measure to most others. It was unhesitatingly recommended by McDowell and Newell (1987) in their review of measures. On the other hand it has been criticized for the excessive number of sub-items and the lengthy period of administration (Perlman 1987).

THE STANFORD ARTHRITIS CENTER HEALTH ASSESSMENT QUESTIONNAIRE (HAQ)

Fries *et al.* (1980) developed the HAQ on the basis that outcome should be measured in terms of the patient's value system. Functional ability (e.g. the ability to walk) is a component of this but sedimentation rate is not. The framework used for the development of the HAQ was based on the belief that a patient desires to be alive, free of pain, functioning normally, experiencing minimal treatment toxicity, and financially solvent. Patient outcome was thus represented by (1) death, (2) discomfort, (3) disability, (4) therapeutic toxicity, (5) dollar cost.

In the process of developing this measure 62 potential questions were selected from questionnaires in use in the rheumatic-diseases field and elsewhere, including the Uniform Database for Rheumatic Diseases (Fries *et al.* 1974; Convery *et al.* 1977); the Barthel Index (Mahoney and Barthel 1965); the ADL (Katz *et al.* 1963). Testing the measure for reliability and validity with patients with rheumatoid arthritis reduced the measure to 21 questions, grouped into nine components, and graded in ordinal fashion from 0 to 3. Individual items with correlations of 0.85 or higher were eliminated in the interests of conciseness, on the assumption that this suggested redundancy between components. Correlations of remaining items range between 0.35 and 0.65 (Fries *et al.* 1980). The resulting instrument was subsequently administered in more than two dozen settings.

The HAQ is suitable for use in community settings and has been administered to patients with rheumatoid and osteo-arthritis, systemic lupus and ankylosing spondylitis.

It is relatively coherent and concise and is self-administered so does not rely on skilled personnel to administer (it is therefore relatively cheap). Administration takes 5–10 minutes and manual scoring can be completed within a minute.

Content

Functional ability is measured by nine components: dressing and grooming, rising, eating, walking, hygiene, reach, grip, outside activity and sexual activity. Each of these components consists of one or more relevant questions. Pain, discomfort, drug toxicity and financial costs are also assessed. Examples of questions are:

Are you able to:
Dress yourself, including tying shoelaces and doing buttons?
Stand up from an armless chair?
Get in and out of bed?
Walk outdoors on flat ground?
Do chores such as vacuuming, housework or light gardening?

The range of answers is, 'without any difficulty; with some difficulty; with much difficulty; unable to do'.

Scoring

In relation to functional ability, the ordinal scoring of 0–3 is based on the following scale: without difficulty = 0, with some difficulty = 1, with much difficulty = 2 and unable to do = 3. The index is calculated by the addition of scores and then dividing the score by the total number of components answered. The authors reported reluctance among patients to report sexual activity (Fries *et al.* 1980), and thus some investigators omit this item (Fitzpatrick *et al.* 1988).

The scales of pain, discomfort and drug toxicity range from 0 to 3. Questions concerning the severity of pain range from none = 0 to severe = 3. The scale for discomfort comprises better = 1, the same = 2 or worse = 3. The drug toxicity index is composed of questions about the adverse effects from drugs and treatment ranging from none = 0 to severe = 3. Initial tests for validity and reliability revealed weak results, and this component requires further testing (Fries *et al.* 1980).

In the personal–cost section (applicable to private health care systems), medical and surgical costs are calculated for the past year. The number and type of medications, X-rays, surgery, physician and paramedical visits, appliances, number of laboratory tests, and hospitalizations are detailed. The average cost in the area covered by the research team (Stanford, California) was determined and used for the computation of the dollar values. This section can be applied only in countries and areas where costs are known. Social costs are calculated by determining changes in employment, income, the need to employ domestic help, the cost of transport for medical care and all arthritis-related costs over the past twelve months (Fries *et al.* 1980). The cost questions have not yet been satisfactorily tested; initial tests for validity suffered from poor patient recall.

Fitzpatrick *et al.* (1989), in their comparison of the HAQ and the Functional Limitation Profile (FLP) (derived from the Sickness Impact Profile), reported that nothing appeared to be achieved in relation to precision by the complex scoring system utilized by the FLP in comparison with the simpler ordinal assumptions of the HAQ.

Validity

It has been extensively validated. Correlations of the HAQ against observed patient performance ranged from fair to high (0.47–0.88) (Fries *et al.* 1980; 1982; Fries 1983; Kirwan and Reeback 1983).

Several studies have tested the validity of the HAQ, in particular by correlation of the results of the HAQ with the Arthritis Impact Measurement Scales (AIMS) (Fries *et al.* 1982; Brown *et al.* 1984). These two instruments were shown to measure the same dimensions of disability; the correlation coefficient reported by Fries *et al.* (1982) was 0.91. Inter-correlations within the three parts of each instrument relating to physical disability, psychological state and pain were high and those across these three dimensions were weak. Patient self-assessed global arthritis scores were also strongly associated with disability score and less strongly to pain. These correlations are consistent with current knowledge within the speciality of rheumatology, that disability is a large component of arthritic patients' concerns.

The HAQ has been reported by Liange *et al.* (1985) to correlate well with other well-tested scales of health status, such as the Sickness Impact Profile (Bergner *et al.* 1981). A study in the UK by Fitzpatrick *et al.* (1988) of 105 patients with rheumatoid arthritis reported high inter-measure correlations between the HAQ, the Functional Limitations Profile (FLP) (Charlton *et al.* 1983), and between observations of grip strength and the articular index (e.g. the correlations between grip strength and the HAQ on two occasions were -0.73 and -0.68). The HAQ appears to be a valid measure of function in rheumatoid arthritis.

Liange *et al.* (1985) have also reported good correlations between the HAQ and other scales of health status and functional ability, including the Sickness Impact Profile (Bergner *et al.* 1981) and the Functional Status Index (Denniston and Jette 1980; Jette 1980). Principal components analysis has shown factor loadings along the first 'disability' component, which explains 65 per cent of the variance, and a second component with positive loadings for fine activities of the upper extremity and negative loadings for weight-bearing actions of the lower extremity, which explains an additional 10 per cent of the variance (Fries *et al.* 1980; 1982). From this, it was inferred that the resulting disability index (an equal weight sum) is well focused and appropriate for measuring overall arthritis severity.

The HAQ was reported in early studies to be sensitive to change (Fries 1983). Fitzpatrick *et al.* (1989), in their UK study, reported that the HAQ performed better than the FLP in relation to specificity and sensitivity (detection of change over time), although at best this can only be said to be moderate. The large standard deviations in the scores of both measures indicated the presence of many 'false positives' for both improvement and deterioration. Further testing is required for its sensitivity.

Reliability

The earliest tests for reliability were reported by Fries *et al.* (1980). In addition to the reporting of mean values, these included correlations of HAQ scores with the results of direct observations by a nurse of patients' performance of 15 household and personal-care tasks, mobility and grip; and of self-administered and interview-based HAQ completion. These early tests were based on just 20 patient volunteers attending a rheumatoid arthritis clinic. The correlations for individual items for self-administration versus interview-administered HAQ range from average (or 'respectable') at 0.56 to excellent 0.85. The corresponding correlations for the disability score was 0.85, indicating good reliability for this component.

The inter-item correlations ranged from average at 0.47 to excellent at 0.88. The weaker items (e.g. reach) were subsequently reworded to minimize variability in responses – e.g. this question originally read 'reach and get down heavy objects'. People's ideas of 'heavy' varied, so respondents are now asked about a standardized item: 'reach and get down a 5lb. bag of sugar which is above your head'. The authors also compared overall questionnaire and evaluator agreement; these agreed exactly on 59 per cent of the responses and were within one point in 93 per cent of cases (the weighted kappa statistic result, using rank disagreement rates, was 0.52, implying 'moderate' agreement).

Fries et al. (1982) reported mean values from a diverse English-speaking community population of 331 respondents suffering from rheumatoid arthritis. The authors also reported the test-retest correlation of 0.98, based on this population. The mean values showed stability on repeat testing. Responses are similar when the instrument is self-completed, administered by a nurse or doctor. Many studies have since replicated or improved upon these correlations indicating excellent levels of reliability (see review by Ramey et al. 1996).

The HAQ is a good measure of function and has been extensively tested for reliability and validity. It is concise, sensitive to change, can be self- or interviewer-administered and is suitable for use in the community. However, it is really only suitable for use with chronically ill patients and the questions relate to negative health. It has been extensively used among clinicians in the USA and UK (Ramey et al. 1992).

THE ARTHRITIS IMPACT MEASUREMENT SCALES (AIMS)

The original version, AIMS1, and the second revised version, AIMS2, were developed by Meenan et al. (1980) and Meenan and Mason (1990). The AIMS was partly adapted from Katz's Index of Activities of Daily Living, the RAND and BUSH scales (Patrick et al. 1973a; Brook et al. 1979a; 1979b; Ware et al. 1979; Bush 1984). This measure aims to assess patient outcome in arthritis and other chronic diseases. It covers physical, social and emotional well-being. AIMS1 was well tested for reliability and validity, it was sensitive to change, and suitable for use in community settings. A shortened version of the AIMS1 was produced which appears to have retained adequate internal consistency, test-retest reliability and concurrent and predictive validity, similar to those achieved with the longer version (Wallston et al. 1989). As with the HAQ, the disadvantages of AIMS are that it is really only suitable for use with chronically ill patients and the questions relate to negative health. AIMS is extensively used in the USA, but less in the UK and Europe. It is self-administered and takes approximately 15 minutes to complete.

Content

AIMS1

The original AIMS1 had 45 multiple choice items, with nine sub-scales. It assesses nine dimensions of health and functional ability: mobility, physical activity (walking, bending, lifting), activities of daily living, dexterity, household activities (management of money, medication, housekeeping), pain, social activity, depression and anxiety. An additional 19 items cover general health, health perceptions and demographic details (e.g. questions, including a visual analogue item, that assess the effect of arthritis, other medical problems and their treatment). Typical questions from the AIMS are:

Do you have to stay indoors most or all of the day because of your health?
Yes/No

Do you have trouble bending, lifting or stooping because of your health?
Yes/No

Can you easily turn a key in a lock?
Yes/No

How much help do you need in getting dressed?
No help at all/only need help in tying shoes/need help in
getting dressed

During the past month, how much of the time have you
enjoyed the things you do?
All of the time/most of the time/a good bit of the time/
some of the time/a little of the time/none of the time?

During the past month, how much of the time have you
felt tense or 'high strung'?
All of the time/most of the time/a good bit of the time/
some of the time/a little of the time/none of the time?

Some items require just yes/no answers and others
are scaled.

Scoring

To achieve the item scores some recoding is required as the questionnaire items are worded and
coded to avoid response bias. The AIMS instrument is composed of 45 items; these are summed
into nine scales. A 'normalization procedure' converts scores into the range of 0–10, with 0 representing good 'health status' and 10 representing
poor 'health status'.

For each scale, the items are listed in Guttman
order so that a respondent indicating disability on
one item will also indicate disability on section
items falling below it. In scoring AIMS Guttman
characteristics are ignored and each item is scored
separately, with higher scores indicating greater
limitation. Most questions refer to problems experienced within the last month. No item weights
are used. A total health-status score can be derived
by adding the values for the six scales: mobility,
physical activity, household activity, dexterity,
pain and depression. The scale is ordinal in type. It
has been described as superior to other applications
of Guttman scaling (McDowell and Newell 1987).

AIMS2

The authors developed AIMS2 in an attempt to
produce a more comprehensive and sensitive version of AIMS1 (Meenan et al. 1992). The revised
AIMS – AIMS2 – is a 78-item questionnaire (instead of the original 45 items of AIMS1), it has
some new items and others have been revised or

deleted. The three new sections evaluate arm function, work and social support. Sections were added
to assess satisfaction with function, attribution of
problems to arthritis, and self-designation of prio-
rity areas for improvement. The first 57 items form
12 scales: mobility level, walking and bending,
hand and finger function, arm function, self-care
tasks, household tasks, social activity, social support, pain from arthritis, work, level of tension and
mood. The remaining items relate to satisfaction
with health status in each of the areas of functioning
measured, functional problems due to arthritis,
prioritization of the three areas in which the respondent would most like to see improvement,
general health perceptions, overall impact of arthritis in each of the areas of functioning measured,
type and duration of arthritis, medication usage,
comorbidity and socio-demographic characteristics (Meenan and Mason 1990; 1994). Most questions refer to problems experienced within the last
month.

Content

Examples of AIMS2:

How often were you in a bed or chair for most or all of the
day?
Did you have trouble doing vigorous activities such as
running, lifting heavy objects, or participating in stre-
nuous sports?
Could you easily button a shirt or blouse?
How often did you get together with friends or relatives?
How often did you have severe pain from your arthritis?
How often were you unable to do any paid work, house-
work or schoolwork?
All days (1)/most days (2)/some days (3)/few days (4)/no
days (5)
How often have you felt tense or strung up?
How often have you been in low or very low spirits?
Always (1)/very often (2)/sometimes (3)/almost never (4)/
never (5)

Scoring

The AIMS2, like AIMS1, is self-administered, and
takes approximately 20 minutes to complete. Items
are listed in Guttman scale order, so that a respondent who indicates a disability on one item
will also indicate disability on section items falling

below it. Unlike the AIMS1 which had a combination of dichotomous 'yes/no' and scaled response categories, the AIMS2 has mainly scaled response choices; examples include: 'All days' (1) to 'no days' (5); 'always' (1) to 'never' (5) or 'very satisfied' (1) to 'very dissatisfied' (5). Scale scores are summed, the range of scores depends on the number of items in the sub-scale. No item weights are used. A 'normalization procedure' converts scores into the range of 0 to 10, with 0 representing good 'health status' and 10 representing poor 'health status' (AIMS1 and AIMS2). The scale is ordinal in type. As mentioned earlier the original AIMS was described as superior to other applications of Guttman scaling (McDowell and Newell 1987).

Validity and reliability of AIMS2

The scaling properties, validity and reliability of the AIMS2 have been reported to be satisfactory with initial tests. Meenan et al. (1992) reported, on the basis of a study of 408 respondents with rheumatoid or osteo-arthritis, that the internal consistency coefficients for the 12 scales were 0.72–0.91 in the rheumatoid arthritis group and 0.74–0.96 in the osteo-arthritis group. Test-retest reliability at two weeks (postal survey) was 0.78–0.94. All within-scale factor analyses produced single factors, except for mobility level in osteo-arthritis (Meenan et al. 1992). The revised scale awaits further testing.

Validity of AIMS1

Most information on the psychometric properties of AIMS comes from the extensive work carried out on the AIMS1 (Meenan and Mason 1990; 1994). Given that items have been revised, deleted and some new items have been included, and given that most responses are now scaled, it is unlikely that the results from AIMS1 apply to AIMS2. The results for the AIMS1 are reported below.

The AIMS1 was extensively tested for reliability and validity (Meenan et al. 1980; 1982; 1984; Meenan 1982; 1985; Brown et al. 1984). AIMS1 was tested for validity on a sample of 625 English-speaking patients with various rheumatic diseases, drawn from 15 different clinical establishments in 10 US states. No major problems with the administration occurred. All nine of the AIMS1 scales were weakly to moderately correlated (all significant) with two physician-derived general standards of health status – the American Rheumatism Association Function Scale: r = between 0.24 and 0.52 and disease status: r = between 0.14 and 0.52). The AIMS1 scales were also correlated with clinical rheumatology standards: walking time, grip strength, joint count, range of motion. The items measuring physical well-being (mobility, physical activity, dexterity, household activities, activities of daily living) were more highly correlated with these physical standards than were the AIMS psychological and social scales (e.g. dexterity correlated highly with grip strength; mobility and physical activity were most strongly related to walking time).

The authors reported that single-scale factor analyses demonstrated that each set of AIMS1 items except household activities loaded strongly on a single factor. This indicated that the group items represented a coherent scale. The nine AIMS1 items were grouped into three discrete factors in relation to health status: physical function, psychological function and pain. More recent developments by its authors include a four-factor and a five-factor model, developed from studies of 360 rheumatoid arthritis patients, on the grounds that these are more likely to reflect the major dimensions of health status and represent a fuller assessment of health status. In the five-factor model, the physical dimension of AIMS1 exhibits separate upper-extremity and lower-extremity components. The fourth factor, primarily represented by the pain scale, reflects the added arthritis symptom measure (Mason et al. 1988).

The sensitivity of the AIMS1 was assessed by comparing it with standard clinical outcome measures (joint counts for tenderness and swelling, grip strength, physician assessments of disease activity and functional class) in a double-blind, multi-centre clinical drug trial based on 161 patients (Meenan et al. 1984). Using AIMS, differences between treatments were found for physical activity, anxiety, depression, pain and the overall impact using the visual analogue scale item. The findings were consistent with other studies of the same treatments and demonstrated that AIMS is sensitive enough to detect clinically meaningful differences in treatment outcomes. It was as sensitive as traditional clinical measures, and also indicated additional differences not detected by standard approaches.

The AIMS1 was used by Weinberger *et al.* (1990) in a study of 439 patients with osteo-arthritis; they reported a strong association between poor self-esteem and a poor AIMS1 score. A study administering the HAQ and the AIMS1 to patients with rheumatoid arthritis demonstrated that the scales measured similar dimensions of health status. The instruments were highly correlated providing further support for the convergent validity of the scale; the analyses supported the existence of three relatively discrete components of health status: pain, physical disability and psychological status (Brown *et al.* 1984).

Reliability of AIMS1

The AIMS1 was tested for reliability on a sample of 625 English-speaking patients with various rheumatic diseases, drawn from 15 different clinical establishments in 10 US states. No major problems with AIMS emerged with comprehension or administration. Coefficients of scalability and reliability on all nine of the AIMS1 scales exceeded 0.60 and 0.90 respectively for all but the household activity scale (this had a reproducibility coefficient of 0.88). The test-retest correlation across all nine scale items was 0.87. These results indicated good internal consistency, strong hierarchical scale properties and test-retest stability. The tests for reliability and validity were repeated on a variety of subjects in different demographic, functional and diagnostic categories. Most reliability coefficients were reported as meeting or exceeding accepted criteria. The pattern of validity correlations for AIMS1 were maintained (Meenan *et al.* 1980; 1982; Meenan 1982; Brown *et al.* 1984).

While cross-cultural results for reliability and validity are generally supported for the AIMS, its original social activity and activities of daily living (ADL) sub-scales, unlike the remaining sub-scales, did not achieve satisfactory levels of reliability and validity in a study of Hispanics, whites of Eastern European origin, and black people in the USA (Coulton *et al.* 1989).

The AIMS1 has been adapted and used to measure and compare health status across chronic disease groups, although its sub-scales were not all able to distinguish between these groups (Brown *et al.* 1984; Meenan 1985). Since its initial development the three-component model AIMS1 has been used in many studies (Kazis *et al.* 1983; 1988; Meenan *et al.* 1984; Mason *et al.* 1988). Its applications have been predominantly in clinical settings (with arthritis and rheumatism patients) as an assessment of outcome after therapy.

In sum, the AIMS has good measurement properties, has been extensively tested for validity, and the identified dimensions explain the majority of illness impact estimated by patients. AIMS2 promises to be a superior instrument. The AIMS scales are strictly copyrighted. A manual is available for the AIMS2 (Meenan and Mason 1990; 1994).

THE INDEX OF ACTIVITIES OF DAILY LIVING (ADL)

One of the best known and oldest of the disability scales is the Activities of Daily Living (ADL) index developed by Katz *et al.* (1963; 1966; 1968; 1970; 1973; Katz and Akpom 1976). They designed the Index of Activities of Daily Living in order to describe, for clinical purposes, the states of elderly patients.

Content

The index consists of a rating form that is completed by a therapist or other observer. In each of the activities assessed the patient is rated by the observer on a three-point scale of independence for each activity. Examples from the evaluation form are:

Bathing
Receives no assistance (gets in and out of tub by self if tub is usual means of bathing) ———
Receives assistance in bathing only one part of the body (such as back of a leg) ———
Receives assistance in bathing more than one part of the body (or not bathed) ———

Dressing
Gets clothes and gets completely dressed without assistance ———
Gets clothes and gets dressed without assistance except for assistance in tying shoes ———

Receives assistance in getting clothes or in getting dressed, or stays partly or completely undressed ———

Continence
Controls urination and bowel movement completely by self ———
Has occasional accidents ———
Supervision helps keep urine or bowel control; catheter is used, or is incontinent ———

Feeding
Feeds self without assistance ———
Feeds self except for getting assistance in cutting meat or buttering bread ———
Receives assistance in feeding or is fed partly or completely by using tubes or intravenous fluids ———

The authors later developed a survey instrument for obtaining health-status data containing questions about the need for and use of health services and attitudes towards medical care. Five categories of 'need' were defined and ranked: no disability, restricted activity with no chronic conditions, restricted activity with chronic condition, mobility limitations and bed disability. These were chosen to permit comparisons with existing national surveys (Katz *et al.* 1973).

Scoring

Patients are graded on ordinal scales by interviewers in relation to their ability in bathing, dressing, transferring (e.g. to chair), toileting, continence and feeding. Scores on individual scales are summed, all items being treated as equally important, thus yielding a single total score. On the basis of more than 2,000 evaluations of states of patients, the authors observed that these functions decreased in order. They claimed to have a measure of fundamental biological functions, a claim questioned by those using Guttman scales (Williams *et al.* 1976).

The first stage in the scoring involves translating the three-point scales into a dependent/independent classification. The patients' overall performance is then summarized on an eight-point scale:

A Independent in feeding, continence, transferring, going to toilet, dressing and bathing
B Independent in all but one of these functions
C Independent in all but bathing and one additional function

D Independent in all but bathing, dressing and one additional function
E Independent in all but bathing, dressing, going to toilet and one additional function
F Independent in all but bathing, dressing, going to toilet, transferring and one additional function
G Dependent in all six functions
Other Dependent in at least two functions, but not classifiable as C, D, E or F.

Full definitions of activities are given by Katz *et al.* (1970).

The use of a single index means loss of information about variability, because different patterns of restriction, with different implications, can be reduced to the same score.

Validity

Despite the scale's widespread popularity among clinicians worldwide, there is little evidence of the validity of the scale. Katz *et al.* (1970) administered the ADL and other instruments to 270 chronically ill patients. The ADL correlated weakly to moderately with a mobility scale (0.50) and with a house-confinement scale (0.39).

The index of ADL was shown to predict the long-term course and social adaptation of patients with a number of conditions, including strokes and hip fractures, and was used to evaluate out-patient treatment for rheumatoid arthritis (Katz *et al.* 1966; 1968). It has also been shown to predict mortality (Brorsson and Asberg 1984). There is other evidence of its predictive validity, reported by Katz and Akpom (1976). However, such concise indices tend to be insensitive to small changes in disease severity and to focus on physical-performance measures. It is also of limited value in community surveys of elderly people because, like other short scales, it does not take adaptation to environment into account. It apparently underestimates dysfunction in community populations (Spector *et al.* 1987).

Reliability

Little testing for reliability has been carried out; this is again surprising given the popularity of this scale, particularly by clinicians. Katz *et al.* (1963) assessed inter-rater reliability; they reported that discrepancies between raters occurred in one in twenty observations.

A Swedish study of Guttman analyses on 100 patients yielded coefficients of scalability of 0.74–0.88, suggesting that the index is a successful cumulative scale (Brorsson and Asberg 1984). More evidence of the ADL's reliability and validity is required.

The Katz is one of the earliest indices for use in evaluating care of elderly and chronically ill patients. It is a popular and useful index with a restricted range of patients. However, the range of disabilities included in the instrument is not comprehensive and thus the populations to which it can be administered are restricted. The single index also means that the information derived from the index is limited. Although still currently popular, it is an old scale that will probably be used less in the future with the development of more comprehensive and sensitive scales (e.g. the AIMS2). Wade (1992) concluded that while this was once the most popular scale among neurologists, for example, it has been overtaken by the Barthel.

TOWNSEND'S DISABILITY SCALE

Townsend's Disability Scale is a concise index which is frequently used in community surveys of the elderly in the UK. It comprises a list of activities of daily living, derived from early research on the disabled of all ages in the UK and USA (Haber 1968; Sainsbury 1973) and Townsend's own early survey work on the elderly (Townsend 1962; Shanas et al. 1968). It was also used in Townsend's later poverty survey (Townsend 1979). However, little work has been carried out on its reliability and validity apart from initial piloting based on these early studies. Moreover, this early work was not very thorough. Sainsbury (1973) stated that the list of tasks of daily living initially selected was chosen on the basis of a 'subjective' decision 'of the more important daily and social activities'. Its advantages are its brevity and acceptability to elderly people.

Content

The index deliberately focuses on a narrow range of activities, in order that the concepts underlying them are generally applicable to a wide section of the population and for ease of application within a survey framework of the general population:

(a) activities which maintain personal existence, such as drinking, eating, evacuating, exercising, sleeping, hearing, washing and dressing
(b) activities which provide the means to fulfil these personal acts, such as obtaining food, preparing meals, providing and cleaning a home.

The scale asks respondents if they have difficulty doing the following tasks (none = 0, some difficulty = 1 or unable to do alone = 2), washing all over, cutting own toenails, running to catch a bus, carrying heavy shopping, going up/down stairs, doing heavy housework, preparing a hot meal, reaching a jug from an overhead shelf and tying a good knot in a piece of string. It can be self- or interviewer-administered, is easily completed and concise. For example:

Do you or would you have any difficulty (or find it troublesome, exhausting or worrying)

(a) Washing down (whether in bath or not)?
(b) Removing a jug, say, from an overhead shelf?
(c) Tying a good knot in string?
(d) Cutting toenails?

The remaining questions are not asked of children under the age of 10 or the bedfast:

(e) Running to catch a bus?
(f) Going up/down stairs?
(g) Going shopping and carrying a full basket of shopping in each hand?
(h) Doing heavy housework?
(i) Preparing a hot meal?

Scoring

Difficulty with each activity is given equal weighting; changes in individual capacity from day to day and season to season are ignored. 'No difficulty' is scored as zero, 'with some difficulty' is scored as 1, and the score is 2 if the reply was 'unable to do alone'. The overall score has a range of 0–18. Townsend, as a result of early validation work, regards people with a score of zero as having no disability, 1–2 as slightly affected, 3–6 some disability, 7–10 as appreciable disability and 11–18 as severe/very severe. The basis for this does not appear to have been tested any further. It is a limited index, covering a narrow range of activities.

Validity and reliability

Neither of the studies from which the scale is derived provides details of the initial testing of the measure (Haber 1968; Sainsbury 1973).

There are numerous examples in the UK of applications of the scale, particularly by Vetter *et al.* (e.g. Vetter *et al.* 1982; Vetter and Ford 1989). The scale is popular, although further and extensive testing for reliability and validity is still required.

Adaptations

There are numerous adaptations of the scale. Some of the items are not appropriate for use with a frail population, e.g. 'running to catch a bus'. The limitations of this scale have led to adaptation of the scale by many researchers, in terms of adding other activities of daily living and increasing the range of responses: no difficulty with the task, slight, moderate or severe difficulty, unable to do alone, and unable to do at all (even with help) (Bowling *et al.* 1988). Each response is scored from 0 (no difficulty) to 5 (unable to do at all) and the scores are summed to produce a total score. It was initially scored from 1 to 6, but the score of '0' was judged to be more useful as the number of people with no problems with any of the tasks is then evident in the raw total score. The simple scoring method still requires validation. It comprises three main domains: mobility, personal care and domestic, and each domain may also be summed separately. The scale was extended by the latter authors to include all the following tasks:

Mobility:
Getting in/out of bed
Transferring from a chair/wheelchair
Going up/down stairs
Getting on/off toilet
Getting in/out of bath
Getting about indoors
Getting about outdoors
Using public transport

Personal care:
Washing self/shaving (men)
Bathing self
Dressing self
Brush/comb hair
Wash hair
Cutting toenails

Domestic:
Cooking/prepare meal
Housework
Laundry
Shopping
Doing odd jobs

Two other items were initially included, brushing or managing teeth and handling money, but these appeared ambiguous. They were excluded after factor analysis. On the basis of community surveys with 662 people aged 85 and over living in London, and almost 700 people aged 65+ living in Essex and London, inter-item correlations coefficients between tasks ranged from around 0.13 (this was for shopping and managing teeth or dentures which would not be expected necessarily to correlate highly) to around 0.74 (for difficulties with washing self and with dressing self which would be expected to correlate more highly); split half reliability: 0.78–0.91 between samples. The inter-item correlation (alpha) for the personal-care task section was 0.70–0.75; for the domestic-task section was 0.80–0.85; and for the mobility section was 0.81–0.89. Testing of the scale was carried out across the three samples, and results were highly statistically significant indicating that the scale has good reliability. The ADL scale items correlated moderately to well with comparable items on dressing self, trouble with steps/stairs, walking outdoors, and walking indoors from the Nottingham Health Profile (Hunt *et al.* 1986), which was used for a sub-sample (0.635, $p < 0.0001$; 0.565, $p < 0.0001$; 0.350, $p < 0.004$; and 0.472, $p < 0.0001$ respectively).

The scale, and items from it (e.g. difficulties getting about outdoors), was also highly significantly associated with relevant physical health problems (e.g. aches, pains, stiffness in joints, muscles), health and social service use, life satisfaction and mental health, and predictive of worsening emotional well-being, supporting its construct (convergent) and predictive validity (Bowling *et al.* 1992; 1993; 1994a; 1994b). However, although the scale is useful in that needs for particular types of health and social services can easily be inferred from the items, it is still at a crude stage of development.

A similar scale has also been developed by the Institute for Economic and Social Research at York University and used in a wide range of surveys (Morton-Williams 1979). Their scale encompasses a wider range of self-care activities than the original Townsend scale, with rankings of: able to do easily, with a little difficulty, with a lot of difficulty, unable to do without someone helping, unable to do even with someone helping (the latter ranking is not always included). However, testing on this scale is also incomplete.

Another adaptation of the scale has been undertaken by Bond and Carstairs (1982) in their survey of 5,000 elderly people in Scotland. These authors distinguished between functional criteria for dependency (mobility, self-care and home-care capacity) and clinical criteria for dependency (incontinence, mental state), and they attempted to measure these. They selected items from the original Sainsbury scale, on the basis of inter-item correlations, which were then subjected to a Guttman scaling analysis. The items selected were based on a hierarchical concept: having difficulty with an activity is associated with having difficulty with earlier scale items. The items classified as mobility incapacity were difficulty/ability travelling by bus, walking outside, getting up from chair (coefficient of reproducibility: 0.97); self-care incapacity included difficulty/ability washing hair, self, bathing; dressing, put on shoes and socks/stockings (coefficient of reproducibility: 0.99); and home-care incapacity included: difficulty/ability: doing heavy shopping; washing clothes; preparing and cooking meals; ironing clothes; light housework; making bed (coefficient of reproducibility: 0.96).

THE KARNOFSKY PERFORMANCE INDEX

The Karnofsky Performance Index emphasizes physical performance and dependency. It was originally designed for use with lung cancer patients in relation to assessing palliative treatments (Karnofsky *et al.* 1948). It is a simple scale from 0 to 100 (normal–moribund). It was developed for use in clinical settings. The scale is heavily weighted towards the physical dimensions of quality of life, rather than social and psychological dimensions. Patients are assigned to categories by a clinician or other health-care professional. It is widely used in the USA and Europe.

An early literature review, examining the frequency of measurement of quality of life in clinical trials of outcome of care in six international cancer journals, showed that only 6 per cent attempted to measure it, and that the vast majority of this 6 per cent used the original performance criteria of Karnofsky (Bardelli and Saracci 1978).

Content

Examples of some of the classifications, which are made by professionals, and scores, are:

Normal; no complaint; no evidence of disease (index: 100).
Requires occasional assistance from others but able to care for most needs (index: 60).
Disabled; requires special care and assistance (index: 40).
Moribund; fatal processes progressing rapidly (index: 10).
Dead (index: 0).

Scoring

Each of the 11 components of the scale is given a notional percentage score (100 = normal; 0 = dead). The scoring procedure has not been assessed for validity. Various categorizations exist.

There are problems with this method, particularly with the assumption that a patient with a low score due to immobility necessarily has a poorer quality of life than a patient with a higher score, and vice versa. For example, the patient with a poor score may have better social support than a patient with a good score and thus, despite the immobility, may have a better quality of life. Moreover, the Karnofsky ratings are often reported as a mean score, yet there is no evidence that the intervals between the 10 categories represent the same degree of dysfunction (O'Brien 1988). Interpretations of the scale's classifications are likely to vary, particularly as the points cover different conceptual elements.

Validity

The disadvantage of the Karnofsky Performance Index, apart from its crude and therefore limited content, is that it involves categorization of patients by another person. This is a fundamental flaw, given the evidence of discrepancies between patients' and physicians' ratings of functioning and quality of life. In Evans *et al.*'s (1984) study, for example, there were wide discrepancies between patients' self-assessments, based on the Sickness Impact Profile, and physicians' assessments, based on the Karnofsky Performance Index, with the latter rating patients as being less impaired than the former.

Mor *et al.* (1984) used the scale in a national hospice-evaluation study. They reported that the construct validity of the scale was achieved: it was strongly related to two other independent measures of patient functioning (Katz's ADL scale and another quality-of-life assessment). It was also able to predict longevity (0.30) in the population of terminally ill cancer patients, thus indicating that it has predictive validity. The Karnofsky Performance Index is a crude, although successful, predictor of survival. Mor (1987), again in a study of cancer patients (total: 2,046), reported a moderate correlation between the Karnofsky and the Spitzer Quality of Life Index; the correlation was probably moderate because the latter is multi-dimensional. One of its most well-known applications has been in the US National Heart Transplantation Study (Evans *et al.* 1984). Results from this study showed a marked shift in the distribution of Karnofsky scores before and after transplantation. However, it does not measure broader quality of life such as social or emotional well-being and is thus limited as a measure of quality of life.

In a study of 139 lung cancer patients, Schaafsma and Osoba (1994) reported weak associations between observer-rated Karnofsky scores and self-rated quality of life using the core European Organization for the Treatment of Cancer 30-item Questionnaire (Aaronson 1993). They also reported that the Karnofsky Performance Index was limited as an index of Quality of Life in cancer patients. Although popular among clinicians, particularly in cancer studies (see the author's *Measuring Disease* for review in relation to oncology), it is a limited measure. In addition, Yates *et al.* (1980) carried out the first objective validation of the scale and concluded that the index is not appropriately scaled and that scale values may bear no relation to clinical significance.

Reliability

The results of testing for inter-rater reliability have varied widely, with some studies reporting low reliability at 29–43% with Cohen's kappa, and others reporting higher (Pearson's) correlations of 0.66–0.69 (Hutchinson *et al.* 1979; Yates *et al.* 1980). Mor *et al.* (1984), on the basis of a national hospice evaluation, reported that the inter-rater reliability coefficient of the 47 interviewers employed at test-retests at four-month intervals was 0.97.

Slevin *et al.* (1988) reported a study involving 108 cancer patients in which two different groups of patients filled in the same collection of instruments, including the Karnofsky index, on a single day, and then daily for five consecutive days. Although the Karnofsky was more robust than the other measures tested (Spitzer's Quality of Life Index, the Hospital Anxiety and Depression scale and LASA visual analogue scales), the same score was achieved on only 54 per cent of occasions, despite the fact that only the five top points on the Karnofsky were covered.

The reliability and validity of the index have only recently begun to be examined (Hutchinson *et al.* 1979). The scale's 'numeric' status has not been seriously challenged, and it has generally been uncritically accepted and applied in a large number of clinical settings (Schag *et al.* 1984). It has even been used in settings where its applicability must be questioned (bone-marrow transplantation in children) (Hinterberger *et al.* 1987).

Other versions of the scale have been developed, but with no obvious improvements in effectiveness over the original version (Zubrod *et al.* 1960; World Health Organization 1979; Nou and Aberg 1980). These are described in the author's *Measuring Disease*.

THE BARTHEL INDEX

The Barthel Index was developed by Mahoney and Barthel (1965). It is based on observed functions.

The index was developed to measure functional ability before and after intervention treatment, and to indicate the amount of nursing care required. It was designed for use with long-term hospital patients with neuromuscular or musculo-skeletal disorders. It has been used more generally to evaluate treatment outcomes since. The Barthel Index is based on a rating scale completed by a therapist or other observer. The scale takes approximately 30 seconds to score.

Content

The scale covers the following dimensions:

Feeding
Mobility from bed to chair
Personal toilet (washing, etc.)
Getting on/off the toilet
Bathing
Walking on level surface
Going up/down stairs
Dressing
Incontinence (bladder and bowel)

A score of zero is given where the patients cannot meet the defined criterion. It omits tasks of daily living such as cooking and shopping and other everyday tasks essential for life in the community. It thus appears suitable only for institutionalized populations (for whom it was designed).

Granger et al. (1979); Fortinsky et al. (1981) and Granger and McNamara (1984) have developed extensions of the Barthel Index, covering 15 topics, although insufficient evidence of the reliability and validity of these extensions exists.

Scoring

Different values are assigned to different activities. Individuals are scored on 10 activities which are summed to give a score of 0 (totally dependent) to 100 (fully independent). The authors of the scale provide detailed instructions for assessing and scoring patients; for example:

Doing personal toilet: 5 = patient can wash hands and face, comb hair, clean teeth, and shave. He may use any kind of razor but must put in blade or plug in razor without help as

well as get it from drawer or cabinet. Female patients must put on own make-up, if used, but need not braid or style hair.

A modified scoring method gives a maximum score of 20 to patients who are continent, able to wash, feed and dress themselves and are independently mobile (Collin et al. 1988).

The scores are intended to reflect the amount of time and assistance a patient requires. However, the scoring method is inconsistent in that changes by a given number of points do not reflect equivalent changes in disability across different activities.

Moreover, as its authors point out, the scale is restricted in that changes can occur beyond the end points of the scale. The scale is also limited to physical activities and does not take mental status or social well-being into account. It is restricted to measuring one aspect of quality of life.

Validity

The original Barthel Index has been tested for validity by Wade et al. (1985, 1992) and Collen et al. (1990), in their evaluations of therapies for stroke patients. The results have been more fully described by Wade (1992). Mattison et al. (1991) used the Barthel Index with 364 patients attending day centres for the physically disabled. They compared it with the PULSES Scale and the Edinburgh Rehabilitation Status Scale (ERSS) (Affleck et al. 1988) and reported that the correlation between the Barthel and these two scales was 0.65 and r = −0.69 respectively. Good results were reported by Wade and Collin (1988). Most studies of its validity compare it with the PULSES profile, which give correlations of −0.74 to −0.90 (Granger et al. 1979). The Barthel Index has been reported to have predictive validity as it correlates well with various prognostic scores of stroke patients (Kalra and Crome 1993), length of hospital stay and mortality (Wylie and White 1964). Factor analysis has confirmed that it measures a single domain, and it has been reported to be sensitive to recovery (Wade and Langton-Hewer 1987).

The original scale, and the more recent adaptations of it, is a popular measure in neurology. Despite its moderate to good results for validity, and its wide use in institutional settings, it is not a comprehensive measure of functioning (e.g. it omits domestic, social and other role functioning) and is less suitable for use in the community, and has been reported to be insensitive to clinical change to elderly patients attending a day hospital (Rodgers *et al.* 1993; Parker *et al.* 1994). As the Barthel Index is a measure of what the patient actually does, rather than ability, scoring may be location dependent (McMurdo and Rennie 1993). It may not be sensitive to improvements of deteriorations beyond the end points of the scale ('floor' and 'ceiling' effects) (McDowell and Newell 1987).

Reliability

Sherwood *et al.* (1977) reported alpha reliability coefficients of 0.95 to 0.97 for three samples of hospital patients, suggesting that the scale is internally consistent. Collin *et al.* (1988) tested it for reliability on 25 stroke patients, and analysed observer agreement, using groups of 2, 3 and 4 observers. They reported that difficulties in agreement were lower for the middle category, and consequently they refined the instructions for observers. Granger *et al.* (1979) reported a test–retest reliability of 0.89 with severely disabled adults, and an inter-rater agreement exceeding 0.95. However, other studies of doctors' and nurses' ratings of elderly nursing home patients have reported poor agreement, particularly for patients with some degree of cognitive impairment (Ranhoff and Laake 1993).

In sum, while simplicity is an attraction of the scale, it also poses a major limitation on its use. Further testing is required before its use can be recommended for widespread use in community surveys and evaluations. Despite its acknowledged limitations, there is an increasing body of literature supporting its use with specific groups of patients such as those with neurological disability (Collin *et al.* 1988; Wade and Collin 1988).

Several modified versions of the scale have been developed (Fortinsky *et al.* 1981; Granger 1982; Granger and McNamara 1984; Shah *et al.* 1989; Gompertz *et al.* 1993a; 1993b). These have been described in the author's *Measuring Disease*. However, Granger and his colleagues now regard their early modifications of the scale to be obsolete and have replaced it with the Functional Independence

Measure (18 items) and Functional Assessment Measure (12 items) (FIM+FAM) (Stineman *et al.* 1994). This is similar in scope to the original measure, concentrating on personal care, mobility and walking, communication and cognition to the neglect of domestic functioning. It has not yet been fully evaluated for its psychometric properties.

THE QUALITY OF WELL-BEING SCALE (QWBS)

The Quality of Well-Being Scale was developed to operationalize 'wellness' for a general health-policy model. This was an attempt to develop an alternative to economic cost-benefit analysis for resource allocation, for example, by comparing the health status of groups of individuals for the evaluation of health-care programmes (Kaplan *et al.* 1976; Bush 1984).

It can be used with general populations and applied to any type of disease. The items in the interview schedule were drawn mainly from the US Health Interview Survey and from the Social Security Administration Survey, but the schedule has been extensively tested on large groups of nurses and graduate students and revised. The QWBS combines mortality with estimates of the quality of life. The scale quantifies the health output of a treatment in terms of years of life, adjusted for their diminished quality, that it is responsible for. It is based on a three-component model of health. First, the assessment of health begins with an assessment of functional status, based on the individual's performance. The authors listed all the ways by which a disease or injury can affect a person's behaviour and performance (Kaplan *et al.* 1976). Second, a value reflecting the relative desirability (utility) is assigned to each functional level (Fanshel and Bush 1970).

Responses to a branching questionnaire are used to assign subjects to one of a number of discrete function states. It is based on a model of health which encompasses symptom/problem, mobility, physical activity and social activity. The QWBS has been used in many evaluative studies of pulmonary disease and in drug trials (Toevs *et al.* 1984; Bombardier *et al.* 1986; Kaplan 1994). Several areas of application have been reported by Bush (1984), most of which are unpublished. The scale includes death. This avoids the problem inherent in other indices where, as death is frequently ignored, the death of a disabled person appears to improve the population estimate of health status (Kaplan *et al.* 1994). Third, information is also collected about future changes (prognosis). This permits a distinction between two people with equal functional disability but one of whom is terminally ill.

The interview schedule is long, and a 30-page manual is purchasable from the authors. The questionnaire takes 10–15 minutes to administer. The QWB is administered by trained interviewers. It can be administered to proxies where people are not able to reply (e.g. stroke victims).

Content

The Quality of Well-Being Scale consists of three ordinal scales on dimensions of daily activity. Combinations of each of the three scales of mobility, physical and social activity were initially taken to define 29 function levels. Subsequent modification has increased the number of function levels to 43. Each function level can be linked with a separate classification of symptoms and problems. Questions are based on performance, not capacity. Four aspects of function are covered, mobility/confinement, physical activity, social activity (e.g. work, housekeeping) and self-care. The categories on each scale range from full independence to death. The physical ability scale has four categories and the others have five.

Respondents are given a list of 22 'symptom/problem' complexes and asked to identify all that applied to them during the preceding six days. They are then asked to indicate which of these has 'bothered them most'. Next, they are asked about mobility, physical and social activity. Actual ability rather than capacity to perform is asked about. Examples of the scale items are:

Mobility
Drove car and used bus or train
Did not drive or had help to use bus or train

Physical activity
Walked without physical problems
Walked with physical limitations

Social activity
Did work, school, or housework and other activities
Limited in amount or kind of work, school or housework

Scoring

Respondents' functional status is classified for each day on the scales of mobility, physical and social activity. The QWBS score is calculated by combining this information with the symptom/problem responses, using a set of preference weights. The latter were developed on the basis of interviews with 800 respondents in a household survey in which respondents were asked to rate different health states on a 10-point scale ranging from death to perfect health. The ratings were used in a multiple regression analysis to obtain weights for different responses. Scores are calculated separately for each of the six days, and the QWBS score is expressed as the average of these. The final score ranges from 0 (equated with death) to 1 (perfect health) (Patrick *et al.* 1973a; 1973b). For each of the 43 function levels a 'preference weight' has been established empirically, ranging from 1 (complete well-being) to 0 (death). The appropriate preference weight is assigned to the respondents' functional-ability level, and the resulting score is known as the Quality of Well-Being score. The authors noted that it is possible to provide a score below zero to represent a state 'worse than death' (Kaplan and Bush 1982). The weights assigned represent preferences of the relative importance that members of society assigned to each functional level. The third stage of rating involves adjusting for prognosis (Kaplan *et al.* 1976; 1979). The authors are currently developing a new self-administration version of the scale. Further testing for the validation of the scaling technique has been reported by Kaplan and Ernst (1983). The means and variances of preferences for attributes of quality of life did not change over time (Kaplan *et al.* 1978).

Validity

The content validity of the QWBS has been stated by Kaplan *et al.* (1976). It is able to successfully predict outcome among people with HIV infection (Kaplan *et al.* 1995). Its content validity as an index of disability is enhanced by incorporating death. Kaplan *et al.* (1976) report correlations of -0.75 between the QWBS and number of reported symptoms, and of 0.96 between the QWBS and the number of chronic health problems. The correlation between the QWBS and the number of physician contacts in the preceding eight days was 0.55. It correlates well (0.76) with self-rated quality of life. A review of the literature has shown that it correlates with functional ability and broader health status scales from 0.17 to 0.71, with most correlations at 0.50 or more (Revicki and Kaplan 1993). Thus it is said by its authors to have convergent validity. Its predictive value has been reported to be between 0.95 and 0.98 and sensitivity at 0.90, on the basis of data from 1,324 subjects with a range of diseases and injuries. It is able to discriminate between changes in life quality over time (Kaplan *et al*. 1976).

The Quality of Well-Being Scale was used by Leighton Read *et al*. (1987) in a study of 400 outpatients in Boston, Massachusetts, USA. The authors tested this scale, the SIP and the Rand Corporation's General Health Rating Index (GHRI) for convergent-construct validity, content and discriminant validity. The findings for convergent-construct validity were similar to those achieved by the developers of the scales – the correlations between scales were moderately high (0.46–0.55). They reported the GHRI to be the easiest to use, as they found both the SIP and the QWB scales required a major commitment to interviewer training. All were equally acceptable to respondents. The QWBS contained more items than the others on specific symptoms; in contrast the SIP contained more detail on dysfunction. The authors concluded that each scale was a valid measure of health status.

Reliability

The reliability coefficient obtained when judges reassessed scale values for 29 function levels was 0.90 (Kaplan and Bush 1982). Test-retest reliability is between 0.93 and 0.98 (Kaplan *et al*. 1978; Bush 1984). The internal consistency reliability estimates for the QWBS overall score have been reported for four populations and reliability estimates have exceeded 0.90. The scale is sufficiently reliable for use in making group comparisons.

While the QWBS is advantageous in that it incorporates mortality, its main disadvantages are its complexity, and the requirement that it needs to be administered by trained interviewers. Kaplan (1994) and Kaplan *et al*. (1994) recommended that the scale is useful for policy analysis and clinical research because of its unidimensionality, but its unidimensional approach makes it less informative for clinical studies, where a multi-dimensional scoring approach is preferable, although less convenient. While the complexity of the scale has generally inhibited its use in clinical research on health outcomes, at the other extreme it has also been used with patients where its appropriateness is questionable (e.g. with paediatric cancer patients (Bradlyn *et al*. 1993)).

THE CRICHTON ROYAL BEHAVIOUR RATING SCALE (CRBRS)

The Crichton Royal Behaviour Rating Scale was developed by Robinson (1968) and refined and tested for reliability and validity by Wilkin and Jolley (1979), on the basis of samples of people in residential homes for the elderly, geriatric and psychiatric wards. The scale has had a wide application in the UK and was used for the evaluation of Department of Health and district health authority-funded nursing homes (Bond *et al*. 1989; Bowling and Formby 1990) and for the assessment of residential care of the elderly (Willcocks *et al*. 1987).

The CRBRS was designed for use with elderly people living in institutions. It is completed by a third person who knows the respondent well (e.g. a nurse in a hospital ward would complete it on behalf of a patient well known to him/her). The modified CRBRS contains ten items, five relating to functional ability (mobility, feeding, dressing, bathing, continence) and five relating to mental disturbance (memory, orientation, communication, co-operation, restlessness). The confusion sub-scale can be used independently of the functional-ability scale.

As the scale was designed for use with populations resident in institutions, home-care activities were excluded. Although the research reports containing evidence of the scale's reliability and validity are now out of print, a brief description of the scale has been published by Wilkin and Thompson (1989). Interviewer training is required.

Notes of guidance are provided for interviewers to elicit the appropriate questions. The interviewer is expected to probe and ask for examples of behaviour before a classification is made. The emphasis of the scale is on behaviour (what the person actually does), rather than on ability. A set of structured questions has been designed by Bond *et al.* (1989) for use with the interviewers' assessments, with high correlations between the two. The interviewer assessment without the structured questions takes approximately three minutes, the assessment with the structured questions can extend the interview to seven to ten minutes (Wilkin and Thompson 1989; Bowling and Formby 1990).

Content

Examples of the rating scale are:

Dressing
0 Correct
1 Imperfect but adequate
2 Adequate with minimum of supervision
3 Inadequate unless continually supervised
4 Unable to dress or to retain clothing

Feeding
0 Correct unaided at appropriate times
1 Adequate with minimum of supervision
2 Inadequate unless constantly supervised
3 Requires feeding

Memory
0 Complete
1 Occasionally forgetful
2 Short-term loss
3 Short- and long-term loss

Orientation
0 Complete
1 Oriented in ward, identifies people correctly
2 Misidentifies but can find way about
3 Cannot find way to bed or toilet without assistance
4 Completely lost

Full details of the CRBRS, together with the full-scale items, interviewer notes and structured questions designed by Bond *et al.* (1989) to accompany the rating scale, are reproduced by Wilkin and Thompson (1989).

Scoring

Each item is scored 0 to 4, except memory and feeding which are scored 0 to 3; thus these two items were designed to make a smaller contribution to the overall score. Individual items are added to obtain the total score. These are grouped into six ranges, although the authors state that they do not

represent levels of dependency: 0–1, 2–5, 6–10, 11–15, 16–20, 21–38. It is unclear what the different scale scores represent.

A sub-scale for confusion can also be derived, consisting of the items relating to memory, orientation and communication. These sub-scale scores are totalled and grouped into four ranges: 0–1 (lucid); 2–3 (intermediate); 4–6 (moderately confused); 7–11 (severely confused) (Evans *et al.* 1981).

Validity

Thompson (1984) used factor analysis to assess the construct validity of the CRBRS. She reported that the ten items reflected two dimensions of dependency: capacity for self-care and ability to walk.

The research reports with details of testing for validity and reliability are out of print, but Wilkin and Thompson (1989) have summarized the results. They reported that total scale scores of 10 or more were associated with a diagnosis of psychiatric disorder. The study reported by Evans *et al.* (1981) suggested that confusion sub-scale scores of 4 or more were associated with a clinical diagnosis of dementia. Total scale scores and the confusion sub-scale scores have been compared with independent clinical assessments and the modified Roth-Hopkins mental-state test (the correlations for the latter range between 0.75 and 0.82) (Vardon and Blessed 1986; Wilkin and Thompson 1989). There has been little work testing the validity of the CRBRS.

Wilkin and Thompson (1989) caution that the scale is insufficiently sensitive as a tool for assessing change over time and should be used to provide population profiles. The problem with using the scale to assess individual change over time is that reliance on different informants to complete the scale may produce bias.

Reliability

The emphasis of the scale on behaviour rather than ability in theory minimizes problems with reliability. In practice, however, it is likely that ratings will reflect the philosophy of the institution; for example, staff working in institutions which encourage independence are likely to assess patients/residents as less dependent than staff in institutions which encourage dependency.

Thompson (1984) assessed the internal reliability of the capacity for self-care dimension of the scale. She reported that reliability can be increased by removing the items relating to feeding, restlessness and co-operation, and by treating mobility as a separate dimension. Wilkin and Jolley (1979) examined inter-rater reliability, using two interviewers to assess the same informant; the correlations obtained were greater than 0.90. Far more testing for reliability is required.

There are some difficulties within the scale which have not yet been resolved; for example, the classification of the use of stairs in the case of a respondent who lives on the ground floor and does not need to use stairs.

Despite the limited evidence about its reliability and validity, the CRBRS is popular in the UK as a measure of functioning for use with elderly people living in institutions. It is fairly concise and easily administered by a trained interviewer. Its popularity in this area is probably partly due to the advantage it has in being specifically designed for use with a third party.

THE CLIFTON ASSESSMENT PROCEDURES FOR THE ELDERLY (CAPE)

The Clifton Assessment Procedures for the Elderly is the most extensively tested measure of dependency in widespread use in the UK, particularly in relation to psychological assessments of the elderly. It was developed for use with elderly people living in institutions, and tested for validity by Pattie and Gilleard (1979). A manual is available which provides details of use and also normative data for a range of patient populations (Pattie and Gilleard 1979). The CAPE consists of two schedules, designed to measure behaviour and cognitive performance, known as the Behaviour Rating Scale and the Cognitive Assessment Scale. The Cognitive Assessment Scale was originally known as the Clifton Assessment Scale, and can be completed by an elderly person in five to fifteen minutes. The Behaviour Rating Scale is a short version of the Stockton Geriatric Rating Scale, designed for use with elderly people in hospital. The whole test can take between five to thirty minutes, depending on the mental and functional ability of the respondent. It is designed to be com-

pleted by a third party who knows the respondent well. Interviewer training is necessary.

Content

The Cognitive Performance Scale consists of a battery of tests which includes items such as the person tracing a circular route with a pencil, avoiding obstacles; the information/orientation items include the usual memory tests of own place of residence, name of the prime minister, date, etc., and, more unusually, knowledge of the colours of the British flag.

The Behavioural Rating Scale contains 18 items. Four items relate to mobility, continence and activities of daily living. The remaining items relate to confused behaviour. The scale asks about current-level functioning. The scale focuses heavily on the behavioural problems of those elderly people who are mentally infirm. The rater is instructed to rate people according to their level of current functioning, and to take into account behaviour over the past two weeks.

The authors suggest that the CAPE relates to four sub-scales: physical disability, apathy, communication difficulties and social disturbance. Examples of the behaviour-rating scale are:

When bathing or dressing, he/she requires:

0 No assistance
1 Some assistance
2 Maximum assistance

With regard to walking, he/she:

0 Shows no signs of weakness
1 Walks slowly without aid, or uses a stick
2 Is unable to walk, or if able to walk, needs frame, crutches or someone by his/her side

He/she is confused (unable to find way around, loses possessions, etc.):

0 Almost never confused
1 Sometimes confused
2 Almost always confused

His/her sleep pattern at night is:

0 Almost never awake
1 Sometimes awake
2 Often awake

Scoring

The 18 items are added to form a total score, or selected items are added to produce sub-scale scores. Each item has a range of scores from 0 (no/few problems) to 2 (frequent/constant problems). Four sub-scales can be created from the items relating to physical disability, apathy, communication difficulties and social disturbance. The total scale range of scores is from 0 to 36. A score of 0–3 indicates independence; 4–7 indicates low dependency; 8–12 indicates medium dependency; 13–17 indicates high dependency and 18–36 is maximum dependency. No item weights are used.

Validity

Early versions of the scale were shown to correlate with clinicians' assessments about appropriate levels of care for females but not males. The sample size was small, 38. The authors also report correlations with other scales such as the Wechsler Memory Scale, but sample sizes were too small to be conclusive. This provides weak evidence of the scale's concurrent validity (Smith *et al.* 1981).

Black *et al.* (1990) compared the diagnostic ability of the CAPE, in relation to dementia, with the diagnosis made by the computer program AGECAT and a clinical diagnosis made by a psychiatrist. The sample was an elderly sample of patients from a general practice (112 were selected from 378 who had been tested three years previously when aged 70+ using a 13-item mental-function test). The authors reported that the sensitivity of the CAPE was low, probably because it identified only the more severe cases. The CAPE only detected about half the number of known cases.

In relation to behaviour, Pattie and Gilleard (1979) have reported that the CAPE can discriminate between elderly people requiring differing degrees of help, with different levels of social adjustment following admission to a residential home, and between mentally infirm people who survive and those who die.

Results of factor analyses showed that two factor structures emerged for three groups of elderly people tested, and no clear factor structure emerged for non-psychiatrically ill elderly people (Pattie and Gilleard 1979). The four sub-scales suggested by the authors for analysing the Behaviour Rating Scale data were not supported. Factor analyses carried out on the CAPE by Twining and Allen (1981), on the basis of 903 people in residential homes for the elderly, also failed to support the four suggested sub-scales.

Reliability

Pattie and Gilleard (1979) report inter-item correlations, and all are fairly high. This suggests that items are consistent and are measuring the same dimensions of dependency. Inter-rater reliability for the four sub-scales was tested on psychiatric and psychogeriatric patients and people in residential homes for the elderly; the correlations were all 0.70 or higher with the exception of the correlation for 'communication difficulties' which was low. Tests for inter-rater reliability for the total scale showed wide variations. Smith *et al.* (1981), in their study of 38 elderly mentally handicapped patients, reported inter-rater a reliability coefficient of 0.58 between two nursing sisters.

Test–retest reliability coefficients range from 0.56 to 0.90 at retests over two to three days with 38 hospital patients aged 65 and over, and at retests over two to three months. The six-month test-retest reliabilities, based on 39 new admissions to homes for the elderly, range from 0.69 to 0.84 (Pattie and Gilleard 1979).

Although this dependency scale has undergone more testing than the Crichton Royal Behaviour Rating Scale, evidence is still limited and for reliability it is weak. The scale, along with others in common use in the UK, has been reviewed by Wilkin and Thompson (1989). They draw attention to ambiguities in the scale wording, for example the terms 'sometimes' and 'frequently' are not defined and therefore likely to be interpreted differently by different raters. The scale has also been reviewed by Mulgrave (1985) who reported its main advantages as being short and easily administered, although further evidence of its reliability and validity is required.

4

BROADER MEASURES OF HEALTH STATUS

Broader measures of health status generally focus on individuals' subjective perceptions of their health. Subjective or perceived health may be defined as an individual's experience of mental, physical and social events as they impinge upon feelings of well-being (Hunt 1988). Many studies in medical sociology have indicated the importance of the perceptual component of illness in determining whether people feel ill or whether they seek help.

While many scales of broader-health status exist and are to be preferred to single-item questions, a popular single-item measure on both sides of the Atlantic consists of asking respondents to rate their health as 'excellent, good, fair or poor'. Some researchers ask respondents to rate this in relation to their age (e.g. Cartwright and Anderson 1981). This single-item measure of self-perceived health status has been found to be related to eventual mortality and to rates of recovery from episodes of ill health (National Heart and Lung Institute 1976; Singer *et al.* 1976). Mortality has been found to be two to three times greater for people who report their health as poor than for those who rate their health as excellent (Kaplan and Camacho 1983). Perceived health has been found to be more closely related to use of health services than medical condition (Goldstein *et al.* 1984). Although the ratings on this question correlate well with subsequent mortality and admission to hospital, it has been subjected to three main criticisms, it provides no information about why people rate themselves as 'excellent', 'good', 'fair' or 'poor'. Also, it provides

only four response choices and around half of a general population sample may rate themselves as in 'excellent' or 'good' health (Bowling and Cartwright 1982; Ware 1984). Some investigators add an extra response category in order to increase sensitivity ('very good') (Ware *et al.* 1993). This measure may be contextual and vary over time with people's varying expectations. Self-ratings of health are often criticized as subjective, but their subjectivity is their strength because they reflect personal evaluations of health.

Given that subjectivity is a major criticism levelled at this type of indicator, it merits some discussion. Health indicators have largely been developed within the era of science based on the logical positivist paradigm. This inevitably leads to suspicion when data are presented which are based on subjective experience. This is despite the research questioning the reliability of 'objective' data. The concordance rate of clinical and pathological diagnoses has been shown to be as low as 45.3 per cent (Heasman and Lipworth 1966), and several studies have reported on the arbitrary nature of normal values in biochemistry (Grasbeck and Saris 1969; Bradwell *et al.* 1974), and of the problem of establishing a dividing line between sick and healthy in relation to diabetes, hypertension and glaucoma (Cochrane and Holland 1971). One Swedish out-patient study also found that there was only 50 per cent agreement between doctors and patients on whether treatment had been successful (Orth-Gomer *et al.* 1979). Similar results have been obtained in relation to low back pain and outcome of surgery, blood-pressure treatment, and results of surgery for peptic ulcer (Hall *et al.* 1976; Thomas and Lyttle 1980; Jachuck *et al.* 1982).

Other measurement formats which are commonly used in studies of health status are symptom checklists. These also have their limitations, but are generally considered to be useful tools if used in conjunction with scaled measurement techniques. There are numerous examples of checklists of symptoms presented to respondents in surveys. Respondents are typically asked to indicate which, if any, they currently suffer from. George and Bearon (1980) give some examples of symptom checklists; other examples can be found in Cartwright's national surveys in the UK (e.g. Dunnell and Cartwright 1972; Cartwright and Anderson 1981; Bowling and Cartwright 1982), and in the Rand Health Insurance Study Questionnaires (Stewart *et al.* 1978). Diagnostic data obtained in population surveys are neither specific nor precise. Questions that ask about symptoms produce a high proportion of affirmative responses (e.g. Dunnell and Cartwright 1972). Items focusing on trivial problems are unlikely to have much discriminatory power in terms of monitoring change between groups over time. They may include not only response errors, but diagnostic errors – many people do not know the specific nature nor cause of their afflictions. Reporting of morbidity may also depend on tolerance levels and pain thresholds; the decision to restrict activities reflects the individual's attitude towards illness and self-care, the expectations and demands of others (family, employer, friends), knowledge and understanding of symptoms experienced and other social and cultural factors.

There is a fundamental question that remains unanswered with measures of health status which should be noted at this point: why are people with poor mental health (e.g. depression) more likely to rate their health status, functional ability and social support as low? In some cases poor mental health will distort perceptions of health and well-being, and poor physical health can also lead to poor mental health and well-being (including reduced social interaction). Researchers need to be aware of this problem, which leads to difficulties in interpreting results.

Given that a subjective measure of health status is required, and it is accepted that single-item measures are limited in value, the issue becomes that of which measure to choose. The researcher also has to decide whether a general and/or specific measure is required, depending on the nature of the study. There is little point in including a health measure if it is unlikely to detect the effects of the treatment or symptoms specific to the condition. Some specific disease-related scales do exist, although the Nottingham Health Profile and the Sickness Impact Profile have also been used as more general measures of quality of life and are apparently successful at distinguishing between patient types.

The case for using general, rather than specific, indicators of health status in population surveys has been clearly argued by Kaplan (1988). For example, detailed information about specific disease categories may appear overwhelming to many respondents not suffering from them. Also the use of disease-specific measures precludes the possibility of comparing programmes (e.g. health promotion) that are directed at different groups suffering from different diseases. Policy analysis requires a general measure of health status. Broader measures of physical, social and psychological functioning exist, but their use in the UK has been limited. If necessary, as in the case of a study of a specific disease group, global measures can be supplemented with disease-effect questions.

The following sections describe the most well-known and best tested measures of broader-health status that are currently available. All were developed in the USA, except the Nottingham Health Profile, and the Functional Limitations Profile (an adaptation of the Sickness Impact Profile) both of which were developed in the UK. Readers will notice that the EuroQol has not been included in this review (EuroQol Group 1990). This is a generic, multi-dimensional health profile which is being developed for use in Europe. It has been excluded because the literature on its psychometric properties is limited, and research indicates that it is highly skewed with large ceiling effects (Brazier *et al.* 1992; 1993). A revised version (EQ-5D) has been issued.

THE SICKNESS IMPACT PROFILE (SIP)

One of the best instruments developed in the USA has been the Sickness Impact Profile (SIP) (Deyo *et al.* 1982; 1983; Bergner, 1988; 1993). The Sickness Impact Profile was developed as a measure of perceived health status, for use as an outcome measure for health-care evaluation across a wide range of health problems and diseases, across demographic and cultural groups. Sickness is measured in relation to its impact on behaviour. The profile emphasizes sickness-related dysfunction rather than disease. It was designed to be sensitive to differences in health status in terms of minor morbidity (Bergner *et al.* 1976a; 1976b; 1981; Gilson *et al.* 1979).

The Sickness Impact Profile concentrates on assessing the impact of sickness on daily activities and behaviour, rather than feelings and clinical reports. The justification was that feelings are difficult to measure and subjective and thus difficult to validate, and clinical reports can be provided only where someone has sought medical care. The authors felt that behavioural reports were less subject to bias than feelings, although reported behaviour can be influenced by perceptual bias and behaviour can be influenced by feelings. The authors acknowledged that the SIP does not measure positive functioning.

The SIP was developed on the basis of a literature review and after extracting statements from health professionals, healthy and ill lay people which described 'sickness related behaviour dysfunction' (Bergner *et al.* 1981).

The populations and patient groups involved in its development varied widely and included inpatients, out-patients, and home-care patients with chronic diseases, patients in intensive care units, patients undergoing hip replacements and arthritis patients. It may be self- or interviewer-administered. It takes 20–30 minutes to complete. Deyo *et al.* (1983) recognized the problem of its length and suggested that attempts to shorten it might augment patient acceptability. A sub-sample of the participants in their study were asked about their opinions of the SIP and, while most said it was acceptable, the few complaints elicited concerned its length and the fact that it was not disease specific. The authors suggest that the sub-scales could be used independently if desired (e.g. the physical function sub-scale consists of only 45 of the 136 items). A study asking interviewers to make ratings of the ease of application of the SIP by Read *et al.* (1987) found that the length of the SIP

was reported to be tedious, largely because of the repetition it contained. They also reported that the SIP involved a major commitment to interviewer training time (at least a week). More optimistic findings were reported by Hall *et al.* (1987). The SIP was used in a general study of patient outcome based in a general practice setting in Sydney, Australia by Hall *et al.* (1987). The SIP was used along with the General Health Questionnaire (see page 82) and the Rand Health Insurance Battery; 160 questionnaires were completed by patients, and only 3 per cent did not complete all the questions across the three scales.

There have been many applications of the SIP to a wide range of patient groups, mainly in the USA, but also in the UK and other parts of the world. One application in the UK was by Fletcher *et al.* (1988) in a randomized controlled trial of outcome of drug treatment of angina patients. The SIP has been widely used in the US heart-transplantation evaluations. Many applications of the SIP have been described by Wenger *et al.* (1984). The advantage this wide application provides is that scores for many population groups are available for comparison.

Given that the length of the SIP (136 items) has been one barrier to its use, there have been attempts to shorten it. de Bruin *et al.* (1993) have constructed a 68-item version using multivariate techniques, claiming that its psychometric properties are similar to the longer 136-item version. Further testing is required.

Content

The SIP incorporates 136 questions, not only on functioning, but also on feelings of emotional well-being and social functioning. This contains 136 items referring to illness-related dysfunction in 12 areas: work, recreation, emotion, affect, home life, sleep, rest, eating, ambulation, mobility, communication and social interaction. A typical set of questions from the SIP requests respondents to tick statements which apply to them on a given day and are related to their state of health:

I spend much of the day lying down in order to rest.
I sit during much of the day.
I am sleeping or dozing most of the time – day and night.
I stand up only with someone's help.

I kneel, stoop, or bend down only by holding on to something.
I am in a restricted position all the time.
I do work around the house only for short periods of time or rest often.
I am doing less of the regular daily work around the house that I would usually do.
I am not doing any of the house cleaning that I would usually do.
I am going out less to visit people.
I am not going out to visit people at all.
I am doing fewer social activities with groups of people.

(© The Johns Hopkins University 1977)

Only those questions to which the respondents answer 'yes' are recorded; thus there is no way of knowing in the analysis whether the columns left blank represent 'no' replies or whether the respondent/interviewer omitted them deliberately or in error.

Scoring

The responses to the 136 items can be summarized by component, by physical or psychosocial dimension or as a single score with a range of 0–100. The lower the score the better the respondents' health status.

The score for the SIP may be calculated using item weights that indicate the relative severity of limitation implied by each statement. The weights were derived from equal-appearing interval-scaling procedures involving more than 100 judges. The judges rated each item on an equal-interval 11-point scale from 'minimally dysfunctional' to 'severely dysfunctional'. The scaling technique has been justified and described by Carter et al. (1976).

The overall score for the SIP is calculated by adding the scale values for each item checked across all categories and dividing by the maximum possible dysfunction score for the SIP. This figure is then multiplied by 100 to obtain the SIP overall score. The two sub-scores (physical and psychosocial) are calculated using a similar formula but limiting the calculations to the relevant items.

Although the many studies using the SIP have ensured the existence of scores for comparison, it is unclear what each score represents. Many other scales also suffer this problem (e.g. the HAQ). It is

known that a normal population may score only 2 or 3 on the SIP, increasing to the mid–30s for terminally ill cancer and stroke patients, but the precise definition of scale points has not so far been tackled.

The study based in Sydney, Australia by Hall et al. (1987) reported that results were skewed towards the healthy end of the SIP scale. Eighteen per cent of patients scored zero on all components. There were no scores above 25 (range of possible scores 0–100). This pattern was repeated within components.

Validity

The early validation studies of the SIP tested it against self-assessments of health status, clinicians' assessments of health status and functional assessment instruments; 278 people were assessed. SIP scores discriminated between four sub-groups divided according to severity of sickness, and correlations between measures were better for patients' self-assessments than physicians' assessments (0.69 with a self-assessment of limitation; 0.63 with a self-assessment of sickness; 0.50 with a clinician's assessment of limitation; and 0.40 with a clinician's assessment of sickness). The combined SIP score was tested against the Katz ADL scale with a correlation of 0.64; and the correlation between the SIP and the National Health Interview Survey Instrument was 0.55 (Bergner et al. 1981).

Convergent and discriminant validity was evaluated using the multi-trait–multi-method technique. Clinical validity was assessed by comparing clinical judgements with SIP scores; all achieved good results. These have been described in some detail by Bergner et al. (1981). More recent evidence pointing to its strong validity properties has been provided by Read et al. (1987). However, the correlations between the SIP score and clinical status have tended to range between 0.40 and 0.60, probably due to the broad nature of the SIP; this may not be a high enough correlation for the successful use of the scale in studies of clinical outcome of health-care interventions (Anderson et al. 1993).

The Australian study by Hall et al. (1987) reported that, with the use of a correlation threshold of −0.30, the SIP correlated with the Rand index. The Rand mental-health index correlated with the SIP items relating to social interaction, emotional behaviour and alertness; and ambulation from the SIP correlated with the Rand physical-abilities scale. Home-management and social-interaction items from the SIP correlated with the role-functioning items on the Rand battery. However, the correlations ranged from 0.32 to 0.54. Other research has reported moderate correlations (0.40–0.60) between the SIP and scales of anxiety and depression, reflecting the behavioural focus of the SIP (Linzer *et al.* 1991).

However, the Sickness Impact Profile has reportedly been used successfully in clinical trials (Bergner *et al.* 1976a; 1976b; 1981) and is valuable for assessing the impact of illness on the chronically ill. It has been used in a randomized controlled trial of early exercise and counselling for patients with myocardial infarction. This study reported that the SIP showed that the group undergoing exercise plus counselling reported better functioning (Ott *et al.* 1983). It has also been used to evaluate treatment for patients with end-stage renal disease, with the result that transplantation patients had better SIP scores (Hart and Evans 1987). In a cross-sectional longitudinal study of 99 women with RA, the SIP was reported to be sensitive to one-year pre- and post-treatment changes showing both improvement and deterioration (Sullivan *et al.* 1990).

More negative results relating to sensitivity were reported by Hall *et al.* (1987) who tested the SIP against the Rand Health Insurance Study batteries. The Rand and the SIP were reported to be measuring different aspects of health. The range of scores for the Rand measures was less skewed than for the SIP. The problem with an instrument which registers high scores is that it may be unable to measure improvements in health. Thus the Rand measures have better discriminative abilities than the SIP.

A follow-up study of 185 stroke patients by Schuling *et al.* (1993) reported that the SIP was 'time consuming and tiring' with these patients, and it was insensitive to improvement in condition at eight weeks, in contrast to the cruder Barthel Index which did detect improvement. Katz *et al.* (1992) also found that the SIP was less sensitive to clinical change among patients undergoing hip replacement than shorter measures, including the SF-36 and a short version of the Arthritis Impact Measurement Scales. A review of studies using the SIP by de Bruin *et al.* (1992) reported research demonstrating that the SIP was insensitive to small

changes and improvements. The SIP's responsiveness to change has not yet been satisfactorily demonstrated. de Bruin *et al.*'s (1992) review also questions the SIP's construct validity as the results of factor analyses have been inconsistent.

Reliability

Work began on the SIP in 1972, and tests for reliability and validity continued to be conducted by its authors for over a decade. Patients studied included those with hypothyroidism, rheumatoid arthritis and hip replacements. The details of the reliability tests conducted on the SIP are reported by Bergner *et al.* (1981). Earlier reliability tests on SIPs of differing lengths before the development of the 136 version are reported by Pollard *et al.* (1976; 1978).

Test-retest reliability was high (0.88–0.92). Internal consistency was also high (0.81–0.97). The interviewer-administered versions scored better in each case than mailed or self-completed versions. Deyo *et al.* (1983) applied the SIP to 79 patients with arthritis and found that test-retest reliability for 23 patients tested was 0.91. It was found to have better reliability than the traditional functional scales of the American Rheumatism Association and patients' self-ratings of function. Test-retest reliability was better for the overall score than for each of the dimensions. Results of studies of the reliability of the SIP throughout Europe and the USA indicate similarly high levels of internal consistency (0.91–0.95), test-retest correlations (0.75–0.85) and also inter-rater reliability (0.87–0.92) (de Bruin *et al.* 1992).

UK adaptations

Although patient acceptance of the SIP was judged by the US authors to be good, it has been rejected for use in evaluations of heart-disease treatment programmes in the UK on the grounds of its length, and the more concise Nottingham Health Profile selected in preference (Buxton 1983; O'Brien 1988).

A modified version of the SIP has been developed at St Thomas's Hospital, London, for a community disability survey. The modified version is called the Functional Limitations Profile

(FLP) (Patrick 1982; Charlton *et al.* 1983). Linguistic changes were made and scale weights were recalculated, although these agreed closely with the original weights of the US version. The translation has been criticized by Hunt *et al.* (1986) on the grounds that language changes alone do not satisfy the requirements for cross-cultural adaptations. The changes made are fairly minimal and the FLP is still 136 items long, is designed to be interviewer-administered and contains the same range of scores from 0 (low) to 100 (high), although the weighting is different.

The authors later reported that FLP and SIP items grouped satisfactorily into five global measures: physical, psychosocial, eating, communication and work. They found the items related to age and number of medical conditions but were poor predictors of service use (Charlton *et al.* 1983).

A UK application of the Functional Limitations Profile was a study of 92 patients with chronic obstructive pulmonary disease by Williams and Bury (1989) who reported poor to good correlations between the FLP physical sub-section and clinical data of 0.38–0.90.

Another application of the FLP has been reported by Fitzpatrick *et al.* (1988) in their study of 105 patients with rheumatoid arthritis assessed over a 15-month period. They used both the FLP and the HAQ, but reported only modest levels of sensitivity and specificity in relation to data on clinical change for each. Although the authors acknowledged that the FLP provided more information and was more precise than the short HAQ, they caution that this has to be weighed against the simpler measurement assumptions and shorter time required to administer the HAQ. Fitzpatrick *et al.* (1988) concluded that the SIP/FLP is less sensitive to improvement than to deterioration. McColl *et al.* (1995) reported that the FLP had a high level of item of non-response and also had ceiling effects.

The conclusion relating to the FLP is that it requires far more testing for reliability and validity before it can be considered the UK alternative to the SIP.

Vetter *et al.* (1989) used their own adaptation of the SIP along with the Barthel Index to assess rehabilitation outcomes among a pilot sample of 59 elderly people receiving either home or day hospital care in Wales. The authors substantially changed the style of the SIP. They reported that respondents found the 'I' format (e.g. 'I dress myself, but do so very slowly') confusing. They became confused about who the 'I' was referring to. The statements were therefore changed to actual questions (e.g. 'Do you dress yourself, but do so very slowly?').

A further problem found with the use of the SIP by these UK researchers was that some questions were not applicable to all patients. Thus the question 'Are you unable to walk up and down hills?' in the original profile could be answered only 'yes' or 'no'. The researchers thus added a 'not applicable' category to avoid confusion, for example, for those who were bed/chairfast. The physical dimension scale of the SIP was found to have acceptable validity and was judged as a suitable measure of outcome (other dimensions are yet to be tested), although the correlations were unreported. The SIP was also found to be a stable measure when repeated eight weeks later on the patients (they were not expected to change in relation to physical state).

The advantages of the SIP and its adaptations are that it can be self-administered or interview based, it can be used with chronically or acutely ill patients, it has been adapted for use in the UK as the Functional Limitations Profile, and it is well tested for reliability and validity. Given its excellent properties of reliability and validity, it has been highly recommended for use as a gold standard by McDowell and Newell (1987) in their review of health-status measures. Its limitations are its length and it can be used only with people who are regarded or who regard themselves as ill; also, its factor structure and responsiveness to change has not been adequately demonstrated. International versions of the SIP have been reviewed by Anderson *et al.* (1993).

THE NOTTINGHAM HEALTH PROFILE (NHP)

The Nottingham Health Profile was developed in the UK and is based on lay perceptions of health status. The conceptual basis of the NHP was that it should reflect lay rather than professional definitions of health. It was developed after interviews with a large number of lay people about the effects of illness on behaviour. Hunt *et al.* (1986) commented that their pilot interviewing to develop the NHP demonstrated that lay people had a limited range of language for describing good health and well-being which would have made the creation of a comprehensive health index difficult. The NHP is not an index of disease, illness or disability but relates rather to how people feel when they are experiencing various states of ill health. As a survey tool it is useful in assessing whether people have a (severe) health problem, although diagnostic data would be required to point to the kind of health problem. The measure was not intended by its developers to measure health-related quality of life, nor to detect health conditions or states of mild symptom severity (Hunt 1984). It is too short to assess the impact of a condition on quality of life. For this, combinations of measures are required: a functional-disability scale, symptom and pain indices, a measure of psychological disturbance, quantitative and more qualitative methods of the impact on social functioning (e.g. work, interpersonal relationships and social support, domestic life, etc.). The NHP can provide only a shallow profile of effects on these aspects.

Pilot work with the NHP led to the identification of relevant concepts. Statements were drawn which exemplified those concepts and, after further piloting, statements were finally categorized into six areas: physical mobility, pain, sleep, energy, emotional reactions and social isolation. The Nottingham Health Profile is designed for self-completion, is concise and easily administered and was the first measure of perceived health which was extensively tested and developed for use in Europe.

Hunt et al. (1986) reported that, when the NHP is based on a postal survey, people are unlikely to return it if they have a high number of zero scores (no problems). People felt they had nothing to contribute to the study. Pilot work has been undertaken with positive items as dummies: 'I sleep soundly at night'; 'I am usually free of any pain'.

In the UK the Nottingham Health Profile has been used to evaluate the outcome of many therapies from the patient's perspective, and to assess the perceived health status of patients before and after undergoing specific surgery (e.g. coronary bypass, varicose veins, haemorrhoids, heart transplantation and various orthopaedic conditions).

The NHP is short and simple, and it can be used with groups of patients or a general population. Although it is suitable for people who are not necessarily unhealthy or ill, like many others it focuses on negative rather than positive experiences. Population norms exist for the instrument, as do scores on individual patient groups (Hunt et al. 1984b).

Content

Part I measures perceived or subjective health status by asking for yes/no responses to 38 simple statements of six dimensions: mobility, pain, energy, sleep, emotional reactions and social isolation. Each dimension has a range of possible scores of 0–100.

Part II asks about any effects of health on seven areas of daily life: work, looking after the home, social life, home life, sex life, interests, hobbies and holidays. Part II items are coded 1 for 'yes' and 0 for 'no' and then scored. Part II is not always a useful addition. For some groups several items do not apply, e.g. the elderly, the unemployed, the disabled, those on low incomes. The authors have recently carried out developmental work on Part II and recommend that Part II should no longer be used.

Examples of the NHP items include:

Part I
This asks about the applicability of statements to the respondent at the present time:

I'm tired all the time.
I have pain at night.
Things are getting me down.
I have unbearable pain.
I take tablets to help me sleep.

A main advantage of the NHP is that its authors have published a book containing a review of the development of the scale, studies of its reliability and validity, the NHP items and a users' manual (Hunt et al. 1986).

Scoring

The NHP is scored with scores ranging from 0 (no problems) to 100 (where all problems in a section are affirmed). The weighted scores are summed for each NHP domain, but an overall score is not obtainable. It has been extensively tested for reliability and validity, and results have been good.

The weights for the NHP were derived using Thurstone's method of paired comparisons. Judgements were obtained from several hundred people and converted into weights using the appropriate formula (McKenna *et al.* 1981).

The NHP scores are not 'true' numbers but are obtained from a scaling technique; thus the appropriate statistical tests for testing hypotheses are non-parametric. Its highly skewed distribution of scores (see column 2) means that careful consideration needs to be given to the application of statistical tests as many assume that the results are normally distributed although statistical transformations can be applied to skewed data, thus permitting the application of parametric statistics.

Part I of the NHP requires respondents to indicate 'yes' or 'no' according to whether the statement applies to them 'in general at the present time'. Relative weights are applied to these. All statements relate to limitations on activity or aspects of distress. Dimension scores of 100 indicate the presence of all limitations listed, and a zero score the absence of limitations, but these two extremes do not reflect the extremes of death or perfect health.

Part II, which has been temporarily withdrawn, relates to seven areas of task performance affected by health. Respondents answer 'yes' if their present state of health is causing problems with the activity. Part II has no weights: a count of affirmative responses is used as a summary statistic.

It is not possible to calculate an overall health-status score, although aggregation within categories is permitted.

There can be problems with the sensitivity of the NHP as a survey instrument because of the zero modal response which means that the NHP does not discriminate for a substantial proportion of the adult population. The problem with using the NHP within a population survey is that the sample would include a large number of relatively fit members who would gain low NHP scores. As it is a severe measure, minor illnesses are not detected by the instrument, and therefore minor improvements over time are unlikely to be detected. This problem was acknowledged by its authors:

> The NHP is clearly tapping only the extreme end of perceived health problems. Such a distribution was built into the NHP during its development. At an early stage it was decided that it would be undesirable to include health problems which would be affirmed by a large proportion of the population.
>
> (Hunt *et al.* 1986)

Hunt (1988) reported the proportion of zero scorers from combined data from several community studies using the NHP:

Section	Proportion of zero scores
Pain	83
Social isolation	82
Physical mobility	78
Energy	75
Emotional reactions	61
Sleep	56

As she admits, this instrument only taps the more extreme end of a distribution.

Kind and Carr-Hill (1987) used the NHP with 1,598 people in a follow-up study of the Rowntree Poverty Survey in York. The sample was weighted towards older and retired adults. Negative responses to all categories of the NHP exceeded 60 per cent, and for social isolation the figure rose to 89 per cent. Three items in particular only received 2 per cent endorsement: 'I find it hard to dress myself', 'I'm unable to walk at all', and 'I feel that life is not worth living'. Also, three of the most often cited items are drawn from the sleep category and three of the least frequently cited items are from the physical-mobility category. The authors argue that the skewness of the distribution of responses does not appear to be based on any logic. For example, nearly half of those who made just one positive response selected 'I'm waking up early in the morning', 17.5 per cent also chose 'I lose my temper easily' but no other item is chosen by more than 5 per cent of this group. In contrast, among those who scored heavily (11 or more positive responses), six items were more popular than 'I lose my temper easily'. They reported no simple relationship between the overall score and the probability of responding to any one item and that there appeared to be considerable redundancy among items. The scale and its scoring system have frequently been criticized for inconsistencies and anomalies (Anderson *et al.* 1993).

Validity

The NHP has been tested for face, content and criterion validity and has been reported to be a satisfactory measure of subjective health status in physical, social and emotional spheres. The face and content validity of the subjective items were established on the basis of the method for devising the scale: the items were drawn from lay experiences and respondents were able to relate to them and understand the relevance of the items (Hunt *et al.* 1986).

There have been numerous applications of the NHP in clinical and community settings. It has been used successfully as an outcome measure with patients undergoing heart transplants in the UK (O'Brien 1988; O'Brien *et al.* 1988) and was found to correlate well with clinical judgements of morbidity and prognosis as well as being simple to administer and analyse.

Jenkinson *et al.* (1988) used both the NHP and Goldberg's General Health Questionnaire on a population of 39 rheumatoid arthritis and 43 migraine patients and reported a correlation of 0.49 between the GHQ and the emotional-reactions scale of the NHP for both samples. The implication is that the NHP is providing no more than a moderately accurate measure in this domain.

Testing for discriminative ability took place with four groups of people aged 65+; 40 people participating in a research exercise programme; 19 patients from a general practitioner (GP's) list who had no known disability or illness and who had not contacted a doctor within the prior two months; 49 people with a variety of health and social problems attending a local authority-run luncheon club; 54 chronically ill patients on GPs' lists; 352 randomly selected patients from GPs' lists. Results showed that the NHP was able to discriminate between groups of 'well' and 'ill' people, and in terms of physiological fitness; high and low GP consulters; social classes, age groups and sexes and that the content of the questions was understood by, and acceptable to, elderly people. Perceived health status was also associated with objective health status (Hunt *et al.* 1980; 1986).

Jenkinson *et al.* (1988) assessed the sensitivity of the NHP with 39 rheumatoid arthritis sufferers and 43 migraine sufferers. The NHP was able to distinguish between the two patient groups: the arthritis patients scored worse in relation to effects on energy levels and mobility. Discriminant analysis showed that the NHP was able to discriminate between 79 per cent of arthritis and 93 per cent of migraine patients.

The NHP has been shown in other studies to be sensitive to change. One unpublished study cited by Hunt *et al.* (1986) was based on a sample of 80 pregnant women. The NHP was administered to the women at three stages during their pregnancy – 18, 27 and 37 weeks. The NHP was sensitive to changes during pregnancy. The NHP was also administered to 141 patients attending a fracture clinic and an equal number of control subjects. Scores were obtained soon after the fracture occurred and eight weeks later. Scores were sensitive to changes in perceived health, concomitant with the healing of the fracture (McKenna *et al.* 1984).

Another application of the NHP was reported by O'Brien *et al.* (1988). The authors used the instrument to measure quality of life before and after combined lung and heart transplantation in the UK. It was again sensitive to changes and correlated well with clinical measures such as exercise capacity (correlation coefficient for the latter not given). The results indicated significant reductions in NHP scores for patients at three months after surgery; no further differences were recorded at six and twelve months postoperatively. In a study of 196 heart transplant patients, the NHP was reported to be sensitive to deterioration in patients' condition prior to transplant and to post-transplant improvement. It was able to predict outcome in relation to length of hospital stay, return to work and leisure activity at three months after transplantation (Buxton *et al.* 1985; Caine *et al.* 1990).

Caine *et al.* (1991) also used the NHP to study the quality of life of 100 males aged under 60 before and after coronary artery bypass grafting. The NHP was sensitive to improvements in health following the procedure (at three months and one year later). The instrument was reported to be sensitive to improvements in patients' condition following treatment in a study of cardiac transplants and in a study of coronary artery bypass surgery (Buxton *et al.* 1985; Wallwork and Caine 1985). Other investigators have also reported good results with the NHP with coronary patients (Permanyer-Miralda *et al.* 1991), and have supported the ability of the NHP to discriminate between a normal population and those with a range of serious medical conditions (van Agt et al. 1993). Modest to good correlations between the NHP dimensions of pain, energy, and sleep and the pain reported by over 1,000 patients with zoster (reactivation of the varicella zoster virus) (of between 0.32–0.50) were reported by Mauskopf et al. (1994) (the other dimensions of the NHP were weaker). However, its performance in relation to respiratory disease, and clinical measures of respiratory function, is variable (Alonso et al. 1992); and it is less stable in relation to rheumatology patients (Fitzpatrick et al. 1992). While the scale appears sensitive to changes following dramatic treatment interventions, its performance with less dramatic, and more minor, treatments is less certain (Hunt et al. 1984a; Brazier et al. 1992).

There has been some criticism that each section does not represent just one dimension (Kind and Carr-Hill 1987; Kind mimeo). In particular, fairly high correlations between the pain and physical-mobility categories were reported. While covariation might be expected for items within categories, covariation between items in different categories raises difficulties in interpretation of a cross-category profile.

Reliability

Two studies have focused on the reliability of the NHP, using the test-retest technique. These were based on 58 patients with osteo-arthritis and 93 with peripheral vascular disease. The questionnaires were repeated with these two groups at four and eight weeks after the first administration respectively. Both demonstrated a fairly high level of reliability with correlations of between 0.71 and 0.88, with the exception of the items on home life (0.64), social life (0.59), interests and hobbies (0.44) for patients with osteo-arthritis; and social life (0.61), looking after the home (0.64) and work (0.55) for patients with vascular disease (Hunt et al. 1981; 1986). Part II of the NHP does not obtain as good results as Part I, which explains its withdrawal. For example, Hunt et al. (1981) reported that the test-retest reliability coefficients on the osteo-arthritis patients ranged between 0.77 to 0.85 for Part I in comparison with a wider range for Part II at 0.44 to 0.86. The authors note that any changes in perceived health between the two administrations

will consequently reduce the correlations (Hunt et al. 1981). The NHP does not meet the requirements for carrying out split-half reliability as it is too short and the items are not homogeneous. The authors also argue that it is not possible to test it against an acceptable gold standard as no suitable measure exists.

A study of its adaptation into French by Bucquet et al. (1990) confirmed the immediate intelligibility of the French version, although it was not without problems. The authors used the same methods of calculating item weights as McKenna et al. (1981) for the original version, based on Thurstone's paired comparisons; their study was based on a quota sample of 625 people ('judges'). However, Bucquet et al. did report that the respondents had difficulties making these ratings, especially in relation to the pain, mobility, energy and sleep sections. They did not all grasp the concept of a 'general view' easily when comparing the health statements. International versions of the scale have been reviewed by Anderson et al. (1993).

In sum, the advantages of the NHP are that it is short, simple and inexpensive to administer, it can be self-administered or interview based, it has been well tested for validity; partly tested for reliability and it is sensitive to change. However, it provides only a limited measure of function, and some disabilities are not assessed at all: e.g. sensory defects, incontinence, eating problems. It also lacks an adequate index of mental distress and requires supplementation if used as a broader measure of health-related quality of life. The measure was not intended by its developers to measure health-related quality of life, nor to detect health conditions or states of mild symptom severity (Hunt 1984). It is too short to test for split-half reliability, and it is a severe measure with a highly skewed distribution – it may not measure minor improvements in health. The result of the focus on severe conditions is that some people who are in distress may not show scores on the profile. Similarly, normally healthy persons or those with few ailments may affirm only a small number of statements on some sections. This makes it difficult to compare their scores over time. People who score zero cannot be shown to improve over time. It is a negative measure of health.

THE MCMASTER HEALTH INDEX QUESTIONNAIRE (MHIQ)

The McMaster Health Index Questionnaire was developed in Ontario, Canada, as a measure of physical, social and emotional functioning. The measure was intended to provide independent measurements of these separate areas, given the authors' recognition that two individuals with the same level of physical disability may differ widely in their social and emotional functioning (Chambers *et al.* 1976). The aim was to produce a health-status questionnaire suitable for administration to general populations that could be used to predict a health professional's clinical assessment of a person's health. It was developed on the basis of a literature review of health-status measurement, brainstorming sessions, and consultation of experts.

The Social Function Index section was developed after consideration of existing scales, including the Spitzer Mental Status Schedule, the Cornell Medical Index and the Katz Adjustment Scale (Brodman *et al.* 1949; Herron *et al.* 1964; Spitzer *et al.* 1964), and a range of survey instruments. Review of sociological studies of leisure and social participation produced an additional list of social function questions.

The selection criteria of items included positive as well as negative discriminators (i.e. good functioning was intended to be identified); general applicability and acceptability; low cost and quick administration; quantifiable responses.

The Health Index of the questionnaire included additional items on physical function and items relating to symptoms (respiratory symptoms) and behaviour (cigarette use). Clinical assessments of social function from 'very poor' to 'very good' were included. The original version contained 172 items. The best 59 items were identified after assessing responsiveness to change, prediction of physician's assessments and multivariate analyses, using physicians' assessments as the criterion variable. These items were tested initially on 70 patients in an acute medical ward and repeated after their discharge. The draft questionnaire was reported to be quick and simple to administer, acceptable to respondents and sensitive to changes in health status (values unreported). Clinical assessments were repeated by an independent physician

on 54 patients. Consistency ratings resulted in a Goodman-Kruskal Index of Agreement value of 0.90.

Further testing with over 200 patients registered with a family physician reported high consistency between social functioning items (dichotomizing responses into good and poor). The sensitivity of the instrument was assessed to be good. Self-completion of the final version of the McMaster Health Index Questionnaire takes 20 minutes.

The McMaster Health Index Questionnaire has been used on a number of different patient populations, including psychiatry out-patients, diabetic patients, respiratory-disease patients, patients with myocardial infarction and patients with rheumatoid arthritis (see review by Chambers 1984).

Content

The final version contains 24 physical-function items (physical activity, mobility, self-care, communication (sight, hearing), global physical function); 25 social-function items (general well-being, work/social role performance/material welfare, family support/participation, friends' support/participation and global social function); and 25 emotional-function items (self-esteem, feelings toward personal relationships, thoughts about the future, critical life events and global emotional function). The MHIQ contains only 59 items as some items cover both social and emotional functions.

All the physical function items are designed to evaluate the patient's functional level on the day the MHIQ is administered. The social-function items are explicitly concerned with a specific time period (usually the present). The agree–disagree emotional-function items are phrased in the present tense. Other emotional-function items refer to the recent past as specifically defined within the question (e.g. within the last year). None of the items ask the respondent to report changes in physical, social or emotional function.

The emphasis is on ability, rather than performance ('Can you . . . ?' rather than 'Do you . . . ?'). The aim was to elicit information on activities that could be observed at the time the MHIQ was completed. Examples of questions are:

Physical:

Today, are you physically able to take part in any sports (hockey, swimming, bowling, golf, and so forth) or exercise regularly?

1 No
2 Yes

Do you have any physical difficulty at all driving a car by yourself?

1 No
2 Yes   Is this because of a physical difficulty?
1 No
2 Yes

Emotional health:

(strongly agree 1 ——— strongly disagree 5)

I sometimes feel that my life is not very useful.
People feel affectionate towards me.

Social health:

(good 1 ——— poor 5)

How would you say your social functioning is today? (By this we mean your ability to work, to have friends, and to get along with your family.)

How much time, in a one-week period do you usually spend watching television? (none ——— more than two hours a day).

Scoring

A score of 1 is given to 'good function' responses for each item, and 0 is assigned to 'poor functioning' responses. The scores are summed, although alternative weighting schemes have been developed (Chambers *et al*. 1982).

Validity

The authors reported, without publishing the values, that the MHIQ correlated well with other scales: the physical-function item correlated well with rheumatologists' and occupational therapists' assessments based on the Lee Index of Functional Capacity; the MHIQ index of emotional, physical and social function correlated well with Bradburn's measures of psychological well-being. The physical-function index also correlated with analogue pain scales and with clinical and biological results (Chambers *et al*. 1982).

Assessments with a group of 96 physiotherapy patients showed a change in MHIQ scores between first visit and discharge, indicating sensitivity to change (Chambers *et al*. 1982) (numbers and values unreported). A subset of the items has been successfully used to predict patient outcome in a randomized controlled trial of patients treated by nurse practitioners and doctors (Sackett *et al*. 1974).

Self-completion has been reported to be superior in terms of sensitivity to change than the other methods (Chambers *et al*. 1987). In addition, 96 patients in a physiotherapy clinic were administered the MHIQ at four points in time. Patients were randomly assigned to different modes of administration: interviewer administered, self-completion, or telephone interview. Self-completion was superior in terms of sensitivity to change than the other methods (Chambers 1984).

Reliability

Chambers (1984) reported that reliability was assessed by asking 30 physiotherapy out-patients to complete the MHIQ on two occasions within a one-week period. Patients were not expected to change in their functional status. The correlation between the physical- and emotional-function values was 0.80. Intraclass correlation coefficients ranged from 0.48 to 0.95 for the physical, emotional and social scores. Internal consistency coefficients between the physical-, emotional- and social-functional indices were 0.76, 0.67 and 0.51 respectively. Reliability was not affected by self- or interviewer-administered scales.

In sum, the advantages of the scale are its flexibility – it can be used in different settings; it is amenable to mathematical scoring contruction; it focuses on present ability; it is positive in orientation; it is simple and inexpensive to administer, and acceptable to patients. It also has an acceptable level of reliability. However, it is of questionable applicability to the very elderly (e.g. question on sports participation in physical index). More studies of its reliability and validity are also needed.

THE RAND HEALTH INSURANCE/MEDICAL OUTCOMES STUDY BATTERIES

The Rand Corporation's health batteries were designed for the Rand Health Insurance Study (HIS), an experiment of health outcome following random allocation to various insurance plans among adults aged 14–61 years. The Medical Outcomes Study (MOS) involved the more detailed assessment of outcome and led to further development of the batteries (Stewart and Ware 1992). The batteries were developed for use in population surveys. More specifically, the Rand Health Insurance Study batteries were developed as an outcome measure to detect changes in health status that might be expected to occur as a result of health-service use within a relatively short period of time. The batteries cover physical health, physiological health, mental health, social health and perceptions of health. The measures were intended to be sensitive to differences in health in general populations (Ware and Karmos 1976; Stewart et al. 1978; 1981; 1989; Ware et al. 1979; 1980; Stewart and Ware 1992).

The HIS is based on a sample of about 8,000 people in 2,750 families in six sites across the USA. The HIS batteries were developed after extensive research into existing measures, and testing of adaptations of existing measures, or of new measures developed on the basis of extensive reviews of the literature. Each section can be used independently.

Apart from the Rand Health Insurance Study, there is an increasing number of other applications of the Rand batteries. One of these applications was carried out in two general practices in Sydney, Australia, by Hall et al. (1987). There is an International Quality of Life Assessment (IQOLA) Project which aims to translate and adapt the widely used short version of the batteries – the SF-36 Health Survey Questionnaire – in 15 countries. The aim of the project is also to validate and provide norms for the new translations, to facilitate their use in international studies of health outcomes (Aaronson et al. 1992).

The measures were developed, then, on the basis of reviews of the literature. Each section can be used independently. The authors have a wide range of publicly available reports of findings to date, and some published papers which show the interrelationships between the HIS batteries (Stewart et al. 1989; Wells et al. 1989). A short 20-item version of the batteries has been developed (Stewart et al. 1988), although this has now been overtaken by a 36-item version (the Short-Form 36), which is attracting international interest and has been tested

in the UK, in other European countries, and in the USA, with acceptable results for reliability and validity (Anderson et al. 1990; Stewart and Ware 1992).

PHYSICAL HEALTH BATTERY

In the Health Insurance Study physical health was operationalized in terms of functional status. A review of the literature revealed six categories of functional activity for which performance has been assumed to reflect physical health: self-care (e.g. feeding, bathing), mobility, physical activities, role activities (e.g. employment), household activities and leisure activities. These six areas were thus incorporated into the Rand battery, called the Functional Limitations Battery. These items in the Functional Limitations Battery were based on items from the US National Health Interview Survey and Patrick et al.'s (1973a; 1973b) work on developing functional ability scales. Performance was measured by three separate batteries of items: functional limitations, physical abilities and disability days.

An advantage of the Rand Functional Limitations Battery over a number of other scales is that it relates the scale to the cause of the physical incapacity.

The Rand Physical Health Battery includes the Physical Abilities Battery in addition to the Functional Limitations Battery. These are similar to each other and were intended to be administered to respondents at different stages of the longitudinal HIS.

Content

Fourteen HIS items assess activities in self-care, mobility, physical, household and leisure activities, and role activities.

Response choices are either 'yes' or 'no' or 'yes, can do', 'yes, can do but only slowly', 'no, unable to do'. Positive responses to problems lead to further items on length of restriction.

Examples from the (revised) Functional Limitations Battery and Physical Abilities Battery are:

Does your health limit the kind of vigorous activities you can do, such as running, lifting heavy objects, or participating in strenuous sports?   Yes   1/No   2

Do you have any trouble either walking several blocks or climbing a few flights of stairs, because of your health? Yes 1/No 2

Do you need help with eating, dressing, bathing, or using the toilet because of your health? Yes 1/No 2

Can you do hard activities at home, heavy work like scrubbing floors, or lifting or moving heavy furniture? Yes 1/Yes, but only slowly 2/No, I can't do this 3

If you wanted to, could you participate in active sports such as swimming, tennis, basketball, volleyball, or rowing a boat? Yes 1/Yes, but only slowly 2/No, I can't do this 3

Many of these items are inapplicable to very elderly people (e.g. strenuous sports activity) or are too general (e.g. asking about several limitations in the same question) to be useful in surveys where discriminative ability is important.

Scoring

Item score ranges vary: 0–3 (none to more severe limitations) for mobility; 0–4 for physical limitations; 0–2 for role limitations. Items can be scored in groups: mobility limitations, role limitations, self-care limitations (the latter included only one item). An overall score – the Functional Status Index – utilizes all items and is an index of the number of categories in which a person has one or more limitations (0–4). This has not been fully tested for validity.

Results from the Rand study showed that the physical health measures yielded skewed distributions: most sample members had no functional limitations or physical disabilities. This is a limitation regarding its suitability for use in population surveys.

Validity

The authors judged the measure to have acceptable content validity as the content of items included in the physical-health measures reflected the range of content reported in the literature. Construct validity was assumed by the authors as associations between the Functional Limitations Battery and the Physical Abilities Battery were moderate to strong (0.49–0.99), indicating an underlying general construct, presumably physical health.

Reliability

Reliability was estimated for the physical-abilities measures using internal-consistency coefficients. The internal-consistency and reproducibility coefficients for HIS measures of physical health were high (0.90 or above); test-retest coefficients (at four months apart) were also high (0.92–0.99).

MENTAL HEALTH BATTERY

As a result of an extensive literature review, ranging from assessments of depression scales to general well-being schedules, the measurement of symptoms of affective (mood) disorders (e.g. depression, anxiety) was considered important, as well as well-being and self-control of behaviour, moods, thought and feelings. The HIS Mental Health Battery contains items hypothesized to measure these constructs. It has been revised since its development in order to extend the range of measurement (particularly with anxiety and depression).

Content

The Revised Mental Health Battery is constructed from the General Well-Being Questionnaire. A new sub-scale has been added defining loss of behavioural/emotional control. The revised version was based on factor analyses. The General Well-Being Questionnaire comprises 46 questions with four to six response choices for each item, ranging from extremely positive to extremely negative evaluations. The Mental Health Battery utilizes 38 of these questions; the remaining eight items are used to estimate socially desirable responses. Examples of items are:

How much have you been bothered by nervousness or your 'nerves' during the past month?

Extremely so – to the point where I could not work or take care of things	1
Very much bothered	2
Bothered quite a bit by nerves	3
Bothered some – enough to bother me	4
Bothered just a little by nerves	5
Not bothered at all by this	6

During the past month, have you had any reason to

wonder if you were losing your mind, or losing control over the way you act, talk, think, feel, or of your memory?

No, not at all	1
Maybe a little	2
Yes, but not enough to be concerned or worried about it	3
Yes, and I have been a little concerned	4
Yes, and I am quite concerned	5
Yes, and I am very much concerned about it	6

In general, would you say your morals have been above reproach?

Yes, definitely	1
Yes, probably	2
I don't know	3
Probably not	4
Definitely not	5

How often have you felt like crying, during the past month?

Always	1
Very often	2
Fairly often	3
Sometimes	4
Almost never	5
Never	6

Scoring

Eight items measure social desirability and should be scored separately from the 38 Mental Health Index items.

Some items are recoded for scoring purposes. Sub-scales can be created relating to a life-satisfaction item; a psychological-distress scale; a psychological well-being scale and the mental-health index. This involves the simple addition of item scores and the recoded scores. High scores are interpreted differently for different sub-scales, according to the scale name; for example, a high score for a negative scale corresponds with an unfavourable score and a high score for a positive scale corresponds with a favourable score. Full details of the scoring method are available from the authors at Rand Corporation, Santa Monica.

Validity

The content validity of the HIS Mental Health Battery was assumed by the authors as it contained items represented in the literature. Construct validity is more questionable as correlations between these scales and those constructed for validity studies ranged from 0–0.01 to 0.94. This reflects doubt about the measurement of a common construct within the scale. The authors use these findings to support their decision to score and interpret separately the four construct specific mental-health scales. An Australian community survey by Hall *et al.* (1987) reported a correlation of -0.76 between the Rand Mental Health Battery and the General Health Questionnaire which largely assesses depression and anxiety.

Reliability

The reliability of the HIS mental-health measures was estimated using internal-consistency and test-retest coefficients. Internal consistency estimates were fairly high (0.72–0.94). Test-retest estimates ranged from 0.70 to 0.80, the time period between administrations being generally less than one week. A more recent development is a brief eight-item depression scale, with initially promising results for reliability and validity (Burnam *et al.* 1988; Wells *et al.* 1989a; 1989b).

DEPRESSION SCREENER

This eight-item, short self-report measure was developed to screen for depression (major depression and dysthymia) in the Rand Medical Outcomes Study (MOS) in the USA. It was developed for use in a screening instrument of three chronic diseases, and it was intended that the whole battery should not take more than 10 minutes to complete (Burnam *et al.* 1988).

The scale was developed on over 5,000 people from a general population sample, mental health service and primary care users. The study measures included the 20-item Center for Epidemiologic Studies Depression Scale (CES-D) (Radloff 1977) which enquired about symptoms and frequency, and two items from the Diagnostic Interview Schedule (DIS) on duration of symptoms (Robins *et al.* 1981). The full Diagnostic Interview Schedule was also used to assess psychiatric disorders (as a gold standard). To select the best items for the screener, logistic regression analyses were employed. The final set of items selected for the screener included six CES-D items and the two DIS items. The latter two items were important predictors of depression and had the largest co-efficients in the final regression model. A six-item screener, with the latter two items removed was also tested – the six-item depression screener. This performed very similarly to the eight-item screener, but the eight-item screener performed slightly better overall.

Content

All the questions relate specifically to depressive symptoms. The response format ranges from yes/no choices for the first three depression questions, to a four-point response choice ranging from 0 = rarely or none of the time to 3 = most or all of the time (the scores are reversed for one positive item in the scale: 'I enjoyed life'). Examples are:

11   In the past year, have you had two weeks or more during which you felt sad, blue or depressed; or when you lost all interest or pleasure in things that you usually cared about or enjoyed?
Yes/no

12A Have you felt depressed or sad much of the time in the past year?
Yes/no

13   For each statement below, mark one circle that best describes how much of the time you felt or behaved this way during the past week.

During the past week:

(b) I had crying spells
(d) I enjoyed life

Rarely or none of the time (<1 day)/some or a little of the time (1–2 days)/occasionally or a moderate amount of the time (3–4 days)/most or all of the time (5–7 days)

Scoring

The individual items carry different weights, and two of the items relate to diagnostically relevant periods. These features distinguish it from other depression scales. There is, however, a complicated scoring equation because of the differential weights applied to the items (see Burnam et al. 1988 for details).

Validity

The test results showed that the screener had high sensitivity and good positive predictive value for detecting recent depressive disorders and those that met full DSM-III criteria (American Psychiatric Association 1987; 1994; Burnam et al. 1988). It was better at predicting depressive disorder in the past month than within the past 6 or 12 months. Varying the cut-off point for the screener improved the sensitivity for longer prevalence periods (6, 12 months and lifetime). Detailed results for the specificity and sensitivity of the instrument by cut-off points have been published (Burnam et al. 1988).

Reliability

The test-retest reliability of the two DIS items from the screener were tested on 230 adults living in the community (baseline interview with the DIS and telephone follow-up of the depression sub-section of the DIS) showed that the overall agreement between the two DIS items asked on a lifetime basis was 86 per cent for two weeks of feeling depressed, and 91 per cent for two years of feeling depressed. The authors stated that the screener is suitable for population surveys and surveys of health-service users. It is a promising development; some minor alteration of wording (e.g. 'blue') will be required, and testing needed, before adoption elsewhere (Burnam et al. 1988).

Modifications of the screener and similar depression screeners from the Rand batteries

Three key items in the screener have been adapted for inclusion in one of the US versions of the SF-36 (the SF-36D). The items relate to (1) depression in the past year for two weeks or more, (2) depression for most days over a two-year period, and (3) depression for much of the time in the past year. The complex scoring of the screener has not been attempted, but instead the patterns of yes/no responses are used to identify patients at risk for major depression or dysthymia. A 'yes' reply to question 1 indicates a risk for major depression, and a 'yes' answer to questions 2 and 3 indicates a risk for dysthymia. Similar questions tested in large community studies identified 89 per cent of adults with a psychiatric diagnosis of major depression or dysthymia (Health Outcomes Institute (previously Interstudy) 1990).

There have been other attempts to develop a short screening questionnaire based on the Rand Health Insurance Experiment Mental Health Inventory. Berwick *et al.* (1991) have developed a five-item screening test which is able to detect the most significant Diagnostic Interview Schedule (DIS) disorders, and it performed as well as the original longer (18-item) version, and as well as Goldberg's (1978) General Health Questionnaire (30-item version).

THE SOCIAL HEALTH BATTERY

The Social Health Battery was developed alongside the other Rand health measures assessing physical and psychological status.

On the basis of the literature again, social health was operationally defined in terms of interpersonal interactions. The Social Health Battery measures social well-being and support, operationalized by measuring social interaction and resources. The two main dimensions of the 11-item battery are the number of social resources a person has, and the frequency with which s/he has contact with relatives and friends.

Content

The 11-item scale covers home, family, friendships, social and community life. It does not cover satisfaction with relationships. The scale has been described by Donald and Ware (1982). Questions include:

About how many close friends do you have – people you feel at ease with and can talk with about what is on your mind? (You may include relatives.)

During the past month, about how often have you had friends over to your home? (Do not count relatives.)

Every day.
Several days a week.
About once a week.
Two or three times in the past month.
Once in the past month.
Not at all in the past month.

And how often were you on the telephone with close friends or relatives during the past month?

Every day.
Several times a week.
About once a week.
Two or three times.
Once.
Not at all.

An additional item asks about frequency of letter writing but the authors advise dropping this item as so few people answer in the affirmative at all.

Scoring

An overall social support score utilizes all the items (except letter writing and a general question asking about how the person gets on with others). This scoring has not been fully tested for validity.

Validity

Data about validity was drawn from 4,603 interviews from the Health Insurance Study. The Social Health Battery is judged by its authors to have content validity insofar as it reflects the two major components of social health identified in the literature: interpersonal interaction and social participation. The authors do not attempt to include any of the other areas of social health; thus content validity is only partial.

Criterion validity was tested by using the items in the scale and a nine-item self-rating of health, a measure of emotional ties and a nine-item psychological-well-being scale. The correlations were low. Further evidence of the validity of the battery is required.

Reliability

The inter-item correlations are low. Test-retest coefficients are moderate and range from 0.55 to 0.68. Further testing for reliability is required.

The results for reliability and validity are not so far convincing. Further testing is required. The large-scale and longitudinal nature of the Rand HIS study offers exciting possibilities for further testing and development of the measure.

SOCIAL SUPPORT SCALE

The Rand social support questionnaire was developed during the MOS (Sherbourne and Hays 1990). It reflects more recent conceptual thought on the subjective components of social support. An early 17-item version was used on almost 2,000 patients with chronic diseases in the Rand MOS study. For this study, social support was operationalized by four multi-item measures of the availability, if needed, of four distinct types of functional support: tangible support, involving the provision of material aid or behavioural assistance; affectionate support, involving expressions of love and affection; positive social interaction, involving the availability of other persons to do pleasurable things with; and emotional/informational support, involving the expression of positive affect, empathetic understanding, and the offering of advice, guidance or feedback (Sherbourne and Hays 1990). The latter was judged to be important to include because the authors felt that this type of support would be beneficial to the health outcomes of people with chronic illnesses.

Although the authors initially used a 17-item scale to represent these dimensions, they subsequently developed a 19-item version, which involved dividing the emotional/informational support domain into two dimensions, and thus the scale then contained five, rather than four, dimensions of social support (Sherbourne and Stewart 1991; Sherbourne *et al.* 1992). The emotional and informational domains were later combined back into the emotional/informational support sub-scale following evaluation by multi-trait correlation matrix, which showed considerable overlap between the items (Sherbourne and Stewart 1991).

In the 19-item version, two single items on the structure of social support are included in order to compensate for the lack of focus on the structure of the network (the number of close friends and relatives, and marital status). The development of the 19-item support scale was based on the same conceptual framework, question type and response format as the 17-item scale, and was described by Sherbourne and Stewart (1991). The 19-item scale is the current version.

The items selected for inclusion were derived from a larger pool of 50 items constructed on the basis of a literature review (Sherbourne and Stewart 1991). The items deliberately reflect subjective impressions of social support, rather than objective network structures (the latter was omitted in order to reduce respondent fatigue).

Content

For each item (in both the 17- and 19-item versions), respondents are asked how often each kind of support was available to them if they needed it. The five-point choice response scale for each item ranges from 'none of the time', 'a little of the time', 'some of the time', 'most of the time' to 'all of the time'. Five points were chosen by the authors on the basis of their review of the research evidence that five to seven response categories are necessary for optimal assessment. Examples from the scale are:

Next are some questions about the support that is available to you.

1 About how many close friends and close relatives do you have (people you feel at ease with and can talk to about what is on your mind)?

Write in number of close friends and relatives:

Circle one number on each line

None of the time (1)	A little of the time (2)	Some of the time (3)	Most of the time (4)	All of the time (5)

2 Someone to help you if you were confined to bed
3 Someone you can count on to listen to you when you need to talk
4 Someone to give you good advice about a crisis
5 Someone to take you to the doctor if you needed it
10 Someone who hugs you
15 Someone to help with daily chores if you were sick
20 Someone to love and make you feel wanted

Scoring

Each response ('none of the time' to 'all of the time') is scored 1 to 5, and summed (the higher the score, the greater the level of social support).

Validity and reliability

Sherbourne *et al.* (1992) used the 19-item scale in a study of the effects of social support and stressful life events, on long-term physical functioning and emotional well-being of 1,402 chronically ill people (with hypertension, diabetes, coronary heart disease or depression) participating in the Rand Medical Outcomes Study. This study supported the scale's construct validity. The authors reported that patients with high levels of social support had better levels of physical functioning and emotional well-being than those with low levels of support, supporting its construct (convergent) validity. In relation to the same sample, the 19 items were reported by Sherbourne and Stewart (1991) to be correlated weakly to moderately with measures of loneliness, health perceptions, mental health and measures of family and social functioning. The authors argue that this supports their construct (discriminant) validity. Standardized factor loadings ranged from 0.76 to 0.93 for the tangible support factor, 0.86–0.92 for the affection factor, 0.82–0.92 for the emotional/informational factor, and 0.91–0.93 for the positive interaction factor. Results of principal components factor analysis of the 19 items also supported the construction of the overall index (the first unrotated factor showed high loadings for each of the items, ranging from 0.67 to 0.88). These results support the scale as containing four dimensions and as providing a common measure of overall support.

Sherbourne and Stewart (1991) reported that the correlations (Pearson's) between the items and the sub-scales were strong. Item-scale correlations ranged from 0.72 to 0.87 for the tangible support scale, 0.80–0.86 for the affection scale, 0.82–0.90 for the emotional/informational scale, and 0.87–0.88 for the positive interaction scale.

The additional item on number of close friends and relatives correlated low to moderately with each of the functional support items (0.18–0.23), indicating its distinct status; marital status was not associated with numbers of close friends or relatives (0.01), but was more highly correlated with the functional support items (0.69–0.82).

Because of its concentration on subjective perceptions, this scale needs to be supplemented with an objective measure of the structure of the network (e.g. size, composition, frequency of contact, geographical proximity, contacts by telephone/mail). Although it requires supplementation, and far more extensive testing, it is a promising scale and merits wider use in order to more fully assess its psychometric properties and cross-cultural applicability. One advantage of this scale is that it contains more health specific items than many of the more generic social support scales that have been developed. Most social support scales were developed in the USA and contain culture specific items which would be unusual in other societies (e.g. about having someone who would loan the respondent a car).

GENERAL HEALTH PERCEPTIONS BATTERY

This asks respondents for an assessment or self-rating of their health in general (Stewart *et al.* 1978; Davies and Ware 1981). These are defined in the HIS with respect to time (perceptions of prior, current and future health) and with respect to three other constructs indicative of general health perceptions, including resistance or susceptibility to illness, health worry and concern, and sickness orientation (the extent to which people perceive illness to be a part of their lives).

A major strength of the General Health Perceptions Battery is ease of administration. Self-administration of this section takes approximately seven minutes. It is of potential use in studies attempting to predict the use of medical services.

Content

The battery contains 29 items, 26 of which were taken from the Health Perceptions Questionnaire developed by Ware and Karmos (1976) for the National Center for Health Services Research.

The items include statements of opinion about personal health (e.g. 'I expect to have a very healthy life'), accompanied by five standardized response categories defining a true–false continuum: definitely true, mostly true, don't know, mostly false, definitely false. These items are used to score six sub-scales assessing different dimensions of health perceptions: past health, present health, future health, health-related worries and concerns, resistance or susceptibility to illness and the tendency to view illness as part of life. Examples of items are:

I try to avoid letting illness interfere with my life.
I will probably be sick a lot in the future.
I don't like going to the doctor.
I'm not as healthy as I used to be.

When I'm sick, I try to just keep going as usual.
I expect to have a very healthy life.
When I think I am getting sick, I fight it.

It is apparent from these questions that analyses need to control for age, especially in relation to expectations about the future and current health status.

Scoring

All items are scored to produce a global figure, although the scoring has not been fully tested for validity. Distributions appear to be fairly normal. Hall *et al.* (1987) reported the Rand measures to be less skewed than the SIP or GHQ.

Validity

The measure of health perceptions was reported by the authors to be correlated with the physical, mental and social health batteries (coefficients unreported). In the Australian study by Hall *et al.* (1987) the Rand batteries relating to general health perceptions were tested on 160 patients along with the Sickness Impact Profile and the General Health Questionnaire. A correlation of −0.30 was considered to be the threshold for assessment of relationships between the three instruments. The Rand mental-health index was reported to correlate weakly to moderately well with three of the SIP components (emotional behaviour): −0.32 to −0.54. To some extent the same constructs are being measured, although these correlations are not high. If 0.50 is taken as the minimum correlation coefficient for validity acceptance for group studies, then the instruments tested do not achieve this (Ware *et al.* 1980). On the other hand, it was reported previously that the GHQ correlated highly with the Rand Mental Health Battery (−0.76) (Hall *et al.* 1987).

The stability of the Health Perceptions Battery has been estimated for intervals of one, two and three years between administrations. The median stability coefficients for one, two and three years for adults are 0.66, 0.59 and 0.56 respectively. Further tests are ongoing for reliability and validity. Preliminary results suggest that it can discriminate between those with and without a chronic disease, is sensitive to individual differences in disease severity, and is sensitive to changes over time in both physical and mental functioning.

Hall *et al.* (1987) reported that of the three instruments used in the Australian study (the Rand instrument, the SIP and the GHQ), the Rand measures had the best discriminative ability and were reported by the authors to be preferred as a general health-status measure in a general population.

Reliability

The reliability of the Health Perceptions Questionnaire scale was estimated using internal consistency and test-retest coefficients. These were tested by its authors using a non-HIS population. Test-retest reliability estimates were based on data collected approximately six weeks apart from the same respondents. Results indicate that the scale was more reliable than single-item measures, although internal-consistency coefficients (unreported) were lower than for test-retest. Internal consistency for the scale generally exceeded 0.50 (sometimes 0.90). More extensive testing of the Rand instruments is still required.

THE SHORT FORM-36 HEALTH SURVEY QUESTIONNAIRE (SF-36)

The Short Form-36 was developed at the Rand Corporation in the USA for use in the Health Insurance Study Experiment/Medical Outcomes Study (HIS/MOS) (Ware *et al.* 1993). It is a concise 36-item health-status questionnaire, and its use across the world has escalated since 1990. The authors of the SF-36 aimed to develop a short, generic measure of subjective health status that was psychometrically sound, and that could be applied in a wide range of settings. Initially, the SF-20 (Short Form 20-item version) was designed. For this, 17 items were taken from the questionnaires used in the HIS and three new items were added (Ware *et al.* 1992). This was used in the MOS. The authors decided to extend the scale to make it more comprehensive and with better psychometric properties. This led to the longer SF-36 item version. The SF-36 is made up of the items which loaded best on factor analyses from 149 items from the longer batteries, based on the results from over

22,000 patients in the Rand HIS/MOS studies. The SF-36 takes 5–10 minutes to complete and is self-administered.

Population norms for the UK have now been presented from a series of postal surveys (Brazier *et al.* 1992; Garratt *et al.* 1993; Jenkinson *et al.* 1993; Ware 1993), results for the rest of Europe are being published (e.g. Bullinger 1995; Sullivan *et al.* 1995) and results for the USA have been reviewed and published in the handbook of the instrument by Ware *et al.* (1993).

The SF-36 was initially solely distributed by the Rand Organization in Santa Monica, where it was developed, and by the Health Outcomes Institute in Bloomington (previously known as InterStudy). Transfers of copyright have led to the sole distributor now being the Medical Outcomes (Study) Trust of the Health Institute at the New England Medical Center, in Boston, where one of its main developers, John Ware, is based. The instrument is known here as the Short Form-36 Health Survey (SF-36 Health Survey). However, Rand still distribute the original instrument, but it is called the Rand 36-item Health Survey. The Health Outcomes Institute also distribute it, in collaboration with Rand, under the title of the Health Status Questionnaire, and have developed an accompanying brief depression screener (the Short Form-36-D), based on Rand items. The versions are virtually identical, but contain minor modifications and differences in scoring, and the Health Outcomes Institute's most recent version (2.0) contains 39 items. Each of the distribution centres provides a manual, including details of scoring, for its version of the instrument, and each aims to improve the questionnaire. The version reviewed here is the SF-36 Health Survey distributed by the Medical Outcomes (Study) Trust (Medical Outcomes Trust 1993; Ware *et al.* 1993). The UK version was developed by Brazier *et al.* (1992). The only changes to the original version include anglicization of some of the language and a slight alteration of the positioning and coding of one of the social functioning items in order to improve reliability in the UK and ease of administration. It is distributed by the UK Clearing House for Information on the Assessment of Health Outcomes; a manual for the UK can be purchased from the Department of Public Health and Primary Care, University of Oxford, OX2 6HE.

Content

The SF-36 contains 36 items which measure eight dimensions: physical functioning (10 items), social functioning (2), role limitations due to physical problems (4), role limitations due to emotional problems (3), mental health (5), energy/vitality (4), pain (2) and general health perception (5). There is also a single item about perceptions of health changes over the past 12 months (in effect, providing a ninth domain). It claims to measure positive as well as negative health.

Two versions are available from the Medical Outcomes Trust with varying time recall referents in the responses to current health-status questions – respondents are asked about their health over the past four weeks (the most commonly used) or (in the case of acute conditions) over the past one week. Examples are:

Does your health limit you in these activities? If so, how much?

(a) Vigorous activities, such as running, lifting heavy objects, participating in strenuous sports
(d) Climbing several flights of stairs
(g) Walking more than a mile
(h) Walking half a mile
(j) Bathing and dressing yourself

Yes, limited a lot/yes, limited a little/no, not limited at all

During the past four weeks, have you had any of the following problems with your work or other regular daily activities as a result of your physical health?

(a) Cut down on the amount of time you spent on work or other activities
(d) Had difficulty performing the work or other activities (e.g. it took extra effort)

Yes/no

How much bodily pain have you had during the past four weeks?

None/very mild/mild/moderate/severe/very severe

Scoring

Each sub-scale employs its own response format; these vary from dichotomous 'yes/no' responses to a six-point scale of 'none' to 'very severe'. While there is no evidence that different response formats produce different results, it is possible that too many different response styles within a single scale can be visually confusing for respondents.

The scoring algorithms adopted for the SF-36 were published after careful study of a number of alternatives. The scoring method selected was chosen for its simplicity and to optimize the ability to make comparisons of results across studies (Ware et al. 1993). Item scores for each of the eight dimensions are summed and transformed, using a scoring algorithm, into a scale from 0 (poor health) to 100 per cent (good health). The coding format requires recoding before each sub-scale can be summed. The sub-scales are not summed together to produce an overall score. The results have conventionally been reported as mean scores for each sub-scale, rather than frequency distribution, despite the well-known tendency of means to distort results by reflecting small numbers of outlying values. The validity of this method, and the common usage of parametric statistics to analyse the SF-36, has been seriously questioned by Julious et al. (1995), given the non-normal distributions of the data.

Validity

The detailed results of the testing of the longer Rand batteries have been published by Stewart and Ware (1992), together with the history of the development of the SF-36 from these instruments. Brazier et al. (1992), on the basis of the results of a postal survey in the UK, reported that the SF-36 was found to be more sensitive to gradations in poor health than the EuroQol (EuroQol Group 1990) and the Nottingham Health Profile (Hunt et al. 1986). The authors cautioned that there was a higher rate of item non-response among older people, a finding confirmed by Sullivan et al. (1995) on the basis of a Swedish postal survey sample (in contrast to interview surveys). However, reports are contradictory, and research in the USA has found good responses among elderly people (Health Outcomes Institute 1990). On a more critical level, Hill and Harries (1994) reported serious flaws in the instrument when used to measure the outcomes of health care for people aged 65 and

over in community settings in the UK. The respondents (who tended to have high levels of co-morbidity and poor physical functioning) often reported during interviews that the SF-36 did not reflect their values. In one district, the median physical functioning score for the group was zero (worst functioning), meaning that the group as a whole were pushed to the margins of the scale. While dramatic improvements in physical functioning in this group, and therefore improvements in scores, were unlikely, the measure was reported to miss some changes that were important to people. These findings support the argument of Hunt and McKenna (1993) who argue that the development and testing of the SF-36 has relied too heavily on psychometric techniques at the expense of serious consultation of lay people for their views about the instrument.

Mangione et al. (1993), in a study of 745 major elective (non-cardiac) patients in Boston, reported that the SF-36 health perception scale had the greatest correlation with the energy and fatigue scale (r = 0.45), correlated moderately with mental health (r = 0.35), social function (r = 0.32), and physical function (r = 0.33), but correlated less well with pain (r = 0.23). These results support the distinctive components of the health perceptions sub-scale although, on the other hand, these moderate to weak correlations among variables that would be expected to be more highly correlated (health perceptions and the various domains of health status) also suggest that the health perceptions battery might have weak construct (convergent) validity.

Mangione et al. (1993) also reported that the SF-36 was able to discriminate between surgical groups (major elective, non-cardiac surgery), and between younger patients and patients who were aged 70 years and over in relation to role function, energy, fatigue and physical function (the older patients had poorer scores on these domains). Ware et al. (1993), in the manual of the SF-36, reported that in tests for validity, the SF-36, was able to discriminate between groups with physical morbidities (the physical functioning sub-scale performed best and the mental-health sub-scale discriminated between patients with mental-health morbidities the best). Investigators in Grampian reported that different common medical conditions (low back pain, menorrhagia, suspected peptic ulcer and varicose veins) achieved a distinct score profile, indicating that the SF-36 can discriminate between conditions (Garratt *et al.* 1993). Further papers by these authors reported the scale means for these patient groups and good responsiveness to change in clinical condition (Garratt *et al.* 1994; Ruta *et al.* 1994a). The mental–health sub-scale has a particularly impressive validity. For example, it was reported to be correlated by between 0.92 and 0.95 with the full Mental Health Inventory from different samples from the HIS (Davies *et al.* 1988; Stewart and Ware 1992). Correlations between the SF-36 and the General Psychological Well-Being measure (Dupuy 1984) ranged from r = 0.19 to r = 0.60, with a median of r = 0.36. Ware *et al.* (1993) presented the data from several studies that show that the correlations for the sub-scales range from weak to strong, but strong correlations were reported between the physical functioning sub-scale and the equivalent sub-scales of the SIP, the AIMS and the NHP (0.52 to 0.85). Strong correlations were reported between the mental–health sub-scale and other psychological sub-scales (the range was r = 0.51 to r = 0.82).

Not all results have been good (see review by Anderson *et al.* 1993). For example, the bodily pain scale has been reported to have poor convergent validity with severity of illness and independent pain scores in the case of knee conditions (McHorney *et al.* 1993). Other studies have reported 'floor' effects in the role functioning scales in severely ill patients, where 25–50 per cent of patients obtained the lowest score possible, with the implication that deterioration in condition will not be detected by the scale (Kurtin *et al.* 1992). The comparable percentage in an HIV population is 63 per cent (Watchel *et al.* 1992). Anderson *et al.* (1993) have also suggested that the item codes can be subject to 'ceiling' effects as they appear too crude to detect improvements. Other investigators have reported that it has little discriminatory power among women receiving different treatments for stage II breast cancer (Levine *et al.* 1988; Guyatt *et al.* 1989). The physical functioning scale also focuses more on mobility at the expense of other pertinent areas of functioning (e.g. domestic), necessitating its supplementation with other scales in studies of people with chronic conditions which affect their functioning (e.g. rheumatoid arthritis). Its sensitivity may vary with disease type.

Reliability

In the UK, Brazier *et al.* (1992) reported internal coefficiency correlations for the eight scales as ranging from 0.60 to 0.81, with a median of 0.76. High inter–item correlations were reported for the sub-scales (e.g. mental health). Jenkinson *et al.* (1993) reported that it has high internal consistency between dimensions, with high Chronbach's alphas being obtained of between 0.76 and 0.90. Garratt *et al.* (1993) reported that the internal consistency between the items exceeded 0.80 with Chronbach's alpha, and inter–item correlations ranged from 0.55 to 0.78. All satisfied statistical criteria of acceptable levels. Ware *et al.* (1993) reviewed 14 studies in the USA which analysed the reliability of the SF-36. The reliability coefficients for internal consistency range from 0.62 to 0.94 for the sub-scales, for test–retest reliability the coefficents range from 0.43 to 0.90, and for alternate form reliability the coefficient was 0.92. In relation to internal consistency, all but 11 coefficients reported in studies in the USA and UK exceeded the 0.70 standard suggested by Nunnally (1978).

Ware *et al.* (1993) also reported the results of a factor analysis of the SF-36, which provided strong evidence for the conceptualization of health underlying the SF-36, and indicated that some scales principally measure physical health, some measure mental health, and others measure both. Garratt *et al.* (1993) also reported the results of a factor analysis which confirmed the distinct scale dimensions.

Ware *et al.* (1993) concluded that the level of reliability achieved by the SF-36 is lower than that achieved by the full length versions of the MOS scales they were constructed to reproduce (e.g. mental health, health perceptions). The minimum reliability standards appear to have been most consistently met with the physical functioning sub-scale.

THE SHORT FORM-12 HEALTH SURVEY QUESTIONNAIRE (SF-12)

Ware *et al.* (1995; 1996a; 1996b), at the Medical Outcomes Trust in Boston, have developed a 12-item version of the SF-36, known as the Short-Form-12 (SF-12). Radosevich and colleagues (Radosevich and Husnik 1995; Radosevich and Pruitt 1995), at the Health Outcomes Institute in Bloomington, have also tested a slightly different 12-item version known as the Health Status Questionnaire-12 (HSQ-12). The 12 items are all contained in each version of the SF-36 distributed by the different centres. Ware *et al.* (1996a; 1996b) reported that the 12 items that were selected for inclusion (with an improved scoring algorithm) were able to reproduce at least 90% of the variance in the physical and mental sub-scales of the SF-36. They argue that, consequently, the population norms for the SF-36 can also be used as norms for the SF-12.

The 12 items for both versions include the self-assessment of health, physical functioning; physical role limitation; mental role limitation; social functioning; mental-health items and pain. Standard four-week and one-week (acute) recall versions are available. These 12 items yield the eight scale profiles of the SF-36, but with fewer levels and with less precise scores, as would be expected with fewer items (e.g. some sub-scales now have just one or two items).

At the Health Outcomes Institute, the items were derived by using regression analysis on the data from over 4,000 respondents to the 39-item version of the questionnaire. Stepwise linear regression was used to select preliminary sets of questions that accounted for approximately 90 per cent of the variability in overall scale scores. The processes and results have been described by Radosevich and Husnik (1995). The authors decided to emphasize items from the physical functioning and mental-health sub-scales as these have been shown to be the most sensitive in distinguishing medical and psychiatric conditions (McHorney *et al.* 1993). The version of the instrument developed by members of the Health Outcomes Institute was then initially tested against their longer 39-item version of the (SF-36) battery among a group of cardiology patients and in a healthy working population (Radosevich and Pruitt 1995). Over 800 respondents took part in the reliability testing. Replicate reliability coefficients for the short (12 items) and long forms (39 items) were above 0.52 for all scales. Seventeen centres are collaborating in a validation exercise of the instrument, based on patients with mental-health conditions, chronic health problems and surgical procedures.

THE DARTMOUTH COOP FUNCTION CHARTS

These charts were developed by a collaborative body of medical doctors in community settings who aimed to produce a simple, concise, valid and reliable instrument which could be used easily during doctor–patient consultations.

The original US version of the charts contains nine sections (or charts): three on functioning (social, physical and role functioning), two on symptoms (pain and emotional condition), three on perceptions (change in health, overall health and quality of life) and one on social support (Nelson *et al.* 1983; 1987; 1990a; 1990b; Nelson and Berwick 1989). The World Organization of Family Doctors (WONCA) selected the charts as an international set of approved self-administration instruments for measuring health and functional status in primary care consultations, and called them the Dartmouth COOP Functional Health Assessment Charts/ WONCA (abbreviated as the COOP/WONCA Charts) (Scholten and van Weel 1992; van Weel *et al.* 1995). A feasibility study was launched in seven countries by WONCA (Landgraf and Nelson 1992). The instrument was revised and comprised six, not nine, charts, and each chart was renamed: physical fitness, feelings, daily activities, social activities, change in health and overall health. The pain, quality of life and social support charts were not included in the WONCA version. Other revisions were made to the question wording and response categories (van Weel and Scholten 1992). The WONCA version of the charts is known as the Dartmouth COOP Functional Health Assessment Charts/WONCA (COOP/WONCA). The history of the development of the charts has been summarized by Anderson *et al.* (1993).

Content

The full, original US version contains three charts on functioning (social, physical and role functioning), two on symptoms (pain and emotional condition), three on perceptions (change in health, overall health and quality of life) and one on social support. As mentioned earlier the WONCA version contains six, not nine, charts, and each chart was renamed: physical fitness, feelings, daily activities, social activities, change in health and overall health.

The original US charts took the last four weeks as the time reference periods for each question, but the WONCA version takes two weeks (e.g. 'During the past two weeks . . . What was the hardest physical activity you could do for at least two minutes?'). Each chart has its own five-point Likert response choices (e.g. in response to the previous example of an item, the responses are: 'very heavy (for example) run, at a fast pace (1)' to 'very light (for example) walk, at a slow pace or not able to walk (5)'; 'no difficulty at all' to 'could not do'; 'much better' to 'much worse'). The problem with this particular chart is that the examples of the activities within each response item (run, jog, walk) do not all fit logically or sensibly with the response item descriptors (very heavy to very light): how does one run in a way that is 'very heavy'? How can the inability to walk logically equate with the response code 'very light'? The response codes conjure up images of strength rather than mobility. This leads to conceptual confusion. The other five charts do not suffer from this problem.

Scoring

The scoring on each has 5 as equalling the worst level of functioning. Each chart represents a distinct domain and the charts are not summed together to form an overall score (Nelson *et al.* 1990a; 1990b). Illustrations (stick figures, faces and symbols plus–minus and arrow signs) are included on each chart, to illustrate the response choices (Nelson *et al.* 1987). They are self-administered. The administration time for the nine charts was five minutes. The charts have been translated into 20 languages. The physical fitness chart (WONCA version) is shown below.

Physical fitness chart:

During the past two weeks . . .
What was the hardest physical activity you could do for at least two minutes?

Very heavy (for example)
run, at a fast pace

Heavy (for example)
jog, at a slow pace

Moderate (for example)
walk, at a fast pace

Light (for example)
walk, at a medium pace

Very light (for example)
walk, at a slow pace
or not able to walk

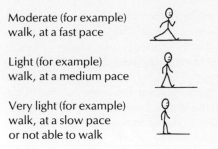

(Dartmouth COOP Functional Health Assessment Charts/WONCA. Copyright © Trustees of Dartmouth/COOP Project 1995.)

The COOP/WONCA charts may be used for research and clinical care. Permission to use the COOP/WONCA charts specifically exclude the right to distribute, reproduce or share them in any form for commercial purposes.

Validity

The charts were initially tested on over 1,400 patients with different groups of conditions from four medical centres in the USA (Nelson *et al.* 1987). In The Netherlands the WONCA version was tested on over 5,000 patients, and their population norms have been published (Scholten and van Weel 1992; van Weel *et al.* 1995). The testing procedures for the WONCA version have been briefly summarized by van Weel and Scholten (1992) and van Weel *et al.* (1995).

In support of their construct (convergent) validity, the charts on functioning and feelings have been reported to correlate well with other measures of physical and emotional functioning respectively, such as the Barthel Index and the Zung Depression Scale (Schuling and Meyboom-de Jong 1992). The psychometric testing of the WONCA version of the scale among two populations in The Netherlands (one with an average age of 43, and the other aged 60 and over) reported that, in the younger age group, the physical fitness chart and the daily activities chart correlated moderately to moderately well with the physical mobility sub-scale of the Nottingham Health Profile, at 0.53 and 0.66 respectively, and with the Rand SF-36 physical functioning sub-scale at 0.52 and 0.55 respectively. The feelings chart correlated moderately well with Goldberg's General Health Questionnaire (0.63) and with the mental-health sub-scale of the Rand SF-36 (0.71). The overall health chart correlated moderately well with the general health sub-scale of the Rand SF-36 (0.62).

The results for the group aged 60+ were weaker. Only the comparisons with the Rand SF-36 was reported for this group. The physical fitness chart and the daily activities chart correlated weakly to moderately with the physical functioning sub-scale of the SF-36 (0.56 and 0.31 respectively); the feelings chart correlated more strongly with the mental-health sub-scale of the SF-36 (0.76); the overall health chart correlated moderately well with the general health sub-scale of the SF-36 (0.67) (van Weel et al. 1995).

The performance of single charts is less precise in detecting differences in functional status than multi-item health-status scales, although the full set of charts perform well together in comparison with the Rand Medical Outcomes Study short-form measures (Meyboom-de Jong and Smith 1990), and show higher levels of sensitivity than Hunt et al.'s (1986) Nottingham Health Profile (Coates and Wilkin 1992). The influence of the illustrations in increasing sensitivity, rather than biasing respondents in some way, particularly in different cultural settings, is uncertain (McHorney et al. 1992).

The evidence on responsiveness to change is limited, although initial studies indicate that the charts are responsive to improvements in elderly patients with a range of conditions (van Weel et al. 1995).

Reliability

Test-retest correlations at four weeks in a German study were reported to be modest at 0.42–0.62 (van de Lisdonk and van Weel 1992). These results echo the low test-retest correlations reported for the original charts (Meyboom-de Jong and Smith 1990). In a Dutch study, with an interval of three weeks, they were were stronger at 0.67–0.82, with a kappa of 0.49–0.59; and over one year they were 0.36–0.72, with a kappa of 0.31–0.38 (Meyboom-de Jong and Smith 1990).

The inter-chart correlations for the WONCA version range between 0.15 and 0.66 (van Weel et al. 1995). Multi-trait–multi-method analysis has reported that the physical and role functioning charts are highly correlated, suggesting a common

domain, while the emotional status and social support charts are more independent, suggesting that they are measuring different domains of functioning (Landgraf et al. 1990).

Despite their popularity in general practice, the charts have not yet been satisfactorily tested for their psychometric properties, and details of the research design on which the testing has been based are often lacking (see review by Anderson et al. 1993). The deliberate omission of pain, social support and quality of life from the short WONCA version, in the interests of brevity, is regrettable, particularly in view of the current emphasis on including a specific self-assessment of quality of life in broader health-status scales. The charts also suffer from the same disadvantage as single-item measures: they are limited in content and therefore their sensitivity is potentially limited. Anderson et al. (1993) concluded that the content validity of the physical fitness chart, for example, is too restricted in scope to be sensitive to disability in older people. However, the psychometric testing of the adapted charts is ongoing under the umbrella of WONCA, who provide a handbook of the scale (van Weel et al. 1995). The COOP/WONCA charts may be used for research and clinical care.

THE CORNELL MEDICAL INDEX (CMI)

The Cornell Medical Index was initially designed for use by physicians in medical-history taking in order to save their time and ensure, where appropriate, that a large body of medical and psychiatric data could be collected. It was intended to serve as a standardized medical history (Brodman et al. 1949). The informal language used on the instrument was intended to be readily translatable into medical terminology. For example: 'Does your heart often race like mad?' (tachycardia); 'Do you have to get up every night and urinate (pass water)?' (nocturia).

In the process of its development, many variations of the CMI items were tested on more than a thousand people in several geographic areas. Those items containing replies substantiated on interview were included in the final version. The final form was tested on 179 medical out-patients and 191 admitted medical patients whose responses were compared with their medical histories taken by participating physicians. Although the index was intended for use as an aid to medical-history taking in clinic and hospital settings, the authors state that it could also be useful in population-health surveys.

One published study of the CMI, based on 5,119 patients reported that, as would be expected, older people reported more physical problems than younger people; and that women reported more problems than men, although they had a similar number of diagnosed disorders (Brodman *et al.* 1953). There are many examples of early applications of the CMI in clinic and institutional settings. Comprehensive references on applications of the index have been compiled by Cornell Medical University and are available on request (Lowe 1975). Abramson *et al.* (1965) summarized the CMI scores reported for 16 samples of people studied in the USA and UK. Reported CMI scores of 30+ ranged between 4 and 82 per cent for female sample members, and between 0 and 79 per cent for males. The populations studied ranged widely from psychiatric hospital out-patients to people labelled as 'healthy'.

The CMI is self-administered. Individuals usually take 10 to 30 minutes to complete it. The authors report that the time taken to complete the CMI depends on people's level of education, and the speed at which they reach decisions. They report the CMI to be acceptable to patients. No training is needed for administration or analysis.

Content

The CMI contains 195 yes–no questions divided into 18 sections relating to physical problems (eight sections), personal habits, frequency of illness (four sections), moods and feelings (six sections). The sections of the CMI are:

A Eyes and ears
B Respiratory system
C Cardiovascular system
D Digestive tract
E Musculoskeletal system
F Skin
G Nervous system
H Genito-urinary system
I Fatigability
J Frequency of illness
K Miscellaneous disease
L Habits

Mood and feelings:

M Inadequacy
N Depression
O Anxiety
P Sensitivity
Q Anger
R Tension

Examples of questions are:

Does your face often get badly flushed?   Yes/No
Do you suffer badly from frequent severe headaches?   Yes/No
Do you usually feel bloated after eating?   Yes/No
Has a doctor ever said you have kidney or bladder disease?   Yes/No
Did anyone in your family ever have a nervous breakdown?   Yes/No
Do you often feel unhappy and depressed?   Yes/No

There are two forms of the CMI, one for men and one for women (differing only in the genito-urinary section). The number of problems admitted are scored and the total number indicates the degree of deviancy.

Scoring

Responses indicating the existence of a problem (the 'yes' replies) are totalled. More than 25 positive responses to items indicate the presence of serious disorder. A medically significant emotional disturbance is considered present if the total score is 30 or more. If the 'yes' replies are chiefly located in one or two sections, the medical problem is localized. If they are scattered throughout the index, the problem is likely to be diffused, usually involving a medical disturbance. More than two or three 'yes' answers on the last page (moods, feelings, attitudes and behaviour questions) suggest a psychological disturbance. However, interpretation of symptoms depends on medical knowledge and thus the index is not a useful diagnostic tool outside medical settings.

Validity and reliability

Although this was a popular early measure, there are few reports of the instrument's reliability and validity. Abramson *et al.* (1965) pointed out that the index is of little value in comparisons of widely divergent cultures within and between societies.

Brodman *et al.* (1954), in a study of 7,527 men undergoing medical examination, including the administration of the CMI, for army training, analysed the follow-up records of 900 of them four months later, after their commencement of training. High CMI scores (50+) were significantly associated with a large amount of reported sickness, hospitalized days, convictions and discharges from the service.

A study of its validity was undertaken by Abramson *et al.* (1965) among 120 randomly selected adults of a Jerusalem housing project. The authors tested its sensitivity and specificity, the former in relation to the proportion of unhealthy persons who gave the defined CMI response ('yes' to items), and specificity in terms of the proportion of healthy persons who did not give this response. Health status was independently assessed by local physicians. The authors reported that the responses to individual CMI questions referring to named disorders were not very valid indicators of the presence of these disorders. Of the people whom physicians reported as having a specific condition, only a half, or in some cases less than a half, of these people themselves reported its presence. The conditions were, on the other hand, rarely reported by people who were assessed by physicians as not having them. Although item responses were not judged to be valid indicators, scores (based on the number of 'yes' responses) were significantly correlated with the physicians' ratings of overall ill health and emotional ill health, although the correlations were weak to moderate (0.26–0.48). Moderate correlations were also obtained between physicians' ratings of emotional and overall health (0.52 for women and 0.57 for men); 78 per cent of the people rated as 'ill' by physicians were also rated by them as emotionally disturbed. In addition, the authors identified the 10 key questions which were the best predictors of physician ratings of emotional ill health; there was a moderate correlation between the number of these items with positive scores and total CMI scores (0.63):

Are you easily upset and irritated?
Do you suffer from severe nervous exhaustion?

Do you usually have great difficulty in falling asleep or staying asleep?
Are you definitely underweight?
Do you often become suddenly scared for no good reason?
Are you considered a nervous person?
Are you constantly keyed up and jittery?
Do you usually feel unhappy and depressed?
Does life look entirely hopeless?
Does every little thing get on your nerves and wear you out?

The general findings of the study that the CMI is of limited value for the detection of specific disorders was also confirmed by a large-scale study in New York by Brodman *et al.* (1959). They compared the results of medical examinations of 5,929 hospital out-patients with computer analyses of the CMI for the same patients. These authors reported that CMI data provided correct diagnoses of 60 common disorders in only 44 per cent of cases known to have these disorders.

The instrument needs further testing if it is to be used in survey research, although evidence of the validity of individual items is not encouraging; it is also fairly limited in so far as it concentrates mainly on symptom reporting regarding mental and physical problems, rather than perceptions of health and well-being.

SPITZER'S QUALITY OF LIFE INDEX (QL)

Spitzer's Quality of Life Index was developed for use by physicians in relation to cancer and chronically ill patients. It is widely used by cancer specialists interested in the health status and quality of life of their patients before and after therapy.

Spitzer *et al.* (1981) aimed to identify the components of quality of life empirically from questioning lay people as well as health professionals. They formed three advisory panels each with 43 members from Sydney, Australia. These consisted of cancer patients and their relatives, patients with chronic diseases and their relatives, healthy people aged between 20–59 and 60+, physicians, nurses, social workers and other health professionals and members of the clergy. One panel received an open-ended questionnaire designed to elicit spontaneous beliefs about factors that could enhance or decrease the quality of life. The second panel received a more structured questionnaire seeking views on various aspects of defined quality of life. The third panel assessed the results from the first two and the relative importance of the main factors. The factors that were rated as the most important formed the first drafts of the QL Index which were tested on 339 people from out-patients' clinics. This resulted in the following dimensions of quality of life being incorporated within the definitive QL Index: activity; performance of activities of daily living; perception of health; support from family and friends; and outlook on life.

Its authors caution that it is not suitable for measuring or classifying the quality of life of ostensibly healthy people (Spitzer et al. 1981). The average completion time is one minute.

Content

The QL consists of five items. Each item represents a different domain of life functioning. The respondents choose the item in terms of the statement's applicability to themselves: activity, daily living, health, support and outlook. These were agreed by a panel of experts to be crucial areas of life functioning. The index is short and easily administered.

The scale also comprises a visual-analogue rating scale and requests the respondent and interviewer to place an X on the line rating quality of life (lowest quality–highest quality).

Respondents are requested to tick statements which apply to them. There are many examples of multiple items within one question and thus this scale confuses several activities within one item:

I am able to eat, wash, go to the toilet and dress without assistance. I drive a car or use public transport without assistance.

I work full time (or nearly so) in my usual occupation or study full time (or nearly so) or manage my own household or take part in as much unpaid or voluntary activity as I wish, whether retired or not.

I have good relationships with others and receive strong support from at least one family member and/or friend.

I am basically a calm person. I generally look forward to things and am able to make my own decisions about my life and surroundings.

Respondents only have the option of one tick per

statement to indicate they can do all of these things, or of not ticking to indicate they cannot do any without assistance. There are problems with interpretation if respondents can do some tasks but not others.

Scoring

The scoring of the Spitzer QL scale is simple. The scale consists of five items, with three options for replies. The item responses comprise scores 0–2, giving an overall score of 0 to 10. The scale can be summed into a single score or each item can be presented separately.

Validity

Spitzer et al. (1981) asked 68 lay people and professionals (e.g. physicians) to assess the scope and format of the instrument; most judged it to be satisfactory and the authors judged the scale to have content validity.

Spitzer et al. (1981) tested the scale for validity, using 150 physicians to rate 879 patients. Fifty-nine per cent of physicians reported that they were 'very confident' of the accuracy of their scores. The analysis of physicians' scores showed that the close clustering of high scores among healthy subjects, the spread of scores among those who were definitely ill, and the low scores of those who were seriously ill, made clinical sense and provided evidence of discriminant construct validity. Convergent validity was judged to be obtained by comparison of physicians' and patients' ratings. When the physicians' ratings were compared to patients' self-ratings, the correlation was moderately high (0.61). The scale is also related to other global-functioning scales (Mor et al. 1984; Morris et al. 1986; Mor 1987). Mor (1987), on the basis of three samples of newly diagnosed cancer patients (total: 2,046), reported a correlation between the Spitzer QL Index and the Karnofsky Performance Scale of 0.63; the correlation was moderate probably because of the multi-dimensional nature of the QL Index. The item correlations of the scale with the Karnofsky Scale ranged from 0.13 to 0.57. The scale and the associated visual-analogue scale has been primarily evaluated in two other main studies which showed a statistically significant correlation with other indices (Spitzer et al. 1981; Gough et al.

1983). However, the correlation coefficients were not high enough to be confident that these scales cover the same dimensions. The scale's reproducibility requires further investigation. The authors reported that the scale was able to discriminate between healthy people and patients with varying conditions.

However, Slevin et al. (1988) concluded on the basis of their analyses that the doctors' ratings of quality of life using the Spitzer scale were of questionable validity. They reported that the Spitzer scale contained inappropriate questions for measuring the quality of life of cancer patients. They suggest that the continued popularity of the Spitzer scale, despite poor reliability and validity of the scales, stems from researchers' tendency to rely on significance values when assessing their scales, rather than on the size of the correlation value.

The Spitzer scale has been reported to be able to predict mortality among cancer patients (Mor et al. 1984, Morris et al. 1986; Mor 1987). It has been used in an Australian study of outcome of breast-cancer patients and was shown to be capable of discriminating between patients on intermittent therapy and those receiving continuous therapy (Coates et al. 1987).

There are numerous applications of this scale in clinical settings. Morris and Sherwood (1987) in the USA administered the QL scale to different samples of cancer patients at different stages of the disease. Over 2,000 patients were included in the study. A strong correlation was reported between the Karnofsky performance-status rating and the QL Index. The QL Index was able to successfully distinguish between cancer patients who were newly diagnosed, those under active treatment and those nearing the terminal stages of the disease. However, the authors did not feel it was sufficiently sensitive for use as an outcome variable in studies evaluating the effect of a treatment or intervention on patients' lives. This was mainly because of the insensitivity of the social-functioning index of the scale.

The QL's reliance on just five items means that it does not adequately account for the different dimensions of quality of life. However, to be fair, the authors did not intend it to be appropriate for measuring global quality of life in healthy populations, and they reported that it does not discriminate adequately among well people (Spitzer et al. 1981).

Reliability

Spitzer et al. (1981), on the basis of 150 physicians' ratings of 879 patients, reported that assessment of internal consistency demonstrated a high coefficient (0.77), and the correlation for inter-rater reliability was high (0.81). The scale has been shown to have reasonable inter-item reliability (Mor et al. 1984; Morris et al. 1986; Mor 1987).

However, there are few other studies of its reliability and validity. Slevin et al. (1988) administered the index along with the Linear Analogue Self Assessment (LASA) quality-of-life visual-analogue scales, the Karnofsky Performance Scale, and the Hospital Anxiety and Depression Scale. The scales were completed by 108 patients and their doctors at the same time. Two different groups of 25 patients filled in the same questionnaires on a single day, and daily for five consecutive days. Reproducibility was not as good as the Karnofsky Performance Index. The Karnofsky, which correlated with the Spitzer Index (patients' rating of quality of life: 0.49), demonstrated greater reproducibility than any of the other scales. The variability in their results from repeated testing calls into question the reliability of the Spitzer QL Index and the other measures administered.

In sum, the initial testing of the scale appeared to show promising results; the scale is able to predict mortality among cancer patients and is related to other global-functioning scales. However, more recent studies of the scale report that it has questionable reliability, and validity (Slevin et al. 1988). Further testing is required; a major disadvantage is the confusion of several dimensions within one item.

LINEAR ANALOGUE SELF ASSESSMENT (LASA)

The Linear Analogue Self Assessment Scale was developed for use with cancer patients and has been used successfully to evaluate quality of life of patients receiving cytotoxic therapy for advanced breast cancer (Priestman and Baum 1976). Although simple, it is apparently lengthy in terms of administration time.

Content

The LASA questionnaire has 25 items, 10 of which relate to the symptoms and effects of the disease and treatment (e.g. pain and nausea); five examine psychological consequences (e.g. anxiety and depression); five measure other physical indices (e.g. ability to perform household chores); and five items are concerned with personal relationships.

The LASA tests employ lines, the length of which are taken to denote the continuum of some emotional or physical experience such as tiredness or anxiety (Priestman and Baum 1976). The lines are usually 10 cm long with stops at right angles to the line at its extremes, representing the limits of the experience being measured. It is a technique that has been easily administered to five-year-old children (Scott *et al.* 1977). Examples of items are:

Ability to perform shopping:
None |_____| Better than ever
Decision making:
Impossible |_____| Excellent
Nausea:
Constant |_____| None
Appetite:
None |_____| Excellent
How would you rate your quality of life?
Very poor |_____| Very good

Scoring

The patient is instructed to mark along the line a point that corresponds to his/her perception of the experience. The distance from the 'none at all' mark to the patient's mark provides a numeric score for the item. The items are summed.

Validity

There are many references in the literature to the validity of LASA in the measurement of pain (Melzack 1983). Slevin *et al.* (1988) in their testing of the scale, however, reported that the LASA scale correlated poorly with the Hospital Anxiety and Depression (HAD) scale. Slevin *et al.* suggested that this was due to the HAD items being less applicable to cancer patients.

The scale has been shown to be capable of discriminating between breast-cancer patients in Australia who receive intermittent therapy and those receiving continuous therapy (Coates *et al.* 1987).

Gough *et al.* (1983) assessed 100 patients with advanced cancer in Australia, using a single LASA item 'How would you rate your general feeling of well-being today?', a 21-item version of the LASA index, self- and interviewer-administered five-item QL Index (Spitzer's) which covered activity, daily living, health, support and outlook. Each patient was evaluated four times at four-weekly intervals for twelve weeks. The correlation coefficients for the four methods ranged from 0.38 to 0.86. The single-item LASA question correlated moderately to well with all three questionnaires (0.38 to 0.67). The LASA-21 correlated from 0.46 to –0.65 with the other items.

Reliability

The test–retest correlations of the LASA were 0.73 (Priestman and Baum 1976). Slevin *et al.* (1988) tested LASA against the Hospital Anxiety and Depression scale, the Karnofsky Index and the Spitzer Quality of Life Index with 108 cancer patients in London and reported that the LASA scale showed similar concordance coefficients when taken as a whole, compared with being divided into four equal parts, i.e. the continuous scale is no more sensitive than the four-point scale. Two different groups of 25 patients also filled in the same forms on a single day, and daily for five consecutive days, during a period when their clinical state was expected to remain stable. Professionals also completed the scales in relation to the same patients. The LASA scale was found to be easily reproducible, and had greater reproducibility than the other scales. Little other information about its reliability has been published.

Although the scale is simple and reported to be reproducible and able to discriminate between groups, it may be problematic to administer because some patients may take some time to accustom themselves to representing their feelings along a continuum. More evidence of its validity is required.

THE MCGILL PAIN QUESTIONNAIRE (MPQ)

This pain scale is not a broader measure of health status but it comprises an important, and often neglected, domain of measurement; it is therefore included here.

Many health-status and disability measures fail to incorporate a comprehensive assessment of pain. Apart from visual-analogue rating scales to assess pain, the most frequently used and most tested of the measures that exist to assess pain is the McGill Pain Questionnaire (MPQ). The McGill Pain Questionnaire consists principally of lists of terms describing the quality and intensity of pain. Melzack and Torgerson (1971) selected 102 words describing pain from the literature, sorted them into the categories of sensory, affective and evaluative words describing intensity; the results were then checked by 20 reviewers. Further testing among 140 students, 20 physicians and 20 patients led to the current 78-item format of the scale and the scale values. The 78 words are grouped in 20 sub-classes of three to five descriptive words, and the 20 sub-classes are grouped in four sections: sensory, affective, evaluative and miscellaneous. Several versions of the scale exist, and a short version of the scale has also been developed which consists of 15 items (Melzack 1987). The completion of the full-length scale takes from 5 to 15 minutes, and the short version takes 2 to 5 minutes, depending on the familiarity of the patients with the words.

Content

Examples of the 78 words respondents are asked to choose from to describe their pain are:

Flickering
Quivering
Pulsing
Throbbing
Beating
Pounding

Tight
Numbing
Drawing
Squeezing
Tearing

In addition to the 78 words describing pain, 9 words also assess course over time and the location of the pain is assessed with a drawing of a body with the words 'external' and 'internal' added.

The short version includes only the items throbbing, shooting, stabbing, sharp, cramping, gnawing, hot-burning, aching, heavy, tender, splitting,

tiring–exhausting, sickening, fearful, punishing–cruel. The short version correlates consistently highly with the long version of the McGill Pain Questionnaire (Melzack 1987).

Scoring

Each description carries a weight corresponding to the severity of the pain, according to evaluations of appropriate ordinal rankings by panels of doctors, patients and students. People then receive pain scores according to the number of descriptive items they select to describe their pain and their assigned weights (0 = no pain; 1 = mild pain; 2 = discomforting; 3 = distressing; 4 = horrible; 5 = excruciating). The McGill Pain Questionnaire generates four sub-scales differentiated by factor analysis. These include sensory and evaluative sub-scales to designate perception of pain, and an affective sub-scale to denote emotional response to pain. The fourth is a miscellaneous sub-scale. These four sub-scales result in four scores. The four scores add up to a total score (the pain rating index). The scale was developed in recognition of these distinct components of pain.

There are four possible and distinct scoring methods ranging from the number of words chosen to the sum of the scale values (based on the scale weights) for all the words selected in a given category or across all categories (Melzack 1975). The scale was published with full details by Melzack and Katz (1992).

Validity

Dubuisson and Melzack (1976) reported that the McGill Pain Questionnaire was able to correctly classify 77 per cent of 95 patients with eight pain syndromes into diagnostic groups on the basis of their verbal description of pain. Other research by Melzack *et al.* (1986) on patients with facial pain has shown that the scale can correctly predict diagnosis for 90 per cent of patients.

Correlations between McGill Pain Questionnaire score and visual analogue ratings for 40 patients ranged from 0.50 to 0.65 (Melzack 1975). There is support from results of principal components analysis for the distinction between affective and sensory dimensions of pain, but less for a distinctive evaluative component (Reading 1979;

Prieto and Geisinger 1983). Love *et al.* (1991) have more recently supported the basic three-factor structure of the scale, using more sophisticated analytic procedures and a large sample.

The specificity of the measure was demonstrated by Greenwald (1987) in a study of 536 cancer patients.

Reliability

Evidence of reliability is sparse (Graham *et al.* 1980). Melzack (1975) reported a test-retest study, based on just 10 patients who completed the scale three times at intervals of three to seven days between each. The average consistency of response was reported to be 70.3 per cent. The test-retest reliability for the 20 categories of pain descriptors, the three specific sub-scales and the total score have been reported to range from weak to moderately good (Reading *et al.* 1982; Love *et al.* 1989).

Although it is difficult to demonstrate that the McGill Pain Questionnaire does reflect the conceptual definition of pain as three distinct dimensions, it is still the leading measure of pain. The short form of the scale has been less frequently used and tested. Cross-cultural applications of the full scale have been reviewed by Naughton and Wiklund (1993), and a list of the languages it has been translated into is given by Melzack and Katz (1992). It is more often used for the measurement of chronic, rather than acute, pain, as it is generally believed that most visual analogue scales work adequately for acute pain (McQuay 1990).

5

MEASURES OF PSYCHOLOGICAL WELL-BEING

There are numerous scales of psychological well-being, in particular those which are aimed specifically at detecting common psychiatric disorders such as anxiety/depression, dementia and mental confusion. The reliability of the classifications of many of these have been questioned. Gold standards for diagnostic categorization have been developed over the years, for example, the revised Diagnostic and Statistical Manual (DSM-IV) of the American Psychiatric Association (1987; 1994) or the International Classification of Diseases (World Health Organization 1992), as well as the previously developed and highly regarded diagnostic instruments Present State Examination and the Research Diagnostic Criteria (Wing *et al*. 1974; Spitzer *et al*. 1978; Wing 1991), although these still fail to account realistically for features of personality or physical illness which may intervene. In the UK the Geriatric Mental State Questionnaire (GMS) has been developed for use with the elderly and is often regarded as a gold-standard survey instrument; the GMS is reviewed in this chapter. A more recently developed and tested assessment schedule for the diagnosis of mental disorder, although again only in relation to the elderly, is the Cambridge Examination for Mental Disorders of the Elderly (CAMDEX) (Roth *et al*. 1986). This also pays special attention to the detection of dementia. However, it is extremely long and unwieldy, and unsuitable for use as a research tool except in a clinical psychiatric survey; it compares unfavourably with other well-developed scales in

relation to cross-cultural applicability and sensitivity (Copeland 1990).

The following sections review the most popular and easily administered scales of common psychiatric disorders in current use in the UK: anxiety/depression and, among the elderly, mental confusion. Some of the broader health-status scales also include sections or batteries on mental health, for example the Rand Batteries (see Chapter 4).

Scales of psychiatric status are generally developed and applied within specific countries. It is often difficult for such scales to have cross-cultural applicability without careful adaptation because of culture specific concepts and values, although some of the more popular scales have been adapted for use outside the UK (e.g. the General Health Questionnaire and the Geriatric Mental State).

DEPRESSION

The term depression is increasingly used to cover a wider range of psychological disturbances. There is considerable confusion about the variety of meanings and this, in turn, has led to conflicting research findings about aetiology and treatment of choice (Snaith 1987). There is little confusion about the recognition of a severe state, sometimes called a psychosis, but milder degrees of the condition lack definition. Sometimes the term 'depressive neurosis' is used but a variety of concepts are associated with this term. In the Present State Examination

Manual, Wing *et al.* (1974) have provided the most succinct definitions of psychopathological terms, and in an attempt to clarify the issues of terminology their definitions of depressive states related to depressed mood, recent loss of interest, self-depreciation, hopelessness and observed depression. There were a number of additional definitions provided for neglect due to brooding, subjective anergia, slowness and underactivity, inefficient thinking, poor concentration, suicidal plans or acts, morning depression, social withdrawal, guilt and other related symptoms.

Wide discrepancies in the early literature on estimates of the prevalence of mental illness in different communities were largely the consequence of the use of different diagnostic criteria. The development and use of standardized research instruments linked to clearly stated diagnostic criteria led to less variation between studies. However, considerable differences still exist between measures with the implication that comparisons between studies can be made only if two studies have utilized the same basic measurement scale.

Many research studies have based the definition of a 'case' of depression on a certain score having been attained on one of the large number of depression-rating scales. The different construction of these scales and the different individual items they include create major difficulties in comparing studies, unless they have been developed in relation to clear criteria such as the DSM-IV (American Psychiatric Association 1994).

The majority of depression-rating scales contain a diverse collection of symptoms, attitudes and feelings and will produce high prevalence rates and a large proportion of false positives if case detection relies upon them (Snaith 1987). Kutner *et al.* (1985), studying depression and anxiety in dialysis patients, found that scales containing disease-related items yielded exaggerated scores.

ZUNG'S SELF RATING DEPRESSION SCALE

The Self Rating Scale was developed by Zung (1965). It was constructed on the basis of the clinical diagnostic criteria most commonly used to characterize depressive disorders. Factor-analysis-derived symptom clusters led to the selection of 20 items covering 'pervasive affect', 'physiological equivalents or concomitants' and 'psychological concomitants'. Altogether over half of the items of this widely used depression scale are composed of feelings or symptoms which do not necessarily indicate the presence of a psychological disorder, and Kutner *et al.* (1985) found that these disease items led to an exaggerated score.

Content

The scale contains 20 statements; 10 are worded symptomatically positive and 10 are worded symptomatically negative. Respondents are asked how the listed statements apply to them. Administration is by self-completion; and completion time is 'a few minutes' (Zung *et al.* 1965). Examples are:

I have trouble sleeping at night.
I eat as much as I used to.
I notice I am losing weight.
I have trouble with constipation.
My heart beats faster than usual.
I feel hopeful about the future.
I find it easy to make decisions.

There are four choices of response category, with numerical values of 1–4 respectively: none or a little of the time; some of the time; a good part of the time; most of the time.

Scoring

Each item scores 1–4. The score values for the 20 items are summed. An index is derived by dividing the sum of the raw scores by the maximum possible score of 80, converted to a decimal and multiplied by 100 (Zung *et al.* 1965). The need to transform the scores has been questioned by Gurtman (1985).

The interpretation of scores is based on norms, which are given in the scale's manual. Below 50 = normal, 50–59 = minimal to mild depression, 60–69 = moderate to marked depression, 69+ = severe to extreme depression. The norms for these scores were based on adults aged 20–64 and may not be appropriate for younger or older people. The cut-off points are not agreed, and investigators have adopted a range of cut-offs from 50 to 60. Zung *et al.* (1965) reported that the mean score on the Zung Scale for out-patients diagnosed as depressive reaction was 64. Zung (1965) reported that the mean score for hospitalized in-patients diagnosed with depressive disorders was 74.

Validity

Zung et al. (1965) tested the scale for validity using the Minnesota Multiphasic Personality Inventory as a gold standard. They administered the scale to new psychiatric out-patients at Duke University (number not specified). The correlations between their instrument and three sub-scales of the Minnesota Inventory were: 0.70, 0.68 and 0.13. The authors commented that the latter correlation was 'unexpectedly low'. Brown and Zung (1972) tested the scale against the Hamilton Depression Scale and reported a correlation of 0.79.

Davies et al. (1975) reported a correlation between the Zung and Hamilton Scale of r = 0.62, between the Zung and the Beck Depression Scale of r = 0.73, and between the Zung and a visual analogue scale of r = 0.62. Biggs et al. (1978) reported a correlation between the Zung and the Hamilton of r = 0.80, although the correlation was lowest at greatest severity levels. In comparison with clinical ratings of severity, Biggs et al. (1978) reported a correlation with the Zung of 0.69, with differences at higher severity. Toner et al. (1988) reported a similar correlation against psychiatric judgements at r = 0.65. The scale is also able to distinguish between patients with a confirmed diagnosis of a depressive state and patients with an initial diagnosis of depression, but subsequently reviewed and given another psychiatric diagnosis (Zung 1965; 1967). Zung et al. (1965) reported the scale was able to distinguish reliably between patients with a psychoneurotic depression and those with an anxiety reaction and found the instrument sensitive to clinical change. However, Toner et al. (1988) reported that the convergent validity of the Zung Scale with physicians' judgements was lower than that of the well-tested Comprehensive Assessment and Referral Evaluation (CARE) scale, 0.65 (kappa: 0.29) in comparison with 0.73 (kappa: 0.46). Arfwidsson et al. (1974) cast doubt on the validity of the scale, suggesting that doctors' ratings are more valid as a means of assessing the degree and quality of depressive symptoms. Also, Carroll et al. (1973) assessed patients known to have varying degrees of depression and reported that the Zung Scale was unable to distinguish between the groups; they reported a correlation of 0.41 between interview-based and Zung ratings. Carroll et al. blame the self-report method rather than the Zung Scale, as the former adopts a different perspective to a psychiatric interviewer. Other studies have found the Zung Scale to be unresponsive to changes in treatment patterns (Hamilton 1976).

The instrument was designed to be unidimensional, although a factor analysis by Morris et al. (1975) confirmed two dimensions: agitation and self-satisfaction. Blumenthal's (1975) factor analysis of the scale yielded four sub-scales: a well-being index, a depressed mood index, an optimism index and a somatic-symptoms index. Cross-cultural applications have been reviewed by Naughton and Wiklund (1993).

Reliability

There is little evidence of the scale's reliability. Zung (1986) reported split half correlations of 0.92. Knight et al. (1983) reported a coefficient of 0.79. The scale has been used successfully with clustering techniques by Byrne (1978). Kaszniak and Allender (1985) suggest that it is unsuitable for use with elderly people because of the large number of somatic items. Also, response rates for self-completed scales may be lower than for administered scales. A comparative study of Zung's Scale with the short version of CARE showed a response rate of 65 per cent for Zung and 100 per cent for CARE. Among the reasons for non-response were visual problems (28 per cent), illiteracy (9 per cent) and lack of motivation (34 per cent) (Toner et al. 1988). These response difficulties apply to all self-rating scales.

The scale is popular because it is short and easy to complete. Zung (1972) developed an observer rated scale to complement the Zung, although Thompson (1989), in line with most reviewers of the scale, reports that it has no advantages.

MONTGOMERY-ASBERG DEPRESSION RATING SCALE (MADRS)

The Montgomery-Asberg Depression Rating Scale was developed by Montgomery and Asberg (1979) on the basis of 54 English and 52 Swedish patients who completed a 65-item psychopathology scale. Analysis identified the 17 most commonly occurring symptoms in depressive illness in the sample. Subsequent analyses, using 64 patients on different types of antidepressive drugs, were then used to create a 10-item depression scale which consisted of those items showing the greatest changes with treatment.

This scale is oriented toward psychic symptoms and covers apparent sadness, reported sadness, inability to feel, difficulty in concentration, inner tension, pessimistic thoughts, suicidal thoughts, lassitude, reduced sleep and reduced appetite. The scale's advantage lies in its brevity.

Content

The scale's 10 items encompass the most commonly occurring symptoms of depressive illness which change in response to treatment (see above). Examples are:

Apparent sadness: representing despondency, gloom and despair (more than just ordinary transient low spirits), reflected in speech, facial expression and posture. Rate by depth and inability to brighten up:

0   No sadness.
1
2   Looks dispirited but does brighten up without difficulty.
3
4   Appears sad and unhappy most of the time.
5
6   Looks miserable all the time. Extremely despondent.

Reduced sleep: representing the experience of reduced duration or depth of sleep compared to the subject's own normal pattern when well.

0   Sleeps as usual.
1
2   Slight difficulty dropping off to sleep or slightly reduced, light or fitful sleep.
3
4   Sleep reduced or broken up by at least two hours.
5
6   Less than two or three hours' sleep.

Lassitude: representing a difficulty getting started or slowness initiating and performing everyday activities.

0   Hardly any difficulty in getting started. No sluggishness.
1
2   Difficulties in starting activities.
3
4   Difficulties in starting simple routine activities which are carried out with effort.
5
6   Complete lassitude. Unable to do anything without help.

Pessimistic thoughts: representing thoughts of guilt, inferiority, self-reproach, sinfulness, remorse and ruin.

0   No pessimistic thoughts.
1
2   Fluctuating ideas of failure, self-reproach or self-depreciation.
3
4   Persistent self-accusation, or definite but still rational ideas of guilt or sin. Increasingly pessimistic about the future.
5
6   Delusions of ruin, remorse or unredeemable sin. Self-accusations which are absurd and unshakeable.

Scoring

Scoring involves computing of scale items. The procedure of arriving at a definition of a case by adding up numbers derived from a severity-grade score of a number of symptoms has a certain attraction until it is realized that one case may be very different from another.

Validity

Montgomery and Asberg (1979) tested scale scores against psychiatrists' judgements, using 18 patients who responded to treatment and 17 who did not. The scale was able to discriminate between the two groups. The scale was also tested against the Hamilton Depression Scale with a reported correlation of 0.70. Kearns *et al.* (1982) reported that the scale was able to distinguish between different levels of severity, and performed as well as the Hamilton Depression Scale. Snaith and Taylor (1985) reported a high correlation between the scale and the depression scale of their self-rated Hospital Anxiety and Depression (HAD) scale (0.81), although the correlation with the anxiety scale of the HAD was low (0.37).

The sensitivity of the scale is questionable. Cooper and Fairburn (1986) found that a group of bulimic and a group of depressed patients had similar scores on the Montgomery-Asberg Depression Rating Scale but different symptoms, or scale items, contributed strongly to the overall score in the two groups.

Reliability

Good results for reliability have been reported by the authors and the scale was found to be robust when used by different professionals in a variety of health-care settings (GPs, nurses, psychologists, psychiatrists) and high inter-rater correlations were produced. Comparisons between two English raters, two Swedish raters and one English and one Swedish rater, rating 11 to 30 patients, produced correlations of between 0.89 and 0.97 (Montgomery *et al.* 1978).

However, 30 per cent of the total score is apparently accounted for by three items which all commonly occur in physical illnesses and states of distress other than depression (Williams 1984; Cooper and Fairburn 1986).

In sum, the scale items and the scoring procedure question the reliability of the scale.

HAMILTON DEPRESSION SCALE

This is a widely used observer scale which includes assessment of cognitive and behavioural components of depression and is particularly thorough in the assessment of the somatic aspects (Hamilton 1967). Like many depression scales, the Hamilton Depression Scale cannot be used to establish a diagnosis of depression, but only to assess severity once depression has already been diagnosed. Interviewer training is required.

Content

The current version of the Hamilton Depression Scale (Hamilton 1959; 1967) consists of 17 items: depressed mood, feelings of guilt, suicidal ideation, work and activities, insight, retardation, agitation, insomnia (early, middle and late), psychic anxiety, somatic anxiety, gastrointestinal symptoms, general somatic symptoms, genital symptoms (loss of libido or menstrual disturbances), hypo-

chondriases and loss of weight. The earlier version of the scale, which is still in use, contained 21 items. Examples of scale items are:

Depressed mood: 0–4

Gloomy attitude, pessimism about the future
Feeling of sadness
Tendency to weep:
   sadness and/or mild depression
   occasional weeping and/or moderate depression
   frequent weeping and/or severe depression
   extreme symptoms

Anxiety, psychic: 0–4

Tension and irritability
Worrying about minor matters
Apprehensive attitude
Fears

Somatic symptoms, gastrointestinal: 0–2

Loss of appetite
Heavy feelings in abdomen
Constipation

Insight: 0–2

Loss of insight
Partial or doubtful loss
No loss

The somatic categories of the scale have been used alone, in conjunction with other depression-rating scales. The somatic items relate to muscular, sensory systems and to cardiovascular, respiratory, gastrointestinal, genito-urinary and autonomic symptoms. For example Martin (1987) used these items without the Hamilton depression (psychosomatic) items together with the Montgomery-Asberg Depression Rating Scale. Although the scale is one of the most widely used in psychiatric research (Freemantle *et al.* 1993), many investigators have modified the scale (Paykel 1985). Potts *et al.* (1990) developed a fully structured interview version (suitable for use with lay interviewers) of the 17-item scale for use in the Rand Medical Outcomes Study. Inter-rater reliability with two psychiatrists rating 20 subjects was good (Pearson's $r = 0.96$), a finding confirmed by other studies (Korner *et al.* 1990). The alpha correlations for internal consistency were 0.82 to 0.83. The test-retest correlations were high at 0.65 for the total score, although the item correlations were variable at −0.04 to 0.77 (15-day retest). They omitted the items with low retest results and drew up a 14-item to replace the 17-item version.

Scoring

Some items are scored 0–4 and others are scored 0–2. Scale items marked 0–4 have the response choices for the rater of absent (0), mild or trivial (1), moderate (2–3), severe (4); and scale items marked 0–2 have the choice of absent (0), slight or doubtful (1), clearly present (2). The items are individually scored by a rater during an interview. The interpretation of categories is described by Hamilton (1967) and reproduced by Williams (1984).

The total scores range from 0–100 (representing the sum of two raters' scores or double the score for one rater). Some studies report total scores with a maximum of 50.

Validity

The scale is reported to have high concurrent validity with good agreement with other scales, particularly the Beck, with correlations reported of over 0.70 (Hamilton 1976). Schwab et al. (1967) compared the Hamilton with the Beck scale on 153 medical in-patients. The correlation between these two scales was 0.75. Knesevich et al. (1977) reported the Hamilton scale correlated 0.68 with a change in global rating on a 10-point scale. Hamer et al. (1991) reported that a threshold score of eight gave a sensitivity of 88 per cent and a positive predictive value of 80 per cent in comparison with diagnoses made with the DSM-III. Tamaklo et al. (1992) also reported that it correlated highly with the Montgomery-Asberg Depression Rating Scale. However, Montgomery and Asberg (1979) reported the scale to be less sensitive than their own, especially at the severe end of the scale, a finding confirmed by Knesevich et al. (1977). Carroll et al. (1973) reported that the Hamilton scale was better able than the Beck Depression Inventory to distinguish between groups of patients known to have varying degrees of depression. They argued that self-report scales, such as the Beck, overweight subjective scores. The Hamilton scale has also been reported to have a greater effect size for change than the Beck

Depression Inventory (Sayer et al. 1993), and is frequently reported to be sensitive to treatment (Tollefson et al. 1993). Hamilton (1967) reported that the scale discriminated between men and women; women generally are more likely to have higher depression scores than men. Factor analysis of the scale has yielded a five-dimensional solution for the scale, although only the first factor (comprising depressed mood, guilt, suicide, work and interests, agitation, psychic anxiety, somatic anxiety and loss of libido) was well defined and clinically interpretable (Gibbons et al. 1993).

Although initial factor analyses gave poor results (Hamilton 1960), later factor analyses gave more satisfactory results (Hamilton 1967; Mowbray 1972; Bech 1981).

Reliability

Its inter-rater reliability is reported to be good: correlations are high ranging from 0.84 to 0.98 (Hamilton 1976; Knesevich et al. 1977; Rehm 1981). However, six of the scale items are symptoms of somatic disturbance and account for 31 per cent of the possible total score; if the insomnia items which so often rate highly in physical illness are included, then 42 per cent of the total is accounted for (Williams 1984). Results for the internal consistency of the scale have been variable (Bech 1981), although Potts et al. (1990) reported research which showed that the scale has a high degree of scale reliability, concurrent, discriminant and construct validity, and is sensitive to treatment changes. However, they did point out that it has been criticized for its lower item reliability and its heavy reliance on the expertise of the interviewer, who is psychiatrically trained.

The Hamilton Scale is the most consistently used measure by investigators (Freemantle et al. 1993). Although popular, the scale should be viewed with caution, given the number of items measuring somatic problems.

THE BECK DEPRESSION INVENTORY (BDI)

If the researcher is interested only in depression, and not more generally in both anxiety and depression, then it is reasonable to use a specially designed scale. The Beck Depression Inventory (BDI) is such a specific scale. It was designed by

Beck *et al.* (1961) and is widely used. It was designed because other widely used scales (e.g. the Minnesota Multiphasic Personality Inventory) were not specifically designed for the measurement of depression or were based on old psychiatric nomenclature. It was developed on the basis of the authors' observations of two samples of 226 and 183 depressed patients' attitudes and symptoms while undergoing psychotherapy. These observations led to the creation of a 21-item inventory; each category describes a specific behavioural manifestation of depression and consists of a series of self-evaluation items which are graded and ranked according to severity (neutral to maximum). A 13-item version of the scale has also been developed (Reynolds and Gould 1981).

The Beck Depression Inventory is generally regarded as better than the Minnesota Multiphasic Personality Inventory and better than similar scales such as the Zung Scale (Hammen 1981). Originally developed to be interviewer administered, it is now a self-rating scale. A large proportion of items relate to somatic disturbance, and this has led to some controversy.

Like the Hamilton, it cannot be used to diagnose depression in the absence of a prior diagnosis – it is only a measure of severity once the clinical diagnosis has been made. This is to exclude people being diagnosed as depressed when they have high BDI scores for situational reasons (e.g. bereavement). It has been reported to have acceptable levels of reliability for use as a research screening instrument with an elderly population (Gallagher *et al.* 1982).

Content

The BDI consists of 21 items, each with four response choices, in the form of statements, ranked in order of severity, from which the respondent selects one that best fits the way s/he feels at 'this moment'. The symptoms and attitudes which the scale aims to measure are sadness, pessimism/discouragement, sense of failure, dissatisfaction, guilt, expectation of punishment, self-dislike, self-accusation, suicidal ideation, crying, irritability, social withdrawal, indecisiveness, body-image distortion, work retardation, insomnia, fatigability, anorexia, weight loss, somatic preoccupation and loss of libido. Examples of items are:

I am not particularly pessimistic or discouraged about the future.
I feel I have nothing to look forward to.
I feel that I won't ever get over my troubles.
I feel that the future is hopeless and that things cannot improve.

I am no more irritated now than I ever am.
I get annoyed or irritated more easily than I used to.
I feel irritated all the time.
I don't get irritated at all by the things that used to irritate me.

I have not lost interest in other people.
I am less interested in other people now than I used to be.
I have lost most of my interest in other people and have little feeling for them.
I have lost all my interest in other people and don't care about them at all.

Scoring

The Beck Depression Inventory is based on a Guttman scale. The original scale permitted selections of four to seven responses which were given a weight of 0 to 3. Revisions to the scale were made in 1974 and in 1978, standardizing the response choices to four for each item; each still carries a weight of 0 to 3.

The numerical values of 0 (low) to 3 (high) which are assigned to each statement indicate the degree of severity. In some categories two alternative statements (2a and 2b) are presented at a given level but are assigned the same weight. In the revised version there is one alternative score for each level (so no statement is assigned the same weight). Items are scored, with a maximum total of 63. Normative data suggest the following categories of severity level: normal 0–9; mild 10–15; mild-moderate 16–19; moderate-severe 20–29; severe > 29 (Steer *et al.* 1986). The BDI is available in a format suitable for computer scoring from National Computer Systems, Minneapolis. The value of the scale is that it can be analysed as continuous data, without artificial cut-off points.

Validity

The scale correlates well with clinicians' ratings of severity of depression and with other depression scales. Beck *et al.* (1961), on the basis of 226 hospital out-patients and admissions, and 183 patients in a replication group, tested the BDI against independent psychiatric diagnoses made by four psychiatrists. Their agreement with the scale was 56 per cent; and agreement within one degree of specificity was achieved in 97 per cent of cases. The authors reported that the scale was able to discriminate between depth-of-depression categories based on clinical ratings for both original and replication groups, the correlations ranging from 0.59 to 0.68. Correlations of 0.66 were obtained between the Beck and Depression Adjective Check Lists and of 0.75 with the Beck and the Minnesota Multiphasic Personality Inventory (Beck 1970). It has been used successfully in clinical and general populations, although most studies have focused on psychiatric patients (Beck *et al.* 1961; Williams 1984). Against the Hamilton, correlations have been reported of 0.58 to 0.82 (Schwab *et al.* 1967; Williams *et al.* 1972; Bech *et al.* 1975; Davies *et al.* 1975; Miller *et al.* 1985). Carroll *et al.* (1973) argue that this camouflages the lack of congruence at severe levels of depression. A review of the literature from 1961 to 1986 by Beck *et al.* (1988) reported that the concurrent validities of the BDI with respect to comparisons with clinical ratings and the Hamilton Scale for Depression were high. The mean correlations with the Hamilton Scale and clinical ratings for psychiatric patients were over 0.70. The respective mean correlations for non-psychiatric patients were 0.74 and 0.60. The Beck was also shown to discriminate between sub-types of depression and to distinguish depression from anxiety. The literature reviewed indicated relationships with the Beck and suicidal behaviour and alcoholism. However, Kearns *et al.* (1982) have reported the Beck to be weak in differentiating moderate from severe depression. Other investigators have reported correlations between the Beck and global severity scores of r = 0.62 to 0.77 (Metcalfe and Goldman 1965; Crawford-Little and McPhail 1973; Bech *et al.* 1975), and there is support for its convergent validity (Moreno *et al.* 1993). The scale has been reported to be associated with perceived social support in a study of carers for elderly confused people (those with lower BDI scores reported that they received greater social support) (Morris *et al.* 1989).

The literature reviewed by Beck *et al.* (1988) also suggests that the BDI represents one underlying general syndrome of depression, comprising three highly intercorrelated factors: negative attitudes to self, performance impairment and somatic disturbance.

Reliability

Reliability was tested by the authors on the basis of 226 hospital out-patients and admissions and 183 patients in a replication group (all adults). Internal consistency was tested using 200 of the cases. The score for each of the 21 items was tested with the total BDI score for each person; all were associated at the $P < 0.0001$ Level. Split-half reliability was tested using 97 of the cases, the correlation between the two halves of the scale was 0.86. Split-half reliability was also assessed using a group of adults by Weckowicz *et al.* (1967); these authors reported a lower figure of 0.53.

Beck *et al.* (1961) carried out test-retest correlations, along with repeated psychiatric ratings in case people remembered their scores or genuinely changed between testings. Consistent relationships between the instrument and clinical ratings were reported, using 38 cases, at two- to five-week intervals. Reliability coefficients were above 0.90 (Beck *et al.* 1961; Beck 1970). Test-retest correlations at 6 and 21 days apart were also carried out by Gallagher *et al.* (1982) on a sample of 159 patients and volunteers from a 'senior centre' in Los Angeles. Test-retest correlations for the total sample, the normal sub-sample and the depressed sub-sample were: 0.90, 0.86 and 0.79 respectively. They also carried out tests for the internal consistency of the scale and reported coefficient alphas of 0.91, 0.76 and 0.73 for these three groups respectively. Lower item inter-correlations of 0.32 to 0.62 were reported by Schwab *et al.* (1967) on the basis of a study of 153 medical in-patients. The extensive review of the literature by Beck *et al.* (1988) reported that a meta-analysis of the BDI's internal consistency estimates yielded a mean coefficient alpha of 0.86 for psychiatric patients and 0.81 for non-psychiatric respondents.

Tests to date indicate that the scale has moderate to good levels of validity and reliability, although most testing has been conducted on psychiatric populations. It is regarded as the scale of choice for researchers in the selection of depressed subjects from a larger population, although, as with most scales, its accuracy depends on people's motivation to report their emotional state accurately (Stehouwer 1985). A comprehensive review of the literature on the reliability and validity of the scale has been published by Beck *et al*. (1988). A version for children and adolescents is available (Kovacs and Beck 1977), and a short 23-item version is available, although less often used (Beck and Beck 1972; Beck *et al*. 1974).

HOSPITAL ANXIETY AND DEPRESSION SCALE (HAD)

The Hospital Anxiety and Depression Scale was developed by Zigmond and Snaith (1983). It is a brief assessment of anxiety and depression, consisting of 14 items divided into two sub-scales for anxiety and depression, in which the patient rates each item on a four-point scale.

Two common problems with questionnaires for the detection of mood disorders are that scores are affected by the physical illness of the patient, and there is insufficient distinction between one mood disorder and another. Zigmond and Snaith developed the Hospital Anxiety and Depression Scale in partial response to this. The scale measures anhedonic depression which the authors take as the best indicator of hypomelancholia and advise the prescription of anti-depressants for those with a high score. Snaith (1987) also recommends the use of a combined researcher-administered and self-assessment scale.

The authors purposefully excluded all items relating to both emotional and physical disorder (e.g. dizziness, headaches), and the items included in the HAD were based solely on the psychic symptoms of neurosis. They also aimed to distinguish between the concepts of anxiety and depression. The seven items comprising the depression sub-scale were based on the anhedonic state. The authors justified this by reference to the evidence that this is probably the central psychopathological feature of that form of depression which responds well to antidepressant drug treatment and is therefore clinically useful information. The seven items comprising the anxiety sub-scale were selected after study of the Present State Examination and

analysis of the psychic manifestations of anxiety neurosis. Severity scales were developed, with ratings from 0 to 3.

Content

Unlike most other scales, the HAD is not derived from factor analysis but from clinical experience. It consists of two sections, with four-point response scales. One section contains the seven items on depression and the other contains the seven items on anxiety. The scale assesses emotional state over the 'past week'. Examples of the scale are:

I feel tense or 'wound up':
Most of the time.
A lot of the time.
From time to time, occasionally.

Worrying thoughts go through my mind:
A great deal of the time.
A lot of the time.
From time to time but not too often.
Only occasionally.

I feel as if I am slowed down:
Nearly all the time.
Very often.
Sometimes.
Not at all.

I get sudden feelings of panic:
Very often indeed.
Quite often.
Not very often.
Not at all.

Scoring

Individual items are scored from 0–3 to 3–0, depending on the direction of the item wording. The item scores represent the degree of distress: none = 0, a little = 1, a lot = 2, unbearably = 3. Items are summed. The higher scores indicate the presence of problems. Using psychiatric diagnoses as a gold standard, HAD depression ratings of 7 or less were considered to be non-cases; scores of 8–10 were considered doubtful cases; and scores of 11+ implies definite cases. Various cut-offs have been used by investigators, but the cut-off of 11+ appears to be preferable in sorting cases from non-cases (Carroll *et al.* 1993).

Validity

The scales were tested for validity on over 100 psychiatric out-patients and hospital staff, with good results (Zigmond and Snaith 1983). Tests on 50 patients reported that the severity ratings correlated highly with psychiatric assessments (r = 0.70 for depression and r = 0.74 for anxiety) (Zigmond and Snaith 1983; and see Snaith and Taylor 1985). There was evidence that the anxiety and depression items were tapping different dimensions. It was easily understood and acceptable to patients. Fallowfield *et al.* (1987) reported a good level of acceptability among general medical patients. Aylard *et al.* (1987) reported correlations with other well-known depression and anxiety scales ranging from 0.67 to 0.77 (Aylard *et al.* 1987). It has been reported to perform better than the General Health Questionnaire (Goldberg 1978) in identifying cases against the criterion of a psychiatric assessment (Wilkinson and Barczak 1988).

It has been reported to be equal to the General Health Questionnaire in ability to detect cases of minor psychiatric disorder (Lewis and Wessely 1990). As a screening instrument, it has a sensitivity of 88 per cent (at a threshold score of 8), when compared with the Structural Clinical Interview for the DSM-III (Hamer *et al.* 1991). It was sensitive to change in a study of treatment of patients with neurotic disorders (Tyrer *et al.* 1988). Further tests by Zigmond and Snaith (1983) showed that physically ill patients, who were not assessed as having mood disorder, had similar scores to the normal sample and scale scores were judged not to be affected by physical illness. A factor analysis of the scale by Andersson (1993) reported that a two-factor solution did not split the items in the way originally intended, and a four-factor solution with three interpreted factors gave a better solution. However, a factor analysis by Moorey *et al.* (1991) did confirm the two-factor structure of the scale, which proved stable when sub-samples as well as the total sample was analysed.

Reliability

Attempts were made to overcome response bias in the scale by alternating the order of responses so that at one item the first response indicates maximum severity and at another item the last response indicates maximum severity. Four possible responses were chosen to prevent people from opting for a middle grade.

The authors tested internal consistency of the scale, using data from 50 patients. The correlations for the anxiety items ranged from 0.41 to 0.76. The analysis of the depression items revealed one weak item which was removed from the scale ('I am awake before I need to get up'), along with the weakest of the anxiety items. The remaining depression items had correlations ranging from 0.30 to 0.60. Higher correlations were reported by Moorey *et al.* (1991).

The criteria were then tested for reliability with a further 50 patients and results judged to be satisfactory (the false positive/negative rates were between 1 and 5 per cent). The severity ratings correlated with psychiatric judgements, with the results for depression: 0.70, and for anxiety: 0.74. Correlations between items and interviewer ratings provided some evidence that the depression and anxiety items were tapping different mood dimensions, rather than the same thing, although some overlap is inevitable. It was apparently easily understood and completed by patients.

Although the authors present the HAD as a reliable and valid instrument on the basis of these tests, far more work on its reliability and validity is required to be carried out before its performance as an indicator can be confidently judged. The depression sub-scale has been reported to have a reasonable specificity and sensitivity in the Urdu language among Asian people living in Britain (Nayani 1989), although the scale was simply translated for this study and not suitably modified for the Asian subjects (see critique by Chaturvedi 1990). Subsequent research has tested the translated scale's conceptual equivalence and reported it to be satisfactory (Mumford *et al.* 1991).

THE SYMPTOMS OF ANXIETY AND DEPRESSION SCALE (SAD)

The Symptoms of Anxiety and Depression Scale assesses anxiety and depression by focusing exclusively on recent symptomatology 'within the last month'. It is a brief self-report measure, empirically derived from two other scales developed by the authors (Bedford et al. 1976).

The SAD has been adapted for use with the elderly (McNab and Phillip 1980). McNab and Phillip (1980) reported their study using the SAD in which 41 people aged 85 and over were visited by health visitors based in one group general practice. The questions were apparently well tolerated by respondents. They reported that 80.5 per cent scored within the normal range, 17.1 per cent were borderline and 2.4 per cent were ill. These scores did not differ significantly from those reported for younger adults by Bedford et al. (1976).

Results from Vetter et al.'s (1982) study of 1,288 people aged 70+ living at home in Wales are broadly consistent with others. They report borderline anxiety in 19 per cent of respondents, and pathological scores in 7 per cent. Females had a higher degree of anxiety than males, although there was no consistent variation of anxiety score with age. In relation to depression, 6 per cent achieved a borderline score and 3 per cent pathological scores. Females again scored higher than males, and there was no consistent variation with age.

Content

The scale consists of seven states of anxiety and seven states of depression. Examples of items, which relate to 'the past week or so', are:

Recently, have you been worried about every little thing?
Recently, have you been so worked up that you couldn't keep still?
Recently, have you had a pain or tense feeling in the back of your neck?
Recently, has worry kept you awake at night?
Recently, have you lost interest in just about everything?

All items' responses are 'no/a little/a lot/ unbearably'.

Scoring

For each question a score of 0–3 is possible, rated according to the degree of distress (none = 0, a little = 1, a lot = 2, unbearably = 3). The scores are

added for the seven questions at each of the two measures, giving a range of 0–21 for each scale, and 0–42 overall.

By comparison with psychiatric opinion, psychiatrically normal scores are judged to be those section SAD scores of 0–2; 3–5 were regarded as borderline; and 6–21 as pathological, indicating extreme dysphoria or clinically significant depression.

Validity

There is some work on the construct and predictive validity of the scale. The SAD has been used by Morgan et al. (1987) in a survey of 979 people aged 65+ living at home in Nottinghamshire. The authors reported a relationship between physical- and mental-health problems, and that emotional disturbance increased the likelihood of medical consultations. However, they also reported a weak correlation between SAD scores and clinical ratings of depression (0.43), and between the SAD and clinical ratings of the severity of depression (0.32). In contrast, Bedford et al. (1976), in tests involving 96 in-patients rated by psychiatrists and psychologists, reported a statistically significant association between patients' depression scores and psychiatrists' ratings of their depression levels.

McNab and Phillip (1980), in their study of people aged 85+, reported that respondents' SAD scores did not differ significantly from health-visitor ratings of the same respondents' mental health, although the degree of concordance was reported to be modest at best.

Vetter and Ford (1989) also used the scale in Wales to predict falls among elderly people and reported a relationship between scale score and the prevalence of falls. On the other hand, as this study was cross-sectional, the long-term predictive ability of the scale was not tested.

Little other published work on its validation exists.

Reliability

Bedford et al. (1976) reported test-retest results at one month for 68 (out of 96 initially assessed) patients rated by psychiatrists and psychologists using the SAD scale. The results showed evidence of a significant change, from an average score of 12.68 to 6.40. The authors cite this change as evidence of its sensitivity to change in mental state rather than as unreliability. Split–half reliability correlations were 0.61 for normal control subjects and 0.69 for the patients.

Again, evidence is scant on its reliability. In sum, although this is an increasingly popular scale for use with elderly populations, far more extensive testing is required before it can be generally recommended.

GOLDBERG'S GENERAL HEALTH QUESTIONNAIRE (GHQ)

The General Health Questionnaire is the most widely applied self-completion measure of psychiatric disturbance in the UK and also has numerous worldwide applications. A major advantage for potential users of the GHQ is the existence of periodically updated handbooks containing its method, a comprehensive review of applications, and studies of reliability and validity (Goldberg 1978; Goldberg and Williams 1988).

The GHQ was developed in London during the 1960s and 1970s and was intended for use in general practice settings. It was derived from various scales, including the Cornell Medical Index. In the construction of the GHQ the concept of psychiatric disorder was thought to be appropriate to general practice settings.

The GHQ is a screening questionnaire for detecting independently verifiable forms of psychiatric illness and does not make clinical diagnoses. If these are necessary, a two-stage strategy must be employed. It is not suitable for the assessment of long-stage (chronic) problems, as it does not detect them. It is a pure state measure, assessing present state in relation to usual state (this question wording is not distortive as most people see their usual state as a normal state) (Goldberg and Williams 1988).

The advantage of the GHQ is that it concentrates on broader components of psychiatric morbidity (particularly anxiety and depression) and is designed to be self-administered. It does not attempt to detect mental subnormality, senile dementia or mania (most of the people within these categories would not be able to complete the questionnaire). It was not intended to be used for the detection of functional psychoses (schizophrenia or psychotic depression), although these conditions are in fact detected. A study of 111 acute geriatric medical in-patients by O'Riordan et al. (1990) showed that there were no significant differences on the GHQ when dementia was the variable (e.g. between normal depressed patients and demented depressed patients), although threshold scores did require raising.

One further advantage of using the GHQ is that short-item versions exist (12, 20, 28, 30), which, although slightly less valid and sensitive than the long version (60 items), are more suitable than the longer versions for use with older frail people. The 28-item version has an additional advantage over the other versions in that it also permits analysis within sub-categories; it was developed mainly for research purposes.

There have been numerous applications of the GHQ in survey research and in clinical settings (e.g. GPs' surgeries). It has been used among 662 people aged 85 and over living in London and was found to be acceptable to respondents, although some required assistance with completion due to poor sight and stiff finger joints (Bowling 1990). The GHQ-30 is popularly used in large social surveys and epidemiological research in the UK (Huppert and Garcia 1991; Stansfeld and Marmot 1992).

Although it has been used extensively in the UK, there have also been many applications of the scale in other countries, particularly in the USA. The 30-item version, for example, was used in a psychological morbidity survey of 1,649 new adult enrollers in a Health Maintenance Organization in the USA (Berwick et al. 1987).

Although the GHQ is culture specific in development, it works well in other settings, e.g. among both white and black residents in Philadelphia, in Calcutta, China, rural Iceland, Brazil and Australia (Tennant 1977; Mari and Williams 1985; for review see Goldberg and Williams 1988). It has been translated into at least 38 languages.

Content

The original version of the GHQ consists of 60 items; shorter versions of 30, 28, 20 and 12 have also been developed. The 12-item version is apparently as efficient as the 30-item version as a case detector.

Examples of questions, which all appear both in the GHQ-30 and the GHQ-60, each of which relate to the past few weeks, are:

Have you recently:

Been able to concentrate on whatever you're doing?
Better than usual, same as usual, less than usual, much less than usual.

Spent much time chatting with people?
More time than usual, about the same as usual, less time than usual, much less than usual.

Felt on the whole you were doing things well?
Better than usual, about the same, less well than usual, much less well.

Been feeling unhappy and depressed?
Not at all, no more than usual, rather more than usual, much more than usual.

Felt that life isn't worth living?
Not at all, no more than usual, rather more than usual, much more than usual.

Scoring

The GHQ consists of a checklist of statements asking respondents to compare their recent experience to their usual state on a 4-point scale of severity. The scoring scale consists of 0 or 1 (the 0–0–1–1 scoring scale, the scores following the sequence of response categories across the page from left to right, is the most commonly used). Some items are negative, others are positive. The overall GHQ is the sum of the item scores. The 0–0–1–1 scoring scale is simply a count of the symptoms and is the simplest and also avoids the problems of middle-user response bias. Goldberg and Williams (1988) demonstrated that very similar results are obtained with the different scoring methods in existence, and little is gained by a Likert severity score.

Threshold scores are defined as equivalent to the concept of 'caseness' that corresponds to the average patient referred to psychiatrists. If the results of a population of GHQ scores are compared with independent psychiatric assessment, it is poss-

ible to state the number of symptoms where the probability that an individual will be thought to be a case exceeds 0.5. This is called a threshold score. The proportion of respondents with scores above this threshold is the probable prevalence of illness. Finlay-Jones and Murphy (1979) have shown that in order to identify 'cases' that correspond to standards derived from the Present State Examination, it is necessary to raise the threshold score.

Since physically ill people score highly on the GHQ, it is not surprising that they are over-represented among false positives. Goldberg and Williams suggest raising the thresholds for use with severe physical illnesses. Goldberg (1978), in the manual for the administration of the GHQ, points to the necessity of manipulating the threshold score to enhance discrimination in different populations.

It is possible to compare the amount of psychiatric disturbance in two populations by comparison of the central tendency (mean, median) and dispersion (SD, inter-quartile range) of scores in each population. Also a given population can be tested on different occasions to assess the changes in psychiatric disturbance over time.

Because of the nature of its response scale, the GHQ is likely to miss very long-standing disorders, since respondents answer 'same as usual' (and thus score zero) for symptoms they are experiencing and have been experiencing for a long time. However, Goldberg and Williams (1988) point out that the loss of cases is minimal as many people cling to a concept of their 'usual self' as being without symptoms. They suggest including questions on medication taking and whether the person thinks s/he has a nervous illness to detect chronic patients. However, Goodchild and Duncan Jones (1985) have suggested an ingenious scoring method which may increase the sensitivity of the GHQ and makes it more likely to detect long-standing illness. This consists of dividing the GHQ questions up into items detecting caseness (negative, e.g. feeling constantly under strain) and those indicating health (positive, e.g. enjoying day-to-day activities). This method assigns a score to those replying 'same as usual' to any of the negative items (so the score for negative items becomes 0111, and for positive items 0011). This method gives superior validity coefficients against caseness over the normal GHQ scoring method (0011) as measured by the Present State Examination. A further advantage is that the scores are more normally distributed and the scale is a more sensitive indicator when used over time. Given the recent development of this method, Goldberg and Williams suggest that this method should be used in addition to previous methods, rather than instead of.

Validity

There is good evidence that assessments of the severity of psychiatric illness are directly proportional to the number of symptoms reported on the GHQ (Goldberg and Huxley 1980). The predictive validity of the GHQ in comparison with other well-known scaling tests of depression is also good (Goldberg 1985; Williams 1987).

The principal components and item analysis used during the development of the GHQ ensured that it has content validity; its construct validity was demonstrated in the principal components analysis which showed that there was a large general factor found in all the analyses reported.

Berwick et al. (1987) carried out a factor analysis of responses which disclosed six factors (anxiety/strain, confidence, depression, energy, social function and insomnia) and a strong tendency for items of similar wording (positive phrasing) to cluster together.

Over 50 validity studies have been conducted of the GHQ. Although not perfect, it correlates well with psychiatric diagnoses of morbidity and depression (Finlay-Jones and Murphy 1979; Williams 1987). The GHQ-30 has been the most widely validated. For example, 29 such studies were reported by Goldberg and Williams (1988). Correlations with other gold standards have established the criterion validity of the GHQ. Using standardized psychiatric interviews as a gold standard, reported sensitivities range between 0.55 and 0.92, and specificities between 0.80 and 0.99, depending on the choice of threshold score (Vieweg and Hedlund 1983). Comparisons of GHQ scores with a structured clinical interview (e.g. the Present State Examination or the Clinical Interview Schedule) report correlations from 0.45 to 0.83. The GHQ-60 had the highest correlations and the GHQ-30 the poorest (see Goldberg and Williams 1988 for review).

Also a study in the USA found a correlation of 0.72 between the Beck Depression Index and the GHQ-30 (Cavanaugh 1983), and an Australian study reported a correlation of 0.57 between the Zung depression scales and the 30-item GHQ (Henderson et al. 1981b). Bowling and Browne (1991), on the basis of surveys with 662 people aged 85+ and almost 800 aged 65+ living at home in London and in Essex, reported correlations with the GHQ and Neugarten's Life Satisfaction Scale A of 0.47 in each case (Essex data is unpublished). This is a moderate correlation, reflecting the different dimensions of emotional well-being tapped by these two scales. Functional ability was also predictive of changes in GHQ score in a follow-up study by this research team, supporting the scale's construct (convergent) validity (Bowling et al. 1992). Watson and Evans (1986), in their study of the health of a multi-cultural sample of mothers with young children in London's East End, reported that mothers' GHQ scores correlated well with interviewers' ratings of the mothers' distress. A further application was undertaken by Jenkinson et al. (1988). The 30-item GHQ and the Nottingham Health Profile (NHP) were administered to people suffering from either migraine or arthritis. Correlations between the emotional-reactions subsection of the NHP and the GHQ were moderate (0.49) for both groups of patients.

Although the GHQ was not developed as a predictive tool, some studies have reported findings demonstrating predictive validity, although two studies have reported negative results. Criterion validity was established using health services as the criterion. Those with the highest GHQ scores have been reported to have the highest use of services (e.g. general practitioner services) (Goldberg and Williams 1988). Berwick et al. (1987) provided further evidence of the predictive validity of the GHQ: elevations of GHQ scores, over two administrations at seven-month intervals, were strongly associated with the probability of both mental-health and non-mental-health care within 12 months of enrolment.

The GHQ is sensitive for transient disorders, detecting symptoms of at least two weeks' duration. It is as sensitive to depression disorders as any of the specially designed depression scales (such as the Beck or HAD) and detects anxiety disorders as well, so it is suitable for use when the researcher wants a broader measure. Numerous surveys indicate that the GHQ is suitable for use with younger and older men and women in community and primary health-care settings (Sims and Salmons 1975; Tarnopolsky *et al.* 1979; Benjamin *et al.* 1982; Cleary *et al.* 1982; Banks 1983; Hobbs *et al.* 1983; 1984; Goldberg and Williams 1988).

Another example of the application of the GHQ was by Watson and Evans (1986) with a multicultural sample of mothers with young children. While they found that mothers' GHQ scores correlated well with interviewers' ratings of the mothers' distress, an analysis of the translation of the questionnaire into Bengali for the Bengali mothers did reveal some problems. The questionnaire was back-translated by an independent translator. There was a high level of agreement between one translation and the original, with the exception of the item: 'Have you recently been feeling nervous and strung up all the time?' which was translated as 'Did you suffer from mental breakdown and mental anxiety?' The other translation had problems with the item 'Have you recently been finding life a struggle all the time?' which was translated 'Are you thinking yourself a struggler?'

They also found that not all items were applicable to mothers with young babies, e.g. 'Have you recently been having restless disturbed nights?'; 'Have you been getting out of the house as much as usual?'; 'Have you spent much time chatting with people?' Because young mothers are more likely to have false positive scores with these items, the authors recommend raising the threshold score, using the 30-item version, from 4 or 5 to 8.

There can be other problems in administration which may affect reliability. Very elderly people with failing eyesight and arthritic fingers may have difficulty completing the GHQ independently and will require varying degrees of assistance from an interviewer (e.g. reading out the items or recording responses). It is unknown whether this produces any social desirability bias; this is a problem potentially affecting all self-rating scales (Bowling 1990).

Reliability

Split-half and test-retest correlations have been carried out on the GHQ with good results. Split-half reliability has been carried out with 853 completed questionnaires, and the correlation achieved was 0.95. Internal consistency, using Cronbach's

alpha, has been reported in a range of studies with correlations ranging from 0.77 to –0.93. Test-retest reliability correlations have been reported ranging from 0.51 to 0.90, the correlations being higher with clinically defined groups with a high prevalence of disorder (Goldberg and Williams 1988). A problem posed by test-retest reliability is one of distinguishing between true change and unreliability. Goldberg and Williams state that the definitive test-retest reliability study of the GHQ remains to be done.

THE GERIATRIC MENTAL STATE (GMS)

The problem of recognizing depression in the elderly is exacerbated because it may present with features similar to dementia; the two conditions may also coexist. This has led to many researchers in psychiatry turning to instruments of high validity and reliability in relation to the elderly, e.g. the Comprehensive Assessment and Referral Evaluation interview schedule (CARE) (Gurland 1980) and the Geriatric Mental State Examination (Henderson *et al.* 1983).

Copeland *et al.* (1976) reported the development of the Geriatric Mental State (GMS) which was derived from British and US instruments: the Present State Examination (PSE) devised by Wing *et al.* (1974) and the Psychiatric Status Schedule (Spitzer *et al.* 1970). They scaled this down to a form suitable for use in community settings, and they used it within a broader semi-structured interview schedule called the Comprehensive Assessment and Referral Evaluation (CARE) interview (Gurland *et al.* 1983; Copeland *et al.* 1987a; 1987b). The CARE interview is broad and covers psychiatric, medical, nutritional, economic and social problems. Interviewer training is required for CARE and for the GMS.

The psychiatric diagnosis derived from the GMS has since been standardized by the application of computer methods and called AGECAT (Dewey and Copeland 1986). AGECAT was used on a sample of general practitioners' elderly patients in Liverpool and produced diagnosis of depressive neurosis in 8 per cent of cases, and of depressive psychosis of 3 per cent (total 11 per cent). If marginal cases were included, the incidence of mild depression was 22 per cent which was close to the 20 per cent found in the early study in Newcastle (Kay *et al.* 1964; Copeland *et al.* 1987a; 1987b).

The GMS is a well-validated and tested scale but is extremely lengthy, although there is a shorter community version available (GMSA), which is still fairly lengthy if used alongside a survey questionnaire. The short version was developed on the basis of data from a random sample of 396 elderly people living at home in London. There is also an even shorter version of this: the SHORT-CARE, which covers only dementia, depression and disability (Gurland *et al.* 1984). The full length GMS is frequently used as a gold standard against which to assess other scales of mental state; it has been chosen as the principal instrument in the three Medical Research Council multi-site studies in the UK and in three similar studies initiated by the World Health and Pan-American Health Organizations (Copeland 1990).

The full GMS takes between 30 and 45 minutes to administer. The CARE, which has 1,500 items concerned with expressed physical symptoms, social problems and the use of services, takes between one-and-a-half to two hours. The short community version (GMSA) takes from 15–20 minutes.

Since 1976 the GMS has been translated into French, Spanish, German, Danish, Dutch and Icelandic. There have been a number of applications of the GMS. The authors of the instrument have also published a number of papers based on analyses of their studies using the GMS (Copeland *et al.* 1986; Dewey and Copeland 1986; Copeland *et al.* 1987a; 1987b; 1988; Davidson *et al.* 1988; McWilliam *et al.* 1988; Sullivan *et al.* 1988; Saunders *et al.* 1989).

Content

The GMS consists of standard tests and interviewer ratings of the degree of confidence in the information. The confusion items are standard (e.g. checks on day of week). Examples of other items are:

Guilt
Do you tend to blame yourself for anything or feel guilty about anything? What?
Code: Obvious self-blame over past and present peccadilloes.
Mentions regrets about past which may or may not be justifiable.

Irritability
Have you been more irritable (angry) lately?
Code: Admits to irritability (anger).

Concentration
Can you concentrate on a television (radio, film) programme? Can you watch it (listen to it) all the way through?
Code: Difficulty in concentrating on entertainment.

Perceptual distortion
Is something odd (strange) going on which you cannot explain?
Code: Puzzled by something odd going on.

Scoring

Detailed instructions on the rating, coding and scoring procedures, which are fairly lengthy, are available from the authors in the Department of Psychiatry at the University of Liverpool.

Validity

The full CARE interview has been tested against psychiatric judgements on 396 subjects in Greater London, with high overall agreement: agreement on depression and dementia reached 88 per cent of cases (Cohen's kappa for overall agreement was 0.7) and AGECAT (a computerized diagnostic system) was judged to provide a reasonable diagnosis (Copeland *et al.* 1986). Other studies by the authors have also reported good levels of agreement (Copeland *et al.* 1987a; 1987b).

The convergent validity of the Zung scale with physicians' judgements was lower than that achieved by CARE, 0.65 (kappa: 0.29), in comparison with 0.73 (kappa: 0.46) (Toner *et al* 1988).

Reliability

Reliability studies were initially undertaken in London and New York, and in Australia and Liverpool with the shorter versions. Inter-rater reliability was 69 per cent for the first study but only 38 per cent in the second, although partial agreement was much higher at between 80 and 85 per cent. No significant differences in the number of positive ratings made between interviewers in the USA or UK were found. In the Australian study, Henderson *et al.* (1983) reported satisfactory inter-rater reliability of the shortened version with average correlations of 0.56 and 0.84.

The GMS has been shown to be reliable between trained psychiatric interviewers, and agreement with clinical diagnosis is acceptable. It has also been shown to be sensitive to change over time (Copeland and Gurland 1978).

The length of the GMS makes it too unwieldy for use in more general surveys, or surveys mainly concerned with issues other than mental health. It is useful in epidemiological and psychiatric surveys focusing entirely or mainly on mental health. For further details, interested readers should consult the references given.

SHORT MENTAL-CONFUSION SCALES

Mental impairment is of such frequent occurrence among very elderly populations that a method of assessment during survey and evaluative research in this population group is now essential.

Mental confusion tests generally have a fairly similar content and vary in length and complexity. There are several short 10-item tests in use worldwide (see the author's *Measuring Disease* for a broader review). Each is culturally specific, although adaptations are minor (e.g. US scales ask about the name of the last President; UK scales ask about the name of the last Prime Minister or name of the Queen).

THE MENTAL STATUS QUESTIONNAIRE (MSQ)

The Mental Status Questionnaire is a concise measure of orientation and memory, drawn partly from standard mental-status examinations. It has been modified in the USA by Pfeiffer (1975) and reduced from 31 to 9 items. It has been widely used in community and clinical populations. It has been successfully used with older people living at home in the USA by Cornoni-Huntley *et al.* (1985) and has been judged to be a useful measure in institutional settings (Ebmeier *et al.* 1988). Wilson and Brass (1973) reported it could be easily administered to 90 per cent of geriatric-ward patients. They indicate that half the questions could be asked without the patient knowing s/he is being tested, and the other half can follow after brief explanation: 'How is your memory, I would like to test it?' They reported that it rarely provoked anxiety

or embarrassment. It can be given without causing fatigue in the very ill.

There are many possible variations to this type of brief testing, e.g. Hodkinson's (1972) abbreviated Mental Test Score based on the longer version of that developed by Blessed *et al.* (1968).

Content

The 10 questions are:

Name of town?
Address/name of place?
Today's date (error of three days on either side of correct date allowed)?
Month?
Year?
Age?
Year of birth?
Month of birth?
Name of Prime Minister?
Name of previous Prime Minister?

Wilson and Brass (1973) found that item one could be excluded, as it contributed little to discrimination. Only the remaining nine items are usually used, and it has become the norm to refer to the scale as having only nine items. The authors caution its use with deaf people and suggest writing down the questions, and acknowledged that it cannot be used with dysphasic patients.

Scoring

The number of correct cases are scored (correct = 1; false = 0). There is no accepted cut-off (normal/abnormal).

Validity

Kahn *et al.* (1960b), on the basis of 1,066 patients in homes for the aged, nursing homes and state mental hospitals in New York City, reported that the MSQ was highly associated with psychiatrists' evaluations of the presence and degree of chronic brain syndrome. However, the authors simply reported percentage differences without significance values.

Wilson and Brass concluded that the MSQ was a powerful measure for detecting and quantifying mental impairment.

Milne *et al.* (1972), in a longitudinal survey of mental health, compared results from the MSQ with the Mental Impairment Measurement, designed by Isaacs and Walkey (1964) and found the MSQ to be less sensitive than the latter.

Reliability

Kahn *et al.* (1960a; 1960b) reported reliability to be satisfactory. In a series of 55 cases, selected because their physical condition seemed likely to remain stable, the MSQ was administered four times at three-week intervals: three-quarters of the scores changed by one or less (Wilson *et al.* 1973). The association between the five items: town, place, age, month born, year born and the five test items: Prime Minister's name and current date, correlate fairly strongly; r : 0.68 (Wilson and Brass 1973).

THE ABBREVIATED MENTAL TEST SCORE (AMTS)

The Abbreviated Mental Test Score (AMTS) was developed by Hodkinson (1972) from the Modified Roth Hopkins Test (Blessed *et al.* 1968). The most discriminating items were incorporated. There was no evidence that patients' performance improved with practice.

Content

The test contains 10 items. These cover the following:

Age
Time (nearest hour)
Year
Name of place
Recognition of two persons
Birthday (date and month)
Date of World War I
Queen's name
Counting 20–1 backwards
Five-minute recall: full street address

Scoring

Scores are totalled. Each correct item scores 1; maximum score: 10. The cut-offs for scoring (normal/abnormal) have varied between studies. Jitapunkul *et al.* (1991) briefly reviewed the literature and reported that investigators have used cut-offs in the range of < 6 to < 10 (a score of 10 = cognitively normal). They carried out a study of 168 acutely ill patients admitted to a ward for the care of the elderly and validated the AMTS against clinical diagnoses plus medical records (based on DSM-IIIR criteria) (tested on admission and one week later), and reported that the best cut-off was 8.

Validity

It has been further tested against the Crichton Royal Behaviour Rating Scale, and clinical diagnosis of dementia by Vardon and Blessed (1986), using 99 residents of homes for the elderly, with a mean age of 82.7. The authors reported that the AMTS does reveal significant cognitive decline which is characteristic of dementias: over 80 per cent of residents allocated a clinical diagnosis of dementia scored 55 per cent or less correct answers on testing. It produced scores closely similar to those obtained on the Modified Roth Hopkins Test (Blessed *et al.* 1968). It has also been tested against a 37-item Roth Hopkins test by Thompson and Blessed (1987). These authors based their research on 52 mentally ill psycho-geriatric day-care patients (mean age: 75). They reported that the 10-item test was better tolerated. The functionally ill scored consistently better than the organically ill. Correlations with longer mental-status scales were 0.91 to 0.96 which were comparable with those reported by Qureshi and Hodkinson (1974) for institutionalized patients (the latter reported correlations with longer mental-test scales of 0.87 to 0.96). Short versions of the AMTS (which include five and seven items) have been tested by Jitapunkel *et al.* (1991) with good results. It also has a higher sensitivity than the original.

Reliability

Its performance has been assessed in institutional and community settings, with good results for inter-observer reliability and repeatability (Qureshi and Hodkinson 1974; Vardon and Blessed 1986; Little *et al.* 1987; Thompson and Blessed 1987), although there are few published data on its reliability.

Jitapunkel *et al.* (1991) developed a short version of the AMTS (AMT7). Its validity, internal consistency and coverage of the relevant domains was comparable to the AMTS but it had a slightly higher sensitivity (81 per cent) (with acceptable specificity: 85 per cent) than the full AMTS. Cronbach's alpha, based on the internal consistency of the AMT7, was 0.85 (it was 0.89 for the full version). The proportion of patients correctly classified was 89.9 (91.1 per cent for the 10-item test).

6

MEASURING SOCIAL NETWORKS AND SOCIAL SUPPORT

SOCIAL-NETWORK ANALYSIS

Network models have been employed in numerous areas of sociology, psychology and anthropology. In research on health–care needs, lack of social support has been associated with increased mortality risk, delayed recovery from disease, poor morale and mental health (Lowenthal and Haven 1968; Berkman and Syme 1979; Lin *et al.* 1979; Bowling and Charlton 1987; Cohen *et al.* 1987; Maes *et al.* 1987; Seeman *et al.* 1987). Studies of premature deaths among males from cardiovascular disease and social networks concluded that the range of the variation explained by social networks was 25–35 per cent (Olsen 1992). However, not everyone fits identical patterns, and research is also contradictory (see reviews by Bowling 1991; 1994). Whatever the nature of the study, measuring social networks and support is fraught with difficulties, as most measures have not been fully tested for validity and reliability.

Social networks and social support are two different concepts. Network analysis was originally developed by sociologists and social anthropologists, although recent methodological advances have been due to the increasing involvement of social psychologists in this area (Mitchell and Trickett 1980). Sociologists believe that the characteristics of the network have some explanatory power of the social behaviour of the people involved (Mitchell 1969). The framework most applicable to the study of social support derives from the theory of social networks. This describes transactions among individuals. Each individual is a node in the network and each exchange a link. Networks are defined as the web of identified social relationships that surround an individual and the characteristics of those linkages. It is the set of people with whom one maintains contact and has some form of social bond. Social contacts and relationships are important ways for the individual to influence the environment and provide pathways through which the environment influences the individual (Saronson *et al.* 1977).

The importance of social networks, and their characteristics, lies in the extent to which they fulfil members' needs. Their functions can be summarized as 'that set of personal contacts through which the individual maintains his social identity, and receives emotional support, material aid, services, information and new social contacts' (Walker *et al.* 1977). House (1981) has suggested that social support involves emotional concern (liking, love); instrumental aid (services); information (about environment) and appraisal (information for self-evaluation). One approach to defining social support proceeds from a consideration of its source, such as who provides it; the functions it serves for people (e.g. material aid); and the intimacy characteristics of the relationship (e.g. whether it is a confiding relationship) (Tolsdorf 1976). Thus social support can be defined as the interactive process in which emotional, instrumental or financial aid is obtained from one's social network.

Cobb (1976) defines social support as 'information leading the subject to believe that he is cared for and loved, esteemed, and a member of a network of mutual obligations'. Thus support exists only if it leads to certain beliefs in the recipient. Thoits (1982) has expanded this model to include instrumental aid. Despite several attempts to conceptualize social support, no agreement has yet been reached; attempts have been criticized as inadequate (Thoits 1982).

Several characteristics of networks appear relevant in terms of support. First, people must have connections with other people (network) in order to receive social support, but social connections do not guarantee access to social support. Finch (1989) also stressed the importance of the type of genealogical relationship, the past pattern of social exchanges, the balance of dependence and independence in the relationship, timing in life, and the quality of the relationship. Sarason et al. (1994) argued that there is a need for theories of social support to incorporate the complexity of those situational, interpersonal and intrapersonal processes that shape people's perceptions of their interactions with others. Other relevant dimensions are:

Size: the number of people maintaining social contact; this can include those who are only called on when needed.

Geographic dispersion: networks vary from those confined by a household, to those in a single neighbourhood, and those that are more widely dispersed. Transport facilities may influence frequency of contact.

Density/integration: the extent to which network members are in each other's networks.

Composition and member homogeneity: friend, neighbour, children, sibling, other relatives; similarities between members (age, socioeconomic status, etc.).

Frequency of contact between members

Strength of ties: degree of intimacy, reciprocity, expectation of durability and availability, emotional intensity.

Social participation: involvement in social, political, educational, church, other activities.

Social anchorage: years of residence in, and familiarity with, neighbourhood, involvement in community.

These structural characteristics of the network will influence:

The availability of instrumental and emotional support, its adequacy, satisfactions with, and perceptions of the network and support/aid obtained.

Networks can thus be operationally defined in terms of size, geographic dispersion, strength of ties, density/integration, composition and member homogeneity (Mitchell 1969; Craven and Wellman 1974; Walker *et al.* 1977).

These structural characteristics are useful in calculating the number and distribution of relationships within a network and their degree of connection. The emerging patterns can then be studied in relation to the particular life situation of the individual. It can be hypothesized that different types of network structure have differing degrees of significance depending on the nature of need to be met.

'Dynamic features of the social network' refers to the positive or negative nature of network interactions. Analyses need to take account of the nature of human emotions involved. The size of the network and calculations of frequency of contact between members are of little value if these interactions are negative and stressful. It is also possible that the existence of a single confidant(e) is of greater value in terms of meeting an individual's emotional needs than a larger number of more superficial friendships. The individual's subjective 'view' of the network takes into account the meaning of relationships and the strength of affectional ties. A different but related dimension is the concept of loneliness. This can be a consequence of perceived or actual poor emotional or social support. This concept and its measurement are discussed at the end of this chapter.

METHODS OF MEASUREMENT

There is currently no assessment scale which comprehensively measures the main components of social network and support with acceptable levels of reliability and validity. Part of the problem stems from lack of agreement on conceptual bases, or even failure to consider these at all.

Many surveys have relied on single-item questions such as marital status, frequency of contact with others and existence of a confidant(e). Single-item measures have been found to be powerful predictors of health status and mortality but alone provide no insight into the dynamics of the network. It is important to match methodology to the empirical issue and correct disciplinary approach. Among the studies using only simple measures of social networks was the Alamada County Human Population Laboratory which provided the most convincing evidence of a link between social networks and mortality (Berkman and Syme 1979) but the precise nature of the relationship is unknown. If more studies used adequate measures, the links may prove to be stronger and the debate about links less controversial.

There is now a trend away from simple totalling of social contacts and single-item questions towards developing scales. Many earlier approaches simply assessed social network and support by questions on marital status and household composition (see review by Hirsch 1981). The implication from the early studies on social ties and mental and physical health is that social ties are important and merit further study. Studies relying on single-item questions and crude or simplistic measures cannot be used to derive substantive implications for practice. It is necessary to differentiate relationships according to their content, process and development. Failure to obtain these data precludes information on how social networks function as social support systems. Survey questions that do not separate social support from network structure do not permit identification of the social conditions under which help and support are provided. It cannot be assumed that having a daughter living nearby will necessarily lead to adequate support and help. Most attempts to measure quality of the network consist of questions asking respondents whom they are close to, in contact with and if they see enough of the mentioned people. Such single items are inadequate as evaluations of the perceived quality of relationships (Adams 1967). Some assessment of satisfaction in relation to social support is essential, given that this has been found to be related to well-being, and its relationship to frequency of contact or perceived support is inconsistent in the literature (Fiore et al. 1986; Seeman and Berkman 1988).

Seeman and Berkman (1988) found that network characteristics do not appear to be so highly correlated with aspects of social support that they are interchangeable. Cohen et al. (1987), on the basis of their study of 155 elderly residents of midtown Manhattan single-room occupancy hotels, reported the results of a factor analysis showing that only 7 of the 19 network variables utilized had sufficient commonality to form a potential scale, suggesting that most variables are independent of each other. The authors criticize the use of scales without prior analysis of scale items and the development of scales without the use of parametric approaches such as factor analysis. As they point out, a possible problem with combining all network variables into one scale is the potential for premature treatment of network variables as unidimensional (i.e. representing one underlying construct). Combining variables which may be independent of each other into a simple scale may attenuate true variance and obscure differences which may be important. Much previous research has been limited to the use of bivariate statistical techniques, therefore making it impossible to control for overlap among variables or to determine the relative strength of variables. Measures of network need to be multi-faceted, taking into account structure and dynamic features of the network, as well as the individual's subjective perceptions of it.

Researchers often assume that measures of network size and frequency of social contacts are fairly 'objective' and stable in comparison with measures of the content and quality of relationships which are likely to be confounded by mental-health status (House and Kahn 1985). Donald and Ware (1982) reported one-year test-retest reliability coefficients of between 0.40 to 0.60 for reports of social contacts. This lack of stability may sometimes reflect the changing nature of relationships, particularly in older populations who experience large network losses through death and illness of (also old) relatives and friends, necessitating caution in the interpretation of results (Bowling and Farquhar 1995). One problem with network scales is that visits to relatives are so routine that they may be taken for granted and unreported as formal social visits (Stueve and Lein 1979). Spouses may also be so taken for granted as part of the network that they too are unreported in network scales (Bowling et al. 1988). Another problem with asking questions about social support is that feelings about the supportive nature of the network (affective component) are influenced by psychological well-being or depression as well as by network structure and functions. Thus people with adequate support may perceive it to be inadequate because they are feeling depressed. This problem has not been resolved. Subjective perceptions are, of course, important, but a measurement schedule should be able to distinguish between subjective and objective elements accurately. Perhaps additional interviews could be carried out with a member of the respondent's social network in order to establish the validity of the information provided by the respondent. Sokolovsky (1986) suggests an ethnographic approach to validate information given: participant observation, life histories, genealogies and informal interviews to probe the social support elements of social networks. An example is Francis's (1984) comparison of the Jewish elderly in Cleveland and England. Francis's methods were based on a comprehensive set of semi-structured questions centring around practical (transportation, shopping, money, etc.) and emotional (advice, visiting, etc.) services. Another example is Wentowski's (1982) study of an urban population in which he elicited examples of support as various events were reported.

In sum, there has been little attempt to test measures of social support for reliability and validity (Tardy 1985). Existing research generally suffers from methodological problems: imprecise definitions, failure to treat social support as a multidimensional concept, and various intervening variables confound studies. The main problem with most studies has been the inadequate conceptualization and operationalization of social support. It is common simply to itemize presence or absence of a spouse, confidant(e), household composition and social activities. Most researchers then total respondents' scores to questions about the structure of social networks and ignore the different dimensions of support. Conceptual definitions are more rarely offered, although sociologists are beginning to offer more developed conceptual statements: that the respondent believes s/he is cared for/loved/esteemed/valued and belongs to a network of significant others.

AVAILABLE MEASURES OF SOCIAL SUPPORT

A selection of the available measures of social support have been optimistically reviewed by Payne and Graham-Jones (1987). These authors felt that existing measures can reasonably measure social support and fall down mainly on lack of testing for criterion validity. They failed to point out that far more evidence of all aspects of their reliability and validity is required before they can be used with confidence. On the other hand, it is encouraging that a start has been made in developing measures of this type. A number of these measures have also been briefly reviewed by Orth-Gomer and Unden (1987). They also reviewed a number of the shorter measures, consisting mainly of single-item questions with little reference to quality of, and satisfaction with, relationships, e.g. Berkman's Social Network Index (Berkman and Syme 1979); House's Social Relationships and Activities Scale (House et al. 1982); Lin's Social Support Scale (Lin et al. 1979) and Orth-Gomer and Johnson's Social Network Interaction Index (Orth-Gomer and Johnson 1987). Although these short-item measures appear to be inadequate in scope and depth, Berkman and Syme's, House's, and Orth-Gomer and Johnson's scale items do predict mortality. On the other hand, the items are insufficiently detailed to indicate precisely what dimensions of poor social support structures are most important. Moreover, there are doubts about the validity of short scales. For example, there is evidence that there is massive item bias in Berkman's Social Network Index, indicating that it cannot be used as a valid measure of social network (Dean et al. 1994).

A review of 33 instruments purporting to measure social support by O'Reilly (1988) reported only modest agreement on conceptual definition and frequently the concepts were not defined or ill defined. In particular, definitional confusion between social network and social support was apparent. Variables used to operationalize these concepts reflected this conceptual confusion. For example, some of the measures he reviews define social support in terms of social-network characteristics (size source and frequency of contact). O'Reilly was less optimistic about the value of existing measures and pointed out that more rigorous standards to establish validity and reliability were required. Several scales, including some of those reviewed here, which were judged to be suitable for use with elderly people, have been briefly described by Oxman and Berkman (1990). There are also several longer scales of social support which have been designed specifically for use with people with mental-health problems. For example, Lehman's (1983) Quality of Life Interview contains a sub-section on frequency and nature of social relationships and contacts, as well as social activities (rating satisfaction using the Delighted–Terrible Faces as the response scale). Bigelow *et al.*'s (1991) Quality of Life Questionnaire also includes a substantial set of questions on social relationships, support and activities including negative–positive aspects of relationships. In both scales, some of the items are specific to people with mental-health problems and they are not recommended for other types of populations. The Team for the Assessment of Psychiatric Services (TAPS) have developed the Social Network Scale as part of their battery of outcome measures, but this is a semi-structured instrument and can take up to an hour to administer (Leff *et al.* 1990; Leff 1993). The full instruments were reviewed by the author in Measuring Disease, and as these sub-scales on social support were developed for use with a specific patient population they are not included in this chapter. Interested readers are referred to the relevant references.

Some of the more general measures of health status and quality of life include items on social support and activities; as these have been reviewed elsewhere in this volume, they will not be reviewed here (e.g. OARS). The Rand Batteries included two promising batteries on network structure (The Social Health Battery) and social support (the Social Support Scale). These were reviewed in the section on the Rand Batteries in Chapter 4 and will also not be repeated here.

INVENTORY OF SOCIALLY SUPPORTIVE BEHAVIOURS (ISSB)

The ISSB is a measure designed by Barrera (1981) for use with a wide range of community populations. Social support was conceptualized as the diversity of natural helping behaviours that individuals actually receive, derived from the previous literature on social support. The authors felt

that most existing scales concentrated on the structure of the network rather than what the members actually did, especially in view of noted discrepancies between actual amount of help provided and subjective perceptions of the amount of help (Liem and Liem 1978).

This scale is operationalized by 40 items generated from the literature to specify the amount of help received in the past month. The average time taken to complete the questionnaire is about 10 minutes.

Content

The ISSB measures four types of support: emotional, instrumental, information appraisal and socializing. The index asks respondents to state how people have helped them in the last month and to respond on a five-point Likert-type scale to each of the 40 items as 'not at all', 'once or twice', 'about once a week', 'several times a week' or 'about every day'. It measures the receipt of support, but not the source. Examples of items include:

Emotional:
Expressed interest and concern in your well-being.
Listened to you talk about your private feelings.
Was right there with you (physically) in a stressful situation.

Items on instrumental appraisal support:
Provided you with a place where you could get away for a while.
Loaned you over $25.
Provided you with some transportation.

Informational appraisal support:
Gave you some information on how to do something.
Gave you feedback on how you were doing without saying it was good or bad.
Helped you understand why you didn't do something well.

Socializing:
Talked to you about some interest of yours.
Did some activity together to help you get your mind off things.

There is a problem with all these statements in that they may or may not relate to real events in people's immediate lives, and some items may measure resources available to the supporter rather than support to the respondents (e.g. items on financial and car loans).

Scoring

The five-point ratings of each item are summed to produce a total score, with higher scores indicating greater support. The author also suggests calculating an average frequency score as this permits a global score to be produced when there is some missing data for items.

A weakness with scales of this type is that, without a distinction between available and enacted support, the scale may simply be measuring the number, type and severity of problems recently experienced by the respondent.

Validity

The validity of the ISSB was tested by correlating results, based on 43 students, with a measure of family relations (Family Environment Scale); the correlation, although significant, was not high: 0.35. The author speculated that this was because the two scales were measuring different dimensions of support. Construct validity was assumed by correlations of the index with a measure of life events: 0.38 to 0.41 (Barrera 1981; Sandler and Barrera 1984). Notes available from the author on the scale summarize the correlations between ISSB and measures of distress from 10 published studies. The correlations range from 0.01 to 0.50, although most were fairly weak. The ISSB has been reported to be significantly related to recovery in stroke patients (Glass and Maddox 1992), supporting its predictive ability.

There is agreement between investigators who have carried out exploratory factor analyses of the scale, and report that the ISSB yields three factors (Barrera and Ainlay 1983; Stokes and Wilson 1984; Walkey *et al*. 1987; Pretorius and Diedricks 1993). A study by Caldwell and Reinhart (1988) is also consistent with these analyses and labels the clusters as Guidance, Emotional Support and Tangible Support.

Reliability

The test-retest reliability correlation coefficient, based on 71 students tested over two days, was 0.88; test-retest reliability coefficients, again using students, over a one-month period were 0.80 and 0.63 (Barrera 1981; Barrera and Ainlay 1983; Valdenegro and Barrera 1983). Internal consistency

reliability coefficients of 0.92 and 0.94 were reported for the first and second administrations of the scale (Barrera 1981). Notes on the ISSB are available from the author at Arizona State University; these report that tests from five studies show the internal consistency coefficients of the scale to be above 0.90.

In sum, there are problems with interpretation of the scale. Also, although preliminary results for reliability testing appear good, far more work on both the reliability and validity of the scale is needed before it can be recommended.

ARIZONA SOCIAL SUPPORT INTERVIEW SCHEDULE (ASSIS)

The ISSB (above) was not designed to provide information on people who supplied resources, nor respondents' subjective appraisals of the adequacy of support. Barrera subsequently designed the Arizona Social Support Interview Schedule (ASSIS) to address this gap. The ASSIS was developed by Barrera (1980; 1981) as an instrument to measure several aspects of support, including procedures for identifying support-network membership and subjects' satisfaction with and need for support. His conceptual definition, based on previous literature, of social network relates to people who provide the functions defined as support. The scale is based on self-report and takes 15–20 minutes to complete.

Content

The scale is operationalized by asking subjects to identify individuals who provide support in the following areas: private feelings, material aid, advice, positive feedback, physical assistance and social participation. In each area, subjects are asked about such support from the named individuals in the past month, and whether the support was sufficient; ratings of satisfaction are made on a three-point scale. Examples of items are:

Private feelings

1 If you wanted to talk to someone about things that are very personal and private, who would you talk to? Give me the first names, initials, or nicknames of the people that you would talk to about things that are very personal and private.
Probe: Is there anyone else that you can think of?

2 During the last month, which of these people did you actually talk to about things that were personal and private?
Probe: Ask specifically about people who were listed in response to 1 but not listed in response to 2.

3 During the last month, would you have liked:
 1 A lot more opportunities to talk to people about your personal and private feelings?
 2 A few more opportunities?
 3 Or was this about right?

4 During the past month, how much do you think you needed people to talk about things that were very personal and private?
 1 Not at all.
 2 A little bit.
 3 Quite a bit.

Social participation

1 Who are the people you get together with to have fun or relax? These could be new names or ones you listed before.
Probe: Anyone else?

2 During the past month, which of these people did you actually get together with to have fun or relax?
Probe: Ask about people who were named in 1 but not 2.

3 During the past month, would you have liked:
 1 A lot more opportunities to get together with people for fun and relaxation?
 2 A few more?
 3 Or was it about right?

4 How much do you think you needed to get together with other people for fun and relaxation during the past month?
 1 Not at all?
 2 A little bit?
 3 Quite a bit?

The interview schedule also includes questions concerning negative interactions, on the basis of the psychiatric literature linking these to mental disturbance (identification of people with whom they have had conflicts in the past month). Finally, subjects are asked about the age, sex and ethnicity of people named.

Scoring

The data obtained allow the calculation of specified scores from the relevant items of total available and total utilized network size, conflict network size, unconflicted network size, amount of support satisfaction and support need. The author reported that the support-satisfaction measure suffers from an extremely skewed distribution in the direction of high satisfaction scores (Barrera 1981). Notes which identify the item scores which should be used in calculations are available from the author at Arizona State University.

Validity

The predictive validity was tested on a sample of 86 pregnant adolescents. It was reported by Barrera (1981) that conflicted network size correlated significantly with depression and anxiety, satisfaction correlated with depression and anxiety, and expressed need correlated significantly with depression and anxiety and somatization (0.23–0.51).

The reported relationship between life events and social support was taken as evidence for the index's construct validity (0.25 to 0.38), although these correlations are at best modest. The ASSIS was administered along with the ISSB. The ISSB showed a modest but significant correlation with total network size (0.32), but was not significantly correlated with satisfaction or need on the ASSIS.

Reliability

The instrument has been tested for test-retest reliability, and results appear moderately satisfactory to good. It was tested on 45 students and total network size produced a correlation coefficient of 0.88 over three days, and studies with a further group of students produced a test-retest correlation over one month of 0.70 (Barrera 1980; Valdenegro and Barrera 1983). Test-retest correlations were 0.54 for size of conflicted network, 0.69 for satisfaction and 0.80 for support need. There was also modest support for predictive and construct validity (Barrera 1981).

Internal consistency correlations for support satisfaction and support need were low to moderate: 0.33 and 0.52 respectively.

A study by Barrera *et al.* (1985) of 36 mental-health out-patients who agreed to supply the name of one network member showed significant kappa coefficients between subjects' and informants' reports of support. Of the 31 cases of non-agreement of ASSIS items, 24 were due to informants stating that they had provided aid when subjects indicated that they had not; and seven were due to subjects reporting that aid was provided and informants did not.

Further testing for both reliability and validity is required. At best the validity of the scale is modest.

PERCEIVED SOCIAL SUPPORT FROM FAMILY AND FRIENDS

This was devised by Procidano and Heller (1983) as a measure of perceived social support. It was designed to assess the functions of social networks specified by Caplan (1974): 'the extent to which an individual perceives that his/her needs for support, information, and feedback are fulfilled by friends . . . and by family'. Thoits (1982) has criticized this definition as inadequate on the grounds that it includes the very term to be defined (support). The scale measures available and received support, especially emotional support. It takes about eight minutes to complete.

Content

It comprises two 20-item self-report measures, derived, after testing with students, from an initial pool of 84 items. One 20-item measure is for perceptions of family support and one 20-item measure is for perceptions of support from/given by friends. Responses require a simple 'yes', 'no', or 'don't know'. Examples are:

Family
I rely on my family for emotional support;
My family is sensitive to my personal needs;
My family gives me the moral support I need.

Friends
My friends enjoy hearing about what I think;
I have a deep, sharing relationship with a number of friends;
I feel that I'm on the fringe of my circle of friends.

A few items refer to support given
My friends come to me for emotional support;
Certain members of my family come to me when they have problems or need advice.

Scoring

Positive item responses are totalled and presented separately for family and friends. An overall score can also be calculated.

Validity

The authors reported that the scale correlated with measures of psycho-pathology and distress (0.85–0.98) therefore demonstrating predictive and construct validity. The sensitivity of scale is unknown.

Reliability

In relation to internal consistency, tests with 222 students produced correlation coefficients of 0.88 and 0.90 respectively for the items relating to family and those relating to friends. Test-retest reliability, using 222 students, was 0.83 over a one-month period (Procidano and Heller 1983). In a study investigating the reliability of the scale among students, the inter-correlations among the sub-scales and between the sub-scales and the total scales were reported to be strong and highly significant (Eskin 1993).

Although the scale has good internal reliability, test-retest reliability and predictive validity, far more testing is required.

SOCIAL SUPPORT QUESTIONNAIRE

This questionnaire was developed by Sarason *et al.* (1983) to measure the availability of, and satisfaction with, social support. The conceptual definition of support was derived from Bowlby's theory of attachment and is based on the existence or availability of people who can be relied upon, who care about, love and value the recipient.

In the construction of the scale, which is based on self-report, 61 items were written to sample the situations in which social support might be important to people. They were administered to 602 students who were asked to list people who provided them with such support. Items that showed low correlations with other items were deleted. Scoring methods were also piloted. The scoring method selected was the simplest – a count of supportive persons. The availability index selected was the number of persons listed divided by the number of items.

Most of the items are concerned with emotional support, so this scale is appropriate for measurement of emotional support only. The scale takes an average of 15 minutes to complete. A short 3-item version and a 6-item version has been developed by Sarason *et al.* (1987b).

Content

The instrument comprises 27 items which ask the subjects (a) to list all the people to whom they can turn in specific situations and (b) to indicate their satisfaction with each of these identified supports on a scale ranging from very satisfied to very dissatisfied. The scale was published in full in Sarason *et al.* (1983). Examples are:

Whom can you really count on to listen to you when you need to talk?
Whom could you really count on to help you out in a crisis situation, even though they would have to go out of their way to do so?
With whom can you totally be yourself?
Whom can you really count on to be dependable when you need help?
Who do you feel really appreciates you as a person?
Whom can you count on to console you when you are very upset?

Scoring

Each item is scored (number of persons listed); the satisfaction score ranges from 1 to 6 (very satisfied to not very satisfied). Two scores are computed by dividing the sum of each of the two scores (number of people; overall satisfaction) by the 27 items: average (per item) number of people, and average level of satisfaction with support.

Validity

Attempts were made by the authors to test the construct validity of the scale. Sarason *et al.* (1983) reported a study of 227 students who were administered the scale along with personality scales (extraversion and neuroticism). The correlations with the Social Support Questionnaire were weak to moderate: −0.02 and −0.43 for availability and satisfaction with support. Another study they reported with 295 students showed an association

between positive life events and number of social supports. And a study with 440 students showed that people with more social supports had more positive self-concepts. They also reported that subjects high in social support were rated as more attractive and skilled socially (Sarason *et al.* 1983; 1985). The authors have published the results of several similar studies supporting the construct validity of the scale (Sarason *et al.* 1987a; 1987b).

Predictive validity was judged to be satisfactory on the basis of correlations with depression (the correlations for 100 men and 127 women for each dimension were from −0.22 to −0.43). The sensitivity of the scale is largely unknown.

Separate factor analyses were performed by the authors for each of the two scores. Each analysis showed a very strong first (unrotated) factor. The first factor accounted for 82 per cent of the common variance for the availability score, and 72 per cent for the satisfaction with support score. All factor loadings exceeded 0.60 and 0.30 for each score respectively. There appeared to be good evidence that one strong factor underlies each score and that they represent different dimensions of the concept. Pretorius and Diedricks (1993) carried out exploratory factor analysis and confirmed that the Social Support Questionnaire contained one factor that represented the structure of the scale.

Reliability

Test-retest reliability over a four-week period, using 602 students, was 0.90 for the availability of support items, and 0.83 for satisfaction with support, using 105 students. The alpha coefficients for internal reliability were 0.97 for availability and 0.94 for satisfaction with support, using 602 university students. Inter-item correlations ranged from 0.37 to −0.71 for availability, and from 0.21 to −0.74 for satisfaction with support. A second study of 227 students showed a correlation between the availability and satisfaction with support scores of 0.31 for men and 0.21 for women (Sarason *et al.* 1983).

In sum, it is a viable measure of support, with good results for internal reliability; construct validity has been demonstrated and predictive validity modest. The development and testing of the scale has led to the authors emphasizing the importance of perceived support, rather than network size *per se*, as the most relevant variable (Sarason *et al.* 1987a). This work has led them to develop a further scale: the Quality of Relationship Index (published in full by Pierce *et al.* 1991). This is not reviewed here and interested readers are referred to the latter reference.

INTERVIEW SCHEDULE FOR SOCIAL INTERACTION (ISSI)

This index was developed by Henderson *et al.* (1980; 1981a). The conceptual definition of support was based on the theory that social relations are based on attachment, social integration, nurturance, reassurance of personal worth, sense of reliability, help and guidance. The scale was developed over a year in pilot studies of 130 people in health centres, out-patient departments in a club for the elderly, and in a general population sample in Canberra. It was reported to be acceptable to both healthy and psychiatrically disturbed respondents.

The scale takes approximately 30 minutes to complete, although reports of 60 minutes have also been published. A short version of the scale has been developed by Unden and Orth–Gomer (1989), with similar levels of reliability, validity and discriminative ability as the full scale.

Content

The scale comprises 52 questions asking about the availability and adequacy of people in specific roles: attachment, provided by close affectional relationships; social integration, provided by membership of a network of persons having shared interests and values; the opportunity for nurturing others; reassurance of personal worth; a sense of reliable alliance; and obtaining help and guidance from informal advisers in times of difficulty. It does not adequately measure the availability and adequacy of attachment and social integration.

A question about the availability of provision is immediately followed by a question on adequacy. Examples are:

How many friends do you have whom you could visit at any time, without waiting for an invitation? You could arrive without being expected and still be sure you would be welcome.

Would you like to have more or fewer friends like this, or is it about right for you?

Three items ask about negative interactions:

How many people whom you have to see regularly do you dislike?

Scoring

The four principal indices yield four scores: availability of attachment, perceived adequacy of attachment, availability of social integration and perceived adequacy of social integration. The following indices are created:

AVAT: the availability of affectionally close relationships (attachments).
ADAT: the perceived adequacy of what comprises these close relationships, expressed as a percentage of what is available.
NONDAT: those who lack close relationships might not be unhappy with their situation. The NONDAT index is a measure of such satisfaction despite the absence of attachment.
ATTROWN: the number of attachment persons with whom the respondents has been having rows in the last month.
AVSI: the availability of more diffuse relationships, as with friends, work associates and acquaintances (social integration).
ADSI: the perceived adequacy of these more diffuse relationships.

The scoring and computing instructions have been published by Henderson *et al.* (1981a).

Validity

The authors judged the scale to have face validity on the basis of its content. They suggested that the items effectively tap the constructs of availability and adequacy of attachment in adulthood and social integration.

Henderson *et al.* (1980) established the construct validity of the scale by analysing its four dimensions in relation to personality assessments (neuroticism and introversion–extraversion as measured by the Eysenck Personality Inventory). The sample comprised 225 members of the general population. Inverse relationships with availability and satisfaction measures and neuroticism were reported (–0.18 to –0.31). Results were less consistent with extraversion. The authors argued that one would predict that a neurotic person would have problems in forming and maintaining social relationships and would consequently be dissatisfied with those relationships. The construct validity of the scale was also supported by findings reported by Magne *et al.* (1992). They found that, of their sample of inpatients who had attempted suicide, social support was associated with marital status and economic activity in the expected directions.

Predictive validity was reported by the authors on the basis of a study of neurosis on 756 residents of Canberra, Australia. The measure was associated with Zung's Self Rating Depression Scale and Goldberg's General Health Questionnaire (–0.15 to –0.96) (Henderson 1981). The study, which was based on baseline data collection from 756 residents in Canberra, with three follow-up interviews with a sub-sample over 12 months, reported that deficiencies in social relationships had an effect on the early development of neurotic symptoms. As both availability and adequacy items correlated significantly and negatively with psychiatric disorder and depression, predictive validity was judged to be satisfactory. The scale was also able to discriminate between new migrants to Canberra and those who had been living there for seven months or more. The strength of this study was that it was carried out on a representative sample of the population and was prospective, not cross-sectional; thus the measures of social ties were less likely to be contaminated by already established neurotic symptoms. The correlations between respondents' ISSI scores and those of someone who was nominated as well informed about their social relationships were weak to moderate, although significant, ranging between 0.26 and 0.59 for the items. This may be an indicator of the difference between actual and perceived support.

Reliability

Test-retest reliability scores for the scale indices over an 18-day period using 51 people from the general population ranged from 0.71 to 0.76; using 756 adults from a general population over an 18-day period, scores ranged from 0.66 to 0.85, and over a 12-month period ranged from 0.66 to 0.85. The problem with this long time period is that support structures might have changed and thus a lower correlation may reflect this rather than the reliability of the measure. Internal consistency reliability coefficients range from 0.67 to 0.81 for the indices.

In sum, although this is a promising scale, again more testing is required.

THE SOCIAL NETWORK SCALE (SNS)

The Social Network Scale was adapted by Stokes (1983), based on Hirsch's (1980) work. This work was based on just 20 recent young widows and 14 older women recently re-entering college studies. Stokes (1983) based the Social Network Scale on four dimensions of network that he judged to be important: network size, number of people the respondent feels close to, number of relatives in the network and network density.

A supplement to the SNS is an eight-item scale which asks people to rate their total social networks, and their networks of friends, on four dimensions: general satisfaction with the network, amount of desired change in the network, satisfaction with assistance in daily activities, and satisfaction with emotional support. The eight ratings are summed to provide a measure of satisfaction.

Content

Hirsch's (1980) conceptual definition of support was based on interaction that affects coping ability: guidance, social reinforcement, aid, socializing, and emotional support. The social support dimension of the scale was operationalized by asking respondents to specify the amount of interaction with network members in five areas of supportive activity, and their degree of satisfaction with the interaction.

The social network dimension of the scale conceptualized social network as a natural support system, based on significant others. This is operationalized by asking people to list in a matrix 'the initials of up to 20 people who are significant in your life and with whom you have contact at least once a month'. People then put an X in those boxes of the matrix that connect people who are significant in each other's lives and who have contact with each other at least once a month. They also indicate which persons in their lists are relatives, and which persons they can 'confide in or turn to for help in an emergency'. This is probably more important in terms of providing effective, satisfying support than network size (Brown *et al.* 1975; Conner *et al.* 1979; Stokes 1983). This yields information on:

1 The size of the network, taking the definition of network as people who are significant in the respondent's life and with whom the respondent interacts regularly.
2 The number of people in the network whom the respondent feels close to – how many one can confide in or turn to for help in an emergency.
3 The number of relatives in the network.
4 Network density (i.e. the degree to which network members are themselves interconnected).

Scoring

Scoring consists of totalling the number of network members, relatives and confidant(e)s. Scoring could also identify the overlap between these categories (e.g. between relatives and confidant(e)s).

A larger number of variables can be computed and scored from the grid:

(i)　　Network size: number of people listed
(ii)　　Relatives: number of relatives listed
(iii)　　Friends: number of people listed who are not relatives
(iv)　　Confidant(e)s: number of people respondents said they could confide in or turn to for help in an emergency
(v)　　Relative confidant(e)s: number of confidant(e)s who are relatives
(vi)　　Friend confidant(e)s: number of confidant(e)s who are not relatives
(vii)　　Percentage relatives: proportion of the network who are relatives (relatives/size)
(viii)　　Percentage confidant(e)s: proportion of the network members who are confidant(e)s (confidant(e)s/size)
(ix)　　Percentage relative confidant(e)s: proportion of confidant(e)s who are relatives (relative confidant(e)s/confidant(e)s)
(x)　　Density: the proportion of the total possible number of relationships which actually exist among members of a social network, excluding the respondent
(xi)　　Relative density: density of the relatives in the social network list

(xii)　　Friend density: density of the friends in the social network list
(xiii)　　Relative–friend density: number of relationships between relatives and friends as a proportion of the total possible number of such relationships.

Validity and reliability

Although the scale has been judged to have face validity, it has not been tested fully for reliability and validity. It is also limited in scope; Stokes has himself supplemented the use of the SNS with other scales measuring the frequency of receipt of support (e.g. the Inventory of Socially Supportive Behaviours (Stokes 1985)). Stokes (1983), on the basis of administering the SNS to 82 students, submitted these dimensions to a principal components analysis and four factors emerged which accounted for over 80 per cent of the variance in the original matrix: size, with emphasis on the number of friends in the network; presence of confidant(e)s; dominance of relatives in the network; and density. Stokes (1983) also reported that the number of confidant(e)s in the social network was predictive of perceived-support satisfaction.

It is not clear what the basis is for limiting social network members to 20. Also, a flaw with calculating the percentage of relatives, confidant(e)s or friends in the network is that this does not take account of size in the presentation: for example, a network composed of 50 per cent relatives could be a network of just two members, one of whom is a relative, or it could be a network size of 20, 10 of whom are relatives. This does not appear to be a satisfactory basis for making comparisons between respondents.

Other main problems with this scale are that it does not have an index of geographical proximity, or frequency of contact, of network members, and it does not distinguish between types of relatives (e.g. sons and daughters are not distinguishable) or the nature of the contact (supportive, instrumental, etc). The value of the scale is the conciseness of the grid, which saves pages of questions, and it is easily supplemented with other structural items and questions on support (Bowling and Farquhar 1995). The structural network features measured by the grid have been reported to have little predictive value in longitudinal studies of psychological morbidity or life satisfaction (Bowling *et al.* 1992;

1993). Moreover, the author's own experience with the scale is that respondents tend to omit their spouses from the network scale – their significance and contact being taken for granted (Bowling *et al.* 1988).

The social support part of the scale has been little tested but was judged to have face reliability; the correlation between respondent and interviewer ratings of satisfaction and support was 0.53 and was judged to be reliable. Inter-item correlations, testing for reliability, ranged from 0.22 to 0.51 (Hirsch 1980).

The sensitivity of the scale is unknown and more evidence of its reliability and validity is required. Generally, it will require supplementation with other items.

THE FAMILY RELATIONSHIP INDEX (FRI)

The Family Relationship Index attempts to measure support from within the family. It has no clear conceptual basis. It was developed by Moos and Moos (1981) and Billings and Moos (1982). It was derived from a 90-item true–false response choice instrument, with 10 sub-scales, called the Family Environment Scale, also developed by the authors. The FRI is composed of the first three sub-scales of the Family Environment Scale. The scale was initially developed with a number of normal and distressed families in different ethnic groups. Over a thousand families were involved.

Content

The FRI sub-scale is composed of three sections (Moos and Moos 1981), taken from the Family Environment Scale. The three sections relate to 'cohesion', 'expressiveness' and 'conflict'. The 'cohesion' section assesses the amount of commitment, assistance and sustenance family members contribute to each other; 'expressiveness' assesses the extent to which family members are encouraged to express their feelings directly; and 'conflict' assesses the extent to which family members express aggression, conflict or anger. The three sections, with examples of item response choices, are:

Cohesion – the degree to which family members are helpful and supportive of each other (e.g. 'There is a feeling of togetherness in our family').

Expressiveness – the extent to which family members are encouraged to act openly and to express their feelings directly (e.g. 'We tell each other about our personal problems').

Conflict – the extent to which the open expression of anger and aggression and generally conflictual interactions are characteristic of the family (e.g. 'We fight a lot in our family').

Scoring

The standardized scores of each sub-scale are averaged to produce a composite score. A manual is available (Moos and Moos 1981; 1994).

Validity

Although there is no reference to the predictive validity of the full scale in the manual, the Family Relationship sub-scale was reported to have predictive validity by Billings and Moos (1982) in their longitudinal study of social support and functioning among 113 patients who had been treated for alcoholism. However, not all correlations achieved statistical significance: the significant correlations reported were those for depression and level and source of reported support (0.19 to 0.74); it is known that people who are depressed tend to perceive their level of support to be lower. There has been little further testing of the scale. The validity and sensitivity of the full scale and the sub-scale are largely unknown.

Reliability

The FRI was reported by Billings and Moos (1981) and Holahan and Moos (1981) to have a high internal consistency (0.89) and to be related to other measures of social support.

Test-retest reliabilities for the full Family Environment Scale's 10 sub-scales at intervals of 8 weeks, 4 months and 12 months ranged between 0.52 and 0.89 (Moos and Moos 1981; Caldwell 1985).

In sum, although tests for reliability appear to be good, the validity of the scale is more questionable, and again the need for further testing is evident. Caldwell (1985), in his critique of the scale, states that the full instrument is useful if used with 'caution', given, in particular, the lack of evidence regarding its psychometric properties.

THE SOCIAL SUPPORT APPRAISALS SCALE (SS-A)
AND THE SOCIAL SUPPORT BEHAVIOURS SCALE
(SS-B)

The Social Support Appraisals Scale was developed
by Vaux et al. (1986a; 1986b). The concept of social
support employed was based on Cobb's (1976)
definition of social support and was designed to tap
the extent to which individuals believe that they are
loved by, esteemed by and involved with family,
friends and others. One of the authors has reported
a relationship between type of network orientation
(e.g. positive or negative) and respondents indicating either secure or anxious attachment styles
(Wallace and Vaux 1993). One main advantage is
the brevity of the scale.

Content: SS-A

The SS-A is a 23-item scale consisting of a list of
statements about relationships with family and
friends. Eight items relate to family relationships,
seven to relationships with friends and eight to
'others' in a general way. Respondents have four
response choices: 'strongly agree', 'agree', 'disagree' or 'strongly disagree'. There is no middle
value. Examples are:

My friends respect me
My family cares for me very much
I am not important to others
I am well liked
I feel a strong bond with my friends
If I died tomorrow very few people would miss me
I feel close to members of my family
My friends and I have done a lot for one another

(Strongly agree/agree/disagree/strongly disagree)

Scoring

Three scores can be computed: SS-A, which is the
sum of all 23 items; SS-A (family) which is the sum
of the eight family items; and SS-A (friends) which
is the sum of the seven friends' items. The limitation of the scale is that it provides no information
about the numbers of people involved in providing
supportive behaviour, nor of who they are (e.g.
spouse, sister, son, etc.).

Validity

Convergent and divergent validity was tested in
relation to five samples of students and five community samples (the total number of respondents
was around a thousand). It was tested against other
measures of social support (the Perceived Social
Support Scale; the Family Relations Index; the
Social Support Questionnaire and two other less
well-known scales; and three single-item questions
on satisfaction with friends). The authors also employed two further scales developed by themselves. One of these was the Social Support
Resources Scale. This was designed to tap many
aspects of the individual's social support network.
Respondents were asked to list up to 10 people who
provided them with five types of support:
emotional support, practical assistance, financial
assistance, socializing and advice/guidance. Respondents provided satisfaction ratings for the five
types of assessed support. Respondents were asked
further questions about the characteristics of the
people identified and the nature of the relationship
(e.g. spouse, friend). Mean scores were computed
for each variable. The final scale tested against the
SS-A was the Social Support Behaviours Scale, also
developed by the authors (see below). The authors
also tested the SS-A against six personality and
depression inventories, including the Affect-
Balance Scale, and the UCLA Revised Loneliness
Scale (see later). The authors provided evidence of
convergent validity with a variety of the support
measures. The vast number of correlation coefficients presented by the authors is too extensive
to reproduce here. However, none of the correlations with other support or personality
measures were very strong (ranging from 0.03 to
−0.51, with one correlation coefficient achieving
−0.72). This is not surprising given the very different theoretical concepts underlying the different
scales.

Reliability

There is no published evidence of reliability.

In sum, the validity of the scale remains
questionable, and evidence of reliability is also
required.

Content: SS-B

The Social Support Behaviours Scale was developed by Vaux *et al.* (1987) to tap five modes of supportive behaviour. It is similar to Barrera *et al.*'s ISSB (see page 94) but does not suffer from the limitation of asking solely about actual rather than potential support (which may simply reflect number of problems). This lists 45 specific supportive behaviours, tapping the five modes of support listed in their Social Support Resources scale: emotional support, socializing, practical assistance, financial assistance and advice/guidance. Respondents indicate how likely their family and friends would be to engage in each of the behaviours in time of need. Examples are:

Would suggest doing something, just to take my mind off my problems.
Would visit with me, or invite me over.
Would give me a ride if I needed one.
Would have lunch or dinner with me.
Would loan me a car if I needed one.
Would go to a movie or concert with me.

(No one would do this/someone might do this/some family member/friends would probably do this/some family member/friend would certainly do this/most family members/friends would certainly do this.)

A problem with these types of scales is that they assume social values, i.e. that respondents all equally value 'a movie or concert', and that other people are in a financial position to, for example, 'loan a car'.

Scoring

The choice of five responses for each type of behaviour itemized ranges from 'no one would do this' to 'most family members/friends would certainly do this' (see above). Items are scored 0 (no one) to 5 (certainly) and summed.

Validity

The predictive validity of the SS-B has been demonstrated in relation to psychological distress and it correlates moderately with other support measures (including SS-A, see page 103) (Vaux and Wood 1985; Vaux *et al.* 1986a; 1986b).

In addition, five methods were used to test the validity of the SS-B as a measure of support: the classification of items by judges; an analogue (role-playing) simulation of samples deficient in each mode of support; tests against a related measure of supportive behaviour (ISSB); an examination of levels of each type of support provided for different problems and confirmatory factor analysis (Vaux *et al.* 1987).

The classification of items according to their content by judges (students) provided some evidence of the content validity of the SS-B. The percentage of items correctly classified by judges ranged from 13 to 100 per cent; in most cases it was over 60 per cent. The unique role-playing exercise with students showed deficits in available support corresponding to their enacted role, providing evidence of sub-scale sensitivity. However, the correlations were weak with the ISSB. This may be because the two measures are based on different concepts of social support – available and enacted respectively. The factor analysis demonstrated that the pattern of item convergence and divergence was highly consistent with predictions and confirmed that the SS-B taps the five modes of support conceptualized very well.

Reliability

Excellent internal consistency was obtained for the SS-B Scale items (the lowest alpha was 0.82).

In sum, the SS-A and SS-B scales are promising but have been little tested for reliability and validity.

INTERPERSONAL SUPPORT EVALUATION LIST (ISEL)

The Interpersonal Support Evaluation List was developed by Cohen *et al.* (1985), on the basis of the theoretical assumption that the buffering effect of social support is cognitively mediated. The testing of this theoretical assumption required an instrument which aimed to measure the perceived availability of support. The items were developed on theoretical grounds to cover the domain of social support that could facilitate coping with stress. It was designed to assess perceived availability of support in four distinct areas: material aid (tangible sub-scale); someone to talk to about one's problems (appraisal sub-scale); comparisons of self with others (self-esteem sub-scale); people to share activities with (belonging sub-scale).

Content

The ISEL consists of a list of 40 (48 in the version for students) statements about the perceived availability of potential social resources. The items are balanced: half the statements comprising the scale contain positive items about social relationships, and half contain negative items.

Respondents are asked to indicate whether each statement is 'probably true' or 'probably false'. Examples of the items are:

There is at least one person I know whose advice I really trust.
There are very few people I trust to help solve my problems.
If I decide on a Friday afternoon that I would like to go to a movie that evening, I could find someone to go with me.
Most people I know don't enjoy the same things that I do.
If I were sick and needed someone to drive me to the doctor, I would have trouble finding someone.
If I had to mail an important letter at the post office by 5.00 and couldn't make it, there is someone who could do it for me.
In general people don't have much confidence in me.
Most people I know think highly of me.

Scoring

The ISEL is scored by counting the number of responses indicating support. There is no information on the validity of this method.

Validity

Cohen *et al.* (1985) reviewed the evidence on the reliability and validity of the scale, most of which was previously unpublished. The scale was tested on over 500 students in Oregon; over 100 students at Carnegie-Mellon University; almost 100 students at Delaware University; over 100 students at Guelph University; and over 100 students at Arizona State University. Four studies were also carried out on the version of the scale for the general population using student samples at the University of California, Carnegie-Mellon University and the University of Oregon (total: over 200 students), and a general population sample participating in the Oregon Smoking Cessation Program (over 60 adults).

The ISEL student scale was found to correlate moderately with other social-support scales: 0.46 with Barrera's ISSB; 0.30 with the total score of the Moos Family Environment Scale; 0.39 with reported network size; 0.46 with number of close friends reported; and 0.42 with number of close relatives reported. The scale for the general population correlated 0.31 with a scale measuring the quality of relationships with partner/spouse. It was expected that the scale would be associated with self-esteem, as this is influenced by feedback from others; the correlation with the Rosenberg Self-Esteem Scale (see page 124) was 0.74. The scale was reported to be significantly associated with depression; social anxiety was controlled to eliminate the possibility that the social support concept was not merely a proxy measure of personality (e.g. social anxiety or social skills). Longitudinal analyses of the groups in the studies showed that the scale was able to predict changes in depressive symptomatology. The latter association indicated that the scale is not simply measuring symptomatology. There was a small but significant association with physical symptomatology and changes in these symptoms. The scale was reported to be a good predictor of smoking cessation and was associated with measures of stress in the direction suggestive of the buffering effects of social support. The authors argue that these data suggest the importance of appraisal support as a protector against the pathogenic effects of stressful life events.

Reliability

Adequate internal and test-retest reliability was reported by the authors. With the scale for students, the internal-reliability alpha coefficient was 0.86, ranging from 0.60 to 0.92 for each sub-scale. The alpha coefficients for the general population scale ranged from 0.88 to 0.90. The sub-scale correlations ranged from 0.62 to 0.82.

The student scales were tested for test-retest reliability at four-week intervals with reported correlations of 0.87 for the total scale, and correlations of 0.71–0.87 for the sub-scales. The general population scale was administered twice with a two-day interval; the reported correlation for the total scale was 0.87, and the sub-scale correlations ranged from 0.67 to 0.84. The six-week test-retest correlations from the smoking-cessation group sample were 0.70 overall, and 0.63–0.69 for the sub-scales. The six-month test-retest correlations for this group were 0.74 for the total scale and 0.49–0.68 for the sub-scales. In sum, although this is a scale which has only recently been developed, and further testing is required, it does cover a wide range of supportive relationships and results of testing for reliability and validity are fairly good. One limitation is that the scale does appear to be orientated towards a young or active population group and so may not be suitable for use with frail elderly people (e.g. questions on advice over job changes, sexual problems and availability of people to give lifts to the airport, etc.). The scale has been used successfully with psychiatric patients living in the community, and the scale was able to discriminate between those who lived independently and those who lived with their families or in group homes (Pomeroy *et al.* 1992).

THE NETWORK TYPOLOGY: THE NETWORK ASSESSMENT INSTRUMENT

Because support can be predictive of outcomes in a range of areas of life, knowing a person's network type can be valuable to health and social services professionals. Also, the aim of social service providers is to develop a care plan for people which supplements, rather than supplants, the care they receive from members of their social network. Therefore, several investigators have attempted to develop frameworks for the assessment of the network for care plans (Kaufman 1990). One of the more successful attempts has been that of Wenger (1989; 1992; 1994) in relation to elderly people.

As a result of qualitative, more anthropological, research with elderly people, Wenger was able to identify different types of social networks and she constructed a typology of support networks (Wenger 1989; Wenger and Shahtahmasebi 1991; Wenger 1994). The typology is based on the theory that the experience of ageing is mediated through, and determined by, the capacity of the support network to respond to change and the nature of the resulting change (Wenger and Shahtahmasebi 1991). The support network is defined by Wenger (1994) as those involved with the person in a sig-

nificant way: as a member of the household, in providing or receiving: companionship, emotional support, instrumental help, advice or personal care.

The Network Typology is developed from the data collected by a questionnaire – the Network Assessment Instrument – which identifies the availability and proximity of family and other 'support ties', the degree of involvement demonstrated by respondents with family, friends, neighbours and community, network density (how many network members know each other), and the size and content of the larger social network. The distinguishing factors between the different types of network are: the availability of local close kin, the level of involvement of family, friends and neighbours, and the level of interaction with the community and voluntary groups. The collection of this data enabled the investigators to identify five types of support networks in relation to the lifestyle and relationship of the elderly person to their network (Wenger 1994):

Local family-dependent support network: This network is mainly focused on close local family ties, with few peripheral friends and neighbours; it is often based on a shared household with, or close to, an adult child, usually a daughter. Nearly all support needs are met by the family. Community involvement is low. The network is small, and the person is more likely to be widowed, older and in poorer health than people with other types of network.

The most numerous members of this network are relatives living within one mile, followed by household members and neighbours.

Locally integrated support network: This includes close relationships with local family, friends and neighbours (the latter two often overlap). These are based on long-term residence and active community involvement in religious/voluntary organizations currently, or in the recent past. These networks are larger than others.

These networks have the highest numbers of neighbours, who are also likely to be friends.

Local self-contained support network: This is characterized by 'arms-length' relationships or infrequent contact with at least one relative living in the same or adjacant community (usually a sibling, niece or nephew). Childlessness is common. Reliance is mainly on neighbours, and the lifestyle is focused on the household. Community involvement, if any, is low key. Networks are smaller than average.

These networks also have more neighbours than other network categories, and the network is predominantly local.

Wider community-focused support network: This network is typified by active relationships with distant relatives, usually children, and high salience of friends and neighbours. The distinction between friends and neighbours is maintained and there is engagement in community or voluntary organizations. There has frequently been retirement migration, absence of local kin, and networks are larger than average. This network is commonly a middle-class or skilled working-class adaptation.

The most numerous membership of these networks are friends who live within a mile away, followed by relatives who live more than 50 miles away, and then equal numbers of friends at 1–5 miles away and neighbours. This membership reflects the absence of local kin.

Private restricted support network: This network is associated with absence of local kin, although a high proportion are married. Contacts with neighbours are minimal, there are few nearby friends and there is a low level of community contacts or involvements. There are two sub-types included in this network: independent married couples and dependent elderly people who have withdrawn or become isolated from local involvement. A low level of social contact often represents a lifelong adaptation. Networks are smaller than average.

The most numerous members of this type of network are relatives who live more than 50 miles away, followed by members of the household or relatives who live 15–50 miles away, reflecting the absence of local kin.

Wenger (1994) reported that most networks can be categorized into one of these types, and that local self-contained and private restricted networks are less robust than other network types, and more vulnerable in the face of ill health or a crisis. The different lifestyles and social characteristics of people represented by the different network types have been described by Wenger (1994).

Content

The Network Assessment Instrument was published in full by Wenger (1994), but it can only be used in conjunction with the appropriate training package developed by Wenger. This is because the identification of the network is the planning aid and is no substitute for professional training on appropriate interventions. A video-based training and resource pack for practitioners and service providers is available (Wenger 1995), and the author has details of training courses. The use of the typology has been piloted with a number of social services teams, and a guide has been published (Wenger 1994).

The Instrument contains eight questions, each with one of three types of 1–3 (coded A,B,C) or 1–6 (coded A–F) point response categories, relating to distance of residence of network member or frequency of interaction/activity (e.g. No relatives (A) to (lives) 50+ miles (F); Never/no friends (A) to (chat/do something) Less often (F); Yes, regularly (A) to No (C)). The questionnaire also contains the information for the interviewer to be able to code (A–F) immediately the type of network from each response code.

Examples of the questions are:

How far away, in distance, does your nearest child or other relative live? (Do not include spouse.)

If you have any friends in this community/neighbourhood, how often do you have a chat or do something with one of your friends?

Do you attend meetings of any community/neighbourhood or social groups, such as old people's clubs, lectures or anything like that?

Scoring

Each item is analysed independently, and the network typology is constructed on the computer, using the response codes and the network type coded by interviewers on the questionnaires.

Validity and reliability

While much descriptive data has been published based on the Network Typology and the Network Assessment Instrument, little information on its reliability and validity has been published to date. It has been piloted with social services practitioners, and Wenger (1994) reported that most of her sample members were able to be classified by the typology. Network type was associated, as predicted, with levels of dependency, reliance on services, informal help, emotional support and social interaction, and survival of respondents over an eight-year follow-up period (Wenger and Shahtahmasebi 1991). These associations suggest that the instrument has construct and predictive validity. Despite changes over time in the network sizes of respondents, the overall frequency distribution of the network type of the sample remained constant (Wenger and Shahtahmasebi 1991), suggesting that the instrument is robust. Conventional data on the psychometric properties (validity and reliability correlations, factor analyses) of the instrument has not yet been published. It has been presented here in view of its potential and increasing use among service providers.

LONELINESS

A further concept requires introduction under the heading of social networks and support: that of loneliness. Loneliness can be defined as an unwelcome feeling of lack or loss of companionship. Weiss (1973) distinguished between situational and personality theories of loneliness. The former emphasize environmental factors as causes of loneliness – e.g. death of a spouse, moving to a new city. Evidence relating to the size and quality of social networks and associations with loneliness is unclear. Apart from a number of psychological studies which are of questionable generalizability as they tend to use student volunteers as subjects, the quality of data on loneliness in relation to the quality of social networks are poor. Most surveys have either been based on small sample sizes or have used crude measures of social network or loneliness (Jones et al. 1985; Bowling et al. 1989).

Although a large number of scales for the assessment of loneliness have been devised, few have been published. The existing scales have been reviewed by Russell (1982). The most widely used scale is the UCLA Loneliness Scale, and this is reviewed below.

THE REVISED UNIVERSITY OF CALIFORNIA AT LOS ANGELES (UCLA) LONELINESS SCALE

The UCLA Loneliness Scale is the most well-known measure of loneliness. It was developed, and later revised, by Russell et al. (1978; 1980). The authors aimed to identify common themes that characterized the experience of loneliness for a broad spectrum of individuals. The UCLA Loneliness Scale was intended to be global.

The scale began with 25 items taken from another measure. The response items, also borrowed, asked individuals to rate how frequently they felt the way described, from 'never' to 'often' on a four-point scale. The scale was tested on clinic volunteers and students. The final loneliness scale consisted of 20 items; selected items all had item-total correlations above 0.50.

One problem with the original version of the scale was that all the items on the measure were worded in the same (lonely) direction. The implication is that tendencies to respond in a certain way could systematically influence loneliness scores. A second potential problem was social-desirability bias, given the possible stigma associated with admissions of loneliness. Thus Russell et al. (1980) revised the scale to take account of these problems, and a set of positively worded loneliness items were included (e.g. 'There are people I feel close to' and 'I have a lot in common with the people around me'). The revised version was tested on 162 students. Testing involved using the original scale and 19 new items, written by the authors, and anxiety and depression measures. The 10 positively and 10 negatively worded items with the highest correlations with a set of items about whether they were lonely were included in the scale. All of the item-criterion correlations were above 0.40.

Content

The scale consists of 20 statements, half of which are descriptive of feelings of loneliness and half descriptive of non-loneliness or satisfaction with relationships. Examples of items are:

I lack companionship.

It is difficult for me to make friends.

There is no one I can turn to.

I feel part of a group of friends.

There are people I feel close to.

Respondents indicate how often each statement applies to them. There are four choices for replies: never (1), rarely (2), sometimes (3) and often (4).

Scoring

The total score of the scale is the sum of all 20 items. Some need to be reversed before scoring (i.e. 1 = 4, 2 = 3, 3 = 2, 4 = 1); these are asterisked on the scale.

Validity

Validity was initially assessed by correlations of the scale with a single-item self-rating of loneliness measure (0.79); a comparison of the scores of two samples of participants (the mean of the clinic sample was 60.1, significantly different from the student group's mean of 39.1); and the loneliness scores were also strongly associated with depression, anxiety, dissatisfaction, unhappiness and shyness. High correlations with other measures of loneliness have been reported (ranging from 0.72 and 0.74). These have been reviewed by Russell (1982). The main limitation of this research is that it has been largely confined to samples of students, raising questions about the validity of the scale in assessing loneliness for other populations. Although there is a need for further testing of the scale on other population groups, initial results do appear encouraging.

Early evidence of the discriminative and predictive validity of the revised scale was provided by studies reporting strong relationships between the scale and measures of depression, and earlier research showed strong relationships between loneliness items and anxiety and self-esteem (Russell 1982).

The revised version of the scale was tested for validity on 162 students, and also using the Beck Depression Inventory. Correlations of 0.32 were obtained with an anxiety index and of 0.62 with the Beck Depression Inventory. The discriminant validity was also assessed by a study of 237 students, with the aim of assessing whether it was measuring a different dimension of well-being to the depression scales. Multivariate analysis was used for this purpose and it was reported that a loneliness index explained an additional 18 per cent of the variance in loneliness scores beyond that accounted for by the mood and personality measures. Concurrent validity was also assessed, and significant associations were reported between solitary activities, having fewer friends and loneliness scores (Russell 1982).

However, the validity of loneliness scales is difficult to assess. In terms of content and face validity, the most face-valid loneliness measures are questions simply asking 'are you lonely?' This then faces the problem of social desirability bias that could limit validity. Problems with the assessment of criterion validity also exist. Loneliness is not synonymous with isolation. There is an absence of external validity criteria for loneliness. Even ratings by others known to the person are not highly reliable.

The scale reportedly has discriminatory ability and has been used in a number of studies of emotional well-being. Stokes (1985) analysed social-network structure and personality factors in relation to loneliness, using the earlier version of the UCLA, in a sample of 97 male and 82 female students. He reported network density to be the most strongly related to loneliness: people with interconnected networks tend to be less lonely. This may be because they feel more sense of community, of belonging to a group. Extraversion and introversion were also related to loneliness.

Mellor and Edelmann (1988) used the revised UCLA loneliness scale in a study of loneliness in 36 people aged over 65. They found that loneliness was associated with having fewer confidant(e)s and with lack of mobility. Riggio et al. (1993) also used the scale and reported that level of social skills predicted perceptions of loneliness.

Factor analyses of the scale have not produced consistent results, with factor structures suggesting either uni- or multi-dimensional (2 to 3) factor structures (Cuffel and Akamatsu 1989; Mahon and Yarcheski 1990; McWhirter 1990).

Reliability

Studies of the original version (which had a different scoring method of 0 to 3) by Russell et al. (1978)

and Perlman and Peplau (1981) have reported good reliability for the scale (alpha: 0.94) and evidence of validity, similarly with the revised version (Russell *et al.* 1980; Russell 1982).

The revised scale has a high internal consistency with a coefficient alpha of 0.96, and a second study of 237 students further confirmed the internal consistency of the scale (0.94) and correlations with other relevant items. As for test–retest reliability,

Jones (cited in Russell *et al.* 1978) found a correlation of 0.73 over a two-month period in a student sample.

In sum, this scale is the most extensively tested of all the loneliness scales available and results so far are encouraging. The main limitation of testing to date has been its reliance on student subjects who may not be representative of the general population.

7

MEASURES OF
LIFE SATISFACTION
AND MORALE

The first population survey of emotional well-being (i.e. life satisfaction and morale) was conducted in 1957 by Gurin *et al.* (1960) in the USA. Respondents were asked: 'Taking all things together, how would you say things are these days – would you say you're very happy, pretty happy or not too happy these days?' Those in the 'not too happy' group were more likely to have psychiatric problems, to be widowed or divorced, to have less education and lower income levels, and to be black. The concept and measurement of well-being, in relation to happiness, life satisfaction and morale, are now receiving increasing attention and more sophisticated measurement scales have been developed, particularly in gerontology. More sophisticated techniques of psychometric testing have also yielded support for the feasibility and validity of measuring well-being using a single instrument (Andrews and Crandall 1976). Indicators of these concepts are useful in assessing the mental health or well-being of people. Life satisfaction, for example, has been related to mental health (Gurin *et al.* 1960; Bradburn 1969).

Measures of well-being are subjective (Campbell 1976). A major methodological problem has been the lack of consistency in the usage of the terms 'happiness', 'life satisfaction' and 'morale' (Stones and Kozma 1980; Stull 1987). While the concepts and measures are related, it has been argued that 'life satisfaction' and 'morale' have a more cognitive component to them, while happiness has a more affective or emotional component (Andrews

and McKennel 1980). The cognitive component implies evaluation, while affect refers to the positive/negative feeling. These concepts relating to well-being are not identical, although many researchers continue to treat these concepts as interchangeable (George and Bearon 1980). Distinguishing between cognitive and affective components of subjective well-being is particularly useful when interpreting data. For example, elderly people often report lower levels of happiness but higher levels of life satisfaction than younger people (Campbell *et al.* 1976; Campbell 1981). This suggests, then, that while cognitive evaluations of life as a whole increase with age, positive affect may decline. Perhaps people become more jaded in their emotions with age, but increase their perceptions of their level of achievement, or adjust their aspirations (Andrews and Robinson 1991). While the differences could simply be due to birth cohort effects (Campbell 1981; Inglehart and Rabier 1986), the example illustrates the value of the different concepts.

HAPPINESS

This has been defined as transitory moods of 'gaiety and elation' that reflect the affect that people feel toward their current state of affairs (Campbell *et al.* 1976). It has also been defined as the extent to which positive feelings outweigh negative feelings (Bradburn 1969). The latter definition often includes the time dimension of 'the past few weeks'. In relation to the construction of the Oxford Happiness Inventory, Argyle *et al.* (1989) defined happiness more comprehensively as the frequency of joy, the average level of satisfaction and the absence of negative feelings. Happiness implies an affective mood or state.

LIFE SATISFACTION

This generally refers to some overall assessment of one's life or a comparison reflecting some perceived discrepancy between one's aspiration and achievement (Campbell *et al.* 1976). Questions regarding overall assessment as well as satisfaction with certain domains are asked. Some explicit or implicit comparison group is usually involved ('compared to others'). In this regard, satisfaction suggests a cognitive process.

MORALE

This is the most poorly defined and measured concept of the three. Kutner *et al.* (1956) defined morale as 'a continuum of responses to life and living problems that reflect the presence or absence of satisfaction, optimism, and expanding life perspectives'. Lawton (1972; 1975) has defined morale as a basic sense of satisfaction with oneself, a feeling that there is a place in the environment for oneself, and an acceptance of what cannot be changed. George (1979) and Stones and Kozma (1980) defined morale as 'courage, discipline, confidence, enthusiasm'.

Lohmann (1977) has shown that many of the major scales of well-being in use are correlated quite substantially. This suggests that all measures are directed towards tapping a common underlying construct. Many of the questions in the scales are similar, accounting for their overlap and inter-correlations. This is particularly true for the Philadelphia Geriatric Center Morale Scale and Neugarten's Life Satisfaction Index A (both scales are reviewed in this chapter). McKennell (1978) has argued that happiness and life-satisfaction measures differentially tap cognitive and affective components, and that correlations between these measures result from loadings on underlying factors that the measures have in common.

The main difficulty for researchers in this area is that of conceptualization – whether or not the dimensions of well-being employed reflect attitudes, personality or mood states and whether or not well-being really is represented by some combination of these.

Two other issues are of concern. Smith (1979) has stated that there appears to be seasonal variation in the global measure of happiness, with happiness highest in the spring, declining in the summer and autumn and dropping to its lowest point in winter. The other is the possibility of positivity bias among some sample members: some people may be reluctant to admit the extent of any unhappiness they may feel on the basis of the assumption that it is socially desirable to be 'happy'.

A further concept which requires inclusion here is self-esteem. Self-esteem is conceptualized slightly differently by psychologists and sociologists. Psychologists refer to self-esteem in relation to a sense of self-worth – a belief that one is a person of value, accepting personal strengths and weaknesses (Rosenberg 1965; Coopersmith 1967; Wells and Marwell 1976). Self-esteem is therefore a self-evaluation. Related concepts include self-regard, self-acceptance, self-concept and self-image. These are all based upon the individual's assessment and evaluation of him/herself (Crandall 1973; Wells and Marwell 1976). High self-esteem is viewed as a component of mental health. Self-concept is the cognitive component of the self and consists of individuals' perceptions of themselves (i.e. what I am really like?). In sociology, the critical role of social interaction and the significance of others in developing self-esteem and its maintenance is emphasized (Wylie 1974). In relation to health and illness, Wilson Barnett (1981) has reviewed the literature on recovery from disease, principally heart surgery, and reports that negative images of the self are associated with delayed or poor recovery.

Available evidence suggests that positive self-esteem is an important component of general assessment of life (Andrews and Withey 1976). Self-esteem may become increasingly salient with the transition from middle to old age (Schwartz 1975). Most self-esteem theorists suggest, with some evidence, that self-esteem is developed and maintained through a successful process of personal interaction and negotiation with the environment

(Rosenberg 1965; Wells and Marwell 1976). As successful negotiations are less likely in later life, self-esteem among older people is less likely to be positive. Schwartz (1975) has thus defined self-esteem as the essential component of quality of life for the aged. If age changes are to be expected, the impact of an intervention could become confounded with developmental changes over time. Evidence is limited and there is no reason why a sensitive measure to assess the impact of interventions should not be attempted. As self-esteem is a dimension of life satisfaction, morale and happiness, scales of self-esteem are reviewed at the end of this chapter. In addition, due to the focus on positive aspects of health and quality of life, some investigators are attempting to develop measures of satisfaction with illness (Hyland and Kenyon 1992) and measures of life satisfaction as a complement to symptom-orientated measures (Frisch *et al.* 1992). These indicators are not included here, but are a welcome development in a field dominated by negative measures of health and health-related quality of life.

GLOBAL MEASURES

Life satisfaction, morale and happiness are all global concepts, referring to life as a whole rather than to specific aspects of it. Global measures are of relevance in assessing well-being, although they may be of limited utility in evaluative research (George and Bearon 1980). Carp (1977) cautions against drawing policy relevant inferences from data which do not reveal why and with what people are satisfied. Specific measures are an alternative (e.g. housing satisfaction in evaluating effect of relocation) (Andrews and Withey 1976; Campbell *et al.* 1976). Global and item-specific measures are appropriate for different research questions.

One of the advantages of using a few global items rather than global or specific scales is brevity: one or two questions rather than a whole battery. However, a positivity bias, for example, respondents' desire to be socially desirable, can be obtained with short items. Also short items lack sensitivity and therefore are of limited predictive value in longitudinal studies. The effect of question order with such items has been relatively unexplored, although the National Opinion Research Centre found that placing a question about marital happiness immediately before a global question of happiness resulted in a more positive response on global happiness (Smith 1979).

A review of the literature indicates that well-being has been measured by three major scales as well as short global items: Life Satisfaction A (Neugarten *et al.* 1961); Bradburn Affect-Balance Scales (Bradburn and Caplovitz 1965; Bradburn 1969); Philadelphia Geriatric Center Morale Scale (Lawton 1975); and global items of happiness and life satisfaction (Robinson and Shaver 1973; Campbell *et al.* 1976; Smith 1979). Other popular scales are the Delighted–Terrible Faces Scale (Andrews and Withey 1976) and the Psychological Well-Being Schedule (Dupuy 1978). These scales produce global scores of well-being (life satisfaction or morale), except the Delighted–Terrible Faces Scale which contains current life specific items that should be analysed separately. These will be reviewed in the following sections. Popular single-item measures, asking respondents to assess their lives as a whole, are the Ladder Scale (Cantril 1967) and items from the Delighted–Terrible Faces scale (Andrews and Withey 1976). Respondents mark a rung on a ladder or select a face with an expression representing how they feel. For examples of single items, readers are referred to Robinson and Shaver (1973) and Andrews and Robinson (1991). Sauer and Warland (1982) and Andrews and Robinson (1991) have reviewed a wider range of measures of life satisfaction, well-being and happiness.

THE LIFE SATISFACTION INDEX A (LSIA) AND INDEX B (LSIB)

The Life Satisfaction Indexes A and B were developed by Neugarten *et al.* (1961) in order to produce a relatively short self-report measure of life satisfaction based on respondents' feelings. The aim of these scales is to measure general feelings of well-being in order to identify 'successful' ageing. Several versions of the LSI exist. All are derived from the five dimensions of past and present life from a life-satisfaction rating obtained by a clinical interview: zest and apathy, resolution and fortitude, congruence between desired and achieved goals, positive self-concept and mood tone.

LSIA and LSIB were first developed in 1956 on the basis of four rounds of interviews on the subject of life satisfaction, with people aged 50–70, based on a stratified probability sample of middle- and working-class people residing in Kansas City. A second sample was interviewed aged 70–90 two years later, based on a quota sample (overall total 177).

All versions of the index are easily administered and rest on a substantial amount of empirical support. The problem with the scale is its global nature which poses uncertainty about what is being measured. Scale A has been further criticized by Liang (1984) for failing to measure transitory effects.

Content

Scales A and B differ only slightly in content but greatly in form. Life Satisfaction Index A has a checklist of 20 items, statements with which the respondent either agrees or disagrees. Life Satisfaction Index B has 12 open-ended questions that are given a score based upon the content of the answers. The two instruments can be used together or separately (Neugarten *et al.* 1961). Index A has been used more frequently than B, probably due to ease of administration and quantification of structured items.

The original LSIA consists of 20 items (12 positive and 8 negative). A second version, adapted by Wood *et al.* (1969) contains 13 of the original 20 items. Another version uses 18 items. An advantage of Scales A and B, and the shorter versions of A, is that they have positive and negative items.

A wide variety of content areas are tapped by each of these scales, for example, ranging from happiness to satisfaction with level of activity. Some items reflect back over past lives or involve comparing the present with the past, as well as assessment of the present.

Respondents agree or disagree with the items on Scale A; each positive response receives a score of 1. Examples of Scale A items are:

Positive items
I have had more luck in my life than most people.
These are the best years of my life.
The things I do today are as interesting to me as they ever were.

Negative items
This is the dreariest time of my life.

Most of the things I do are boring and monotonous.
Compared to other people I get down in the dumps too often.

Examples of the open-ended items on B are:

Positive
What are the best things about being the age you are now?
(1 = positive answer; 0 = nothing good about it.)

What is the most important thing in your life at the moment?
(2 = anything outside of self, or pleasant interpretation of future; 1 = hanging on; keeping health or job; 0 = getting out of present difficulty, or nothing now, or reference to past.)

Negative
Do you wish you could see more of your close friends than you do, or would you like more time to yourself?
(2 = OK as it is; 0 = wish could see more of friends; 0 = wish more time to self.)

How much unhappiness would you say you find in your life today?
2 = almost none; 1 = some; 0 = a great deal.)

Scoring

Scores are summed over all the items; thus ratings of each dimension are combined. The criticism of this is that the separate dimensions are confounded.

There are two scoring methods for the LSI. In the original method, a two-point agree/disagree response choice rated dissatisfaction as 0 and satisfaction as 1. Analysis of 'undecided' responses then led to the use of a three-point scale, rating satisfaction as 2, uncertain as 1, and dissatisfaction as 0 (Wood *et al.* 1969).

The mean LSI score varies slightly between studies, reflecting different population bases. In the original sample the mean score was 12.4, with a standard deviation of 4.4. Others have reported mean scores ranging between 11.6 (a sample of elderly residents in rural Kansas) to 14.1 (a sample of British males in manual and professional occupations) (see review by George and Bearon 1980). For the 13-item three-point response version, Harris (1975) reported mean scores of 26.7 for adults aged under 64 and 24.4 for those aged 65+.

Several studies using factor analysis and multiple

regression models have confirmed the multi-dimensional nature of the scale and have questioned the original conceptual formulation (Hoyt and Creech 1983). In view of its multi-dimensionality the use of a single score blurs the relationships between the items and it should instead be used as a series of sub-scales. Comparisons require caution, given the different scoring systems used.

Validity

Using a sample of 177 people aged 50 and over, Neugarten et al. (1961) reported a correlation of 0.55 between LSIA and the original clinical life satisfaction rating instrument. As the former was derived from the latter, this is not a sound test of the validity of the scale. The correlation of scores on LSIA with judges' ratings was 0.52, and the correlation of LSIB with judges' ratings was 0.59. Details of these and of the item analysis employed to derive the index items have been described by Neugarten et al. (1961).

Criterion validity was established by assessments by a clinical psychologist, although these were 18–22 months after the fourth interview on 80 remaining sample members and were of questionable value. The correlation between judges' and clinical ratings was 0.64 which was regarded as satisfactory in view of these problems.

Correlations between the LSIA and the Affect-Balance Scale and the Philadelphia Geriatric Center Morale Scale have been reported as 0.66 and 0.76 respectively (Bild and Havighurst 1976; Lohmann 1977).

Bowling and Browne (1991), in an interview study of 662 people aged 85 and over living at home in London, reported that the correlation between Neugarten's Life Satisfaction Scale A and the Delighted–Terrible Faces Scale was −0.65, and with the General Health Questionnaire (which assesses mainly anxiety and depression) was −0.47 (i.e. greater life satisfaction was associated with low anxiety and depression). A similar study by the authors (unpublished) of almost 300 people aged 65 and over living at home in Essex, and of almost 400 people aged 65 to 85 living at home in London reported correlations between Neugarten's Scale and the Delighted–Terrible Faces Scale and the General Health Questionnaire of −0.24 and −0.47 (Essex) and −0.57 and −0.41 (London)

respectively. Although the correlations with the General Health Questionnaire were very similar for the three studies (−0.41 to −0.47), it is uncertain why the correlations with the Faces Scale vary between studies (−0.24 to −0.65), or should be weaker with the younger elderly groups. High correlations between these scales would not be expected as they tap different dimensions of well-being, although overlap would be (as is demonstrated). Scale A was reported in follow-up studies to be significantly associated with poor functioning and health, supporting the scale's construct (convergent) validity, and was also shown to be stable over a two and a half year period (Bowling et al. 1993).

Other inconsistencies using the scale have been reported. For example, although the original authors reported that LSIA did not correlate with demographic factors, other studies have indicated that it does. In particular, positive correlations with socio-economic status have been reported by a number of authors (see review by McDowell and Newell 1987).

Reliability

Internal consistency coefficients in various studies range from 0.70 to 0.76 (Dobson et al. 1979) to around 0.79 (Wood et al. 1969; Stock and Okun 1982), depending upon the version used.

Reliability ratings were made by seven pairs of judges who rated descriptions of 177 cases. The coefficient of correlation between the pairs of ratings was 0.79. For the 177 cases life-satisfaction scores for Scale A ranged from 8 to 25, with a mean of 17.8, and a standard deviation of 4.6. There was no significant difference with sex (Neugarten et al. 1961).

This author (Bowling) has found problems with the scale which affect reliability. The final item 'In spite of what people say, the life of the average person is getting worse not better' is often received with puzzlement about a stereotyped 'average person'. This item assumes agreement over an 'average' person. Moreover, respondents' agreement with this item does not inform us whether their own lives are getting 'worse not better'. Also, it makes the scale too diverse in the number of different dimensions of life satisfaction covered. Two other items also require refinement: 'I feel my age but it does not bother me' – this is difficult for respondents to reply to if they feel their age, but it does bother them; and 'Compared to other people my age, I look smart when I am dressed to go out'– this is difficult to reply to in the case of respondents who are housebound or who live in institutions and do not go out. In the author's study of people aged 85 and over in London and aged 65 and over in Essex and London, the alpha reliability coefficients for the scale ranged from alpha 0.73 to 0.80; and the split-half reliability coefficients ranged from 0.65 to 0.74.

THE LIFE SATISFACTION INDEX Z 13-ITEM VERSION (LSIZ)

Validity, reliability and sensitivity

Wood et al. (1969) have derived a 13-item version of Scale A, known as LSIZ, which is probably the most popular, and applications are numerous.

Moderate correlations were obtained between the LSIZ and a scale of social engagement (0.49) and between the LSIZ and the Symptoms of Anxiety and Depression Scale (0.49), the latter suggesting that the scales assess some common aspect of well-being (Wood et al. 1969). The 13-item LSIZ has been extensively used in the USA. It was used by Usui et al. (1985) in a community survey of people aged 60+ in Jefferson County, Kentucky. The authors reported a correlation of –0.22 between number of physical health problems and life satisfaction, and similar correlations with various social activities, income level and life satisfaction; these were confirmed by multiple regression analysis. In contrast to Morgan et al. (1987), in a study of over 1500 people aged 65+ in Nottinghamshire in the UK, they reported that older respondents had higher life-satisfaction scores. Morgan et al. reported that the average score was 17 for people aged 65–74 and 16.4 for people aged 75+; life satisfaction was significantly lower for those aged 75+.

The LSIZ was used by Kozma and Stones (1987), along with other measures of well-being, in a study of 150 people in acute psychiatric or community psychiatric wards, aged between 50 and 82, in Newfoundland. Correlations between the LSIZ and the Philadelphia Geriatric Center Morale Scale (PGCMS) were reported to be high (0.74). The

authors reported that the LSIZ was able to correctly identify 72 per cent of the community-hospital or acute-ward samples, and PGCMS correctly identified 74 per cent. A scale of social desirability was also used, and the authors reported that controlling for social desirability did not enhance the construct validity of the well-being scales.

Wood et al. (1969) reported that the refined 13-item version of the Index shows a split-half reliability of 0.79. Edwards and Klemmack (1973) reported an internal consistency reliability coefficient of 0.90.

It has been found to be sensitive to change in a study of participation in community programmes (Wylie 1970). As it was developed for use with older people, it is appropriate for use with that population. The scoring for this version of the scale ranges from 0 to 26; item scores are satisfaction: 2; dissatisfaction: 1; don't know: 1.

Although the scales are satisfactory in terms of standard tests of reliability and validity, their global and multi-dimensional nature does pose problems. The issue is what is being predicted? However, these scales are the most commonly used to measure well-being in gerontological research (Larson 1978; Stull 1987).

THE AFFECT-BALANCE SCALE (ABS)

Bradburn (1969) described the Affect-Balance Scale as an indicator of happiness or general psychological well-being. It is not concerned with detecting psychiatric or psychological disorders. Bradburn and Caplovitz (1965) hypothesized that subjective well-being could be indicated by a person's position on two independent dimensions: positive and negative affect. Well-being is expressed as the balance between these two. Thus positive factors can compensate for negative feelings. The scale was developed by Bradburn and Caplovitz (1965) on the basis of a sample of 2,006 adults in Illinois, and by Bradburn (1969), in a revision, on 2,787 adults of mixed socio-economic and ethnic groups based on five probability random samples in Detroit, Chicago, Washington and 10 other large US cities. Respondents were reinterviewed 12 weeks apart for the latter study.

This scale has been subjected to a great deal of analysis (Knapp 1976). Originally 12 items, it is now composed of 10 items, 5 referring to 'positive affect', and 5 referring to 'negative affect'. The two sub-scales are independent, although both correlate with happiness (Bradburn 1969). Balance refers to the balance between positive and negative effect reflected by an individual's score on the scale (the balance is the result of an additive process). However, this scale is also confounded by items referring to activation (e.g. the item 'excited' or 'interested' in something). Additionally some of the items also appear to measure accomplishments. The scale is self-administered.

Content

The wording of the questions appears to have varied between studies. Bradburn specified that the time referent should be 'the past few weeks' (originally 'the past week'). Others have used 'the past few months' or even no time referent (see review by McDowell and Newell 1987).

An advantage of using the scale is that some items refer to positive psychological states, reflecting the recent interest in positive health. Examples of scale items are:

Positive items include:

Things going your way.
Excited, interested in something.
Pleased about having accomplished something.

Negative items include:

Upset because someone criticized you.
Very lonely, remote from people.
Bored.

Scoring

Replies are dichotomous (yes/no). Differential weights were tested but did not significantly alter the results and so are not used.

Each yes response to the 10 items in the scale is assigned a value of 1. The five items that reflect positive affect are summed separately to the five that reflect negative affect. The difference between the scores on positive and negative affect is computed and is taken as the final score, indicating the level of psychological well-being. Bradburn (1969) suggested adding a constant (+5) to remove the negative summary scale scores. Results from studies using this scale, and those using the General Well-Being Schedule, suggest that about 10 per cent of the general population may experience a strong sense of positive well-being.

Validity

Correlations with other measures (testing for validity) are around 0.66; this was achieved with an 18-item version of Neugarten's LSIA (Bild and Havighurst 1976). A review of the scale by George and Bearon (1980) reports inter-scale correlations with other morale scales and an 18-item version of the LSIA of between 0.61 and 0.64.

Cherlin and Reeder (1975) have criticized the scale, suggesting that the two-dimensional structure is not correct. They suggested that there is a third component (activation level) included (e.g. 'particularly excited or interested in something'). Borgatta and Montgomery (1987) have also argued that some items also seem to be measuring instrumental aspects (e.g. accomplishments).

It has been reported to be sensitive to change (Bradburn 1969). The scale was used by Berkanovic et al. (1988) in an interview study of distress and help-seeking among 950 respondents in Los Angeles. The authors found no relationship between distress and use of medical care, although they reported that the distressed reported more illnesses. Significant differences on scale scores by sex of respondents have been reported (Kushman and Lane 1980). Possibly the most well-known application of the scale was by Berkman (1971) in the Alameda County survey, although she only used eight of the items. She reported a correlation of 0.48 with a 20-item index of neurotic traits.

Reliability

Internal consistency (inter-item) correlations range from 0.47 to 0.73 for the positive scale and from 0.48 to 0.73 for the negative scale (Cherlin and Reeder 1975; Warr 1978). Inter-scale correlations were modest at 0.24 to 0.26 (Warr 1978). These correlations are considerably higher than the early correlations reported by Bradburn (1969).

Bradburn (1969) tested the scale for reliability and reported a test-retest correlation of 0.76 three days apart; for nine items associations exceeded 0.90 and for the item 'excited or interested' the test-retest correlation was 0.86.

In sum, it has acceptable levels of validity and reliability and has been found to be applicable for use with older people, although it was not developed specifically as a measure for them. It is easily administered. George and Bearon (1980) rate it as the best measure of affect (frequency of experienced feelings and kinds of reported feelings).

THE PHILADELPHIA GERIATRIC CENTER MORALE SCALE (PGCMS)

This scale and its revised version were developed on the basis of the assumption that well-being is multi-dimensional (Lawton 1972; 1975). Lawton viewed morale in terms of general well-being. The scale also takes into account two other properties: applicability to older, institutionalized populations, and optimal scale length allowing reliability without respondent fatigue (Knapp 1976). A preliminary version of the scale with 41 items was tested on 300 people, with an average age of 78. The scale originally contained 22 items, but with subsequent analyses was revised and now contains 17 (Lawton 1975; Morris and Sherwood 1975). It was developed for use with older people and is therefore appropriate for these populations. It is easily administered and can be self- or interviewer-administered.

Content

The reduced items obtain three major dimensions: agitation (six items), attitude towards own ageing (five items) and lonely dissatisfaction (six items). Examples of scale items are:

How often do you feel lonely?
I see enough of my friends and relatives.
I am as happy now as when I was younger.
Life is hard for me much of the time.

Scoring

One point is scored for each response indicating high morale. Most items are dichotomously coded. The scale can be treated as three sub-scales or as an overall scale. Liang and Bollen (1983) have reviewed the various scoring methods.

The range of scores is from 0 (low) to 17 (high), with higher scores indicating greater morale. The

scale, descriptive statistics and details of the scoring are available from Lawton.

Validity

Correlations testing for validity with Neugarten's scales (reported earlier) vary with Neugarten's various indexes from 0.57 to 0.79 (Lawton 1972; Lohmann 1977).

The scale has been criticized by Borgatta and Montgomery (1987) because it includes measures of happiness and life satisfaction; this is alleged to be questionable in a scale purporting to measure 'morale'. This confusion, they argue, is made even more problematic by the use of different time referents (e.g. 'I am as happy now as when I was younger' and 'How satisfied are you with your life today?'). To be fair to the developers of the scale, they did claim to define the concept of morale in terms of general well-being.

There is limited evidence of sensitivity to change (reports exist by Kalson (1976) and Morris (1975)). It has been reported that the scale is able to discriminate between social groups.

The PGCMS has had numerous applications, one of which, using the 17-item version, was by Ward et al. (1984). They excluded two items that they were already measuring in a series of questions about social integration: 'How often do you feel lonely?' and 'I see enough of my friends and relatives'. They used the scale with a sample of people, average age 70.6, living in Albany-Schenectady-Troy, New York, and reported that morale was associated with satisfaction with frequency of contact with others.

It was also used by Noelker and Harel (1978) in their survey of 14 nursing-home residents in the USA. The average age of respondents was 81. The authors reported that twice as many residents who desired to live in the homes had high morale scores (mean: 12.98; standard deviation 4.25), compared to residents who desired to live elsewhere (mean: 10.33; standard deviation 4.96). Morale was also best predicted by functional health status: 39 per cent of the variance in morale scores was explained by self-rated health.

Reliability

Lawton (1972) reported a split-half reliability coefficient of 0.74, a coefficient of internal consistency of 0.81, and test-retest reliability coefficients ranging from 0.75 (after three months) to 0.91 (after five weeks).

Factor analysis has been carried out by Lawton (1975), replicating work carried out by others. Seventeen items formed three factors: agitation (six items), attitude towards one's own ageing (five items) and lonely dissatisfaction (six items). They provided alpha internal consistency coefficients of between 0.81 and 0.85. Lawton recommended that these 17 items be referred to as the 'revised PGC Morale Scale'.

In sum, the scale has acceptable levels of reliability and validity and is widely believed to be the superior of the existing life-satisfaction and morale scales. The criticism of it is that the inclusion of items measuring both happiness and satisfaction is questionable, given the earlier definition of morale (Stull 1987).

DELIGHTED–TERRIBLE FACES (D–T) SCALE

The Delighted–Terrible Faces Scale (Andrews and Withey 1974; 1976) is popular among investigators in mental health, where it has been frequently adapted and used. Elsewhere, the use of the faces as a response format to questionnaire items (usually unattributed to the authors) is increasingly common. The authors have published the items, and suggest that investigators select relevant items for their own questionnaires. This is an affective evaluation of quality of life which involves a cognitive evaluation and some degree of positive/negative feeling (affect).

The D–T Scale was developed in response to the recognition of deficiencies in other scales. Andrews and Withey (1976) report that a survey of well-being by Campbell et al. (1976) reported that a half to two-thirds of respondents selected one of the two most satisfied categories presented to them. They felt that this concentration at the 'satisfied' end of the scale posed statistical and conceptual problems. The inclusion of seven faces on the D–T scale was an attempt to reduce the skew of distributions and improve discrimination between respondents. They also offered a neutral face, as they felt it was important for respondents to 'opt out' if none of the faces represented their feelings. The faces show clear expressions and can be regarded as 'labelled' (each face is represented by an alphabetical letter, ranging from A (delighted) to G (terrible)). This was seen as an improvement on scales which are laid out along a single dimension with only the end categories labelled, leaving the respondent to infer the appropriate meanings for the intermediate categories.

Content

Respondents are shown seven faces ranging from wide smiles to turned down mouths. They are told: 'Here are some faces expressing various feelings (delighted, pleased, mostly satisfied, mixed, mostly dissatisfied, unhappy, and terrible). Below each is a letter. Which face comes closest to expressing how you feel about . . . ?' (specific items and/or 'life as a whole' are asked about). Examples of items which can be included, and which explain 50–62 per cent of the variance in evaluations of life, are self-accomplishment and problem handling, family life, income, fun and enjoyment, accommodation, family togetherness, time to do things one wants to, non-work activities, national government activities, quality of local goods and services, health status and employment.

Andrews and Withey advise researchers to select study-specific items. They have published a wide selection of items which can be incorporated within a scale.

Scoring

The seven faces are given scores from 1 (delighted) to 7 (terrible). While item responses can be summed, each item can also be analysed independently. The latter is more valid given the lack of information about appropriate weighting of items.

A study of 662 people aged 85+ in the East End of London by Bowling and Browne (1991) and Bowling et al. (1993) reported that the D–T Faces Scale was fairly skewed, with about a quarter of respondents choosing the terrible faces, while over half selected a delighted face. Research on stroke patients in the UK by Anderson (1988) also found the measure to be skewed, with 19 per cent of respondents choosing a terrible face and two-thirds choosing a delighted face. However, both studies reported good acceptance of the scale by respondents.

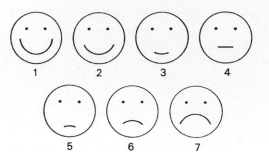

Reproduced with permission from Andrews and Withey, *Social Indicators of Well-being: Americans' Perceptions of Life Quality*.

Validity and reliability

The authors of the scale compared the D–T scale with other similar scales and presented evidence that it was a more valid measure than most other scales assessed; the exception was a visually complex 'circles' scale: different circles had varying numbers of plus signs (these represented good things in life) and minus signs (which represented bad things in life) displayed within them; respondents choose the circles which represent their feelings. Other scales assessed by the authors included a ladder scale in which respondents rated life satisfaction via the ladder rungs; a visual analogue scale with boxes at intervals along the line which represented statements about life satisfaction (delighted–pleased–mostly satisfied – mixed (about equally satisfied and dissatisfied) – mostly dissatisfied – unhappy–terrible), and Bradburn's Affect-Balance Scale. The results are too complex to present here as Andrews and Withey (1976) presented them in model form but are reported in detail by the authors. Few studies using the scale have been published.

It was previously reported by Bowling and Browne (1991) (see section on Neugarten Life Satisfaction Scales), that, on the basis of their samples of elderly people living at home in London and Essex, the correlations between the D–T Faces Scale and Neugarten's Life Satisfaction Scale A fluctuated fairly widely from weak to moderate: from −0.24 to −0.65 (the correlations were in the expected direction – the minus sign reflects the direction of the scoring).

Further analyses (unpublished) of these studies by Bowling and Browne showed reliability coefficients of around alpha 0.80; inter-item cor-

relations were weak to moderate, ranging from 0.30 to 0.59 between studies.

Apart from the original work by Andrews and Withey, which reported good reliability and validity, there have been few published studies reporting usage of this scale in its original form.

THE (PSYCHOLOGICAL) GENERAL WELL-BEING SCHEDULE (GWBS)

The General Well-Being Schedule, sometimes called the Psychological General Well-Being Index (PGWB), is a concise multi-dimensional indicator of subjective feelings of well-being and distress. It was designed for use in the US Health and Nutrition Examination Survey (Dupuy 1978).

The GWBS Index was developed with the aim of providing an index that could be used to measure self-reports of intrapersonal affective or emotional states reflecting a sense of subjective well-being or distress.

Population norms were provided by the national Health and Nutrition Examination Survey (HNS). The most well-known application is the modified version incorporated into the Rand Mental Health Inventory, based on a large community sample of people aged 14–60+ (Brook *et al.* 1979a; 1979b). The Rand Health Insurance Survey provided the most recent national reference standards for the GWBS in the USA: 71 per cent of adults fell into the 'positive well-being' category (scores 73–110), 15.5 per cent showed moderate distress (scores of 61–72), and 13.5 per cent were classified as experiencing 'severe distress' (scores of 0–60). Fifteen of the GWBS items were retained for use in the final version of the Rand Mental Health Inventory. Brook *et al.* (1979a; 1979b) have extensively reviewed the scale.

Content

The initial draft of the instrument contained 68 items, 18 of which were used for the US HNS; these were referred to as the General Well-Being Schedule. A 33–item version was also developed and used (Fazio 1977). One version of the index has 22 items. The items include indicators of both positive and negative affect. It is a self-administered questionnaire; administration time is 12 minutes.

It includes items for six states of being. The

sub-scales used to measure these six states contain three to five items each. The six sub-scales are anxiety (e.g. bothered by nervousness; generally tense; anxious, worried, upset; relaxed, at ease versus highly strung; felt under strain, stress or pressure); depressed mood (e.g. felt depressed; felt downhearted and blue; sad, discouraged, hopeless); positive well-being (e.g. general spirits; happy, satisfied with personal life; interesting daily life; felt cheerful, lighthearted); self-control (e.g. in firm control; afraid of losing control; felt emotionally stable, sure of self); general health (e.g. bothered by illness, bodily disorders, or aches and pains; healthy enough to do things; concerned, worried about health); and vitality (e.g. energy, pep; waking feeling fresh, rested; felt active, vigorous versus dull, sluggish; felt tired, worn-out, used up).

The frame of reference for questions is 'during the last month'. The first 14 questions have six different response choices; and four questions use rating scales, defined by adjectives at each end. Examples of questions are:

How have you been feeling in general (*during the past month*)?

In excellent spirits
In very good spirits
In good spirits mostly
I have been up and down in spirits a lot
In low spirits mostly
In very low spirits

How happy, satisfied, or pleased have you been with your personal life (*during the past month*)?

Extremely happy – could not have been more satisfied or pleased
Very happy
Fairly happy
Satisfied . . . pleased
Somewhat dissatisfied
Very dissatisfied.

How concerned or worried about your health have you been (*during the past month*)?

| 0 | 1 | 2 | 3 | 4 | 5 | 6 | 7 | 8 | 9 | 10 |

Not concerned at all   Very concerned

Scoring

The first 14 questions have six response choices which are scored on a scale of 0 to 5. A value of 0 is allocated for the most negative response and 5 for the most positive response (rating scales are also used; see earlier). The range of scores is from 0 to 110, and the range for the sub-scales is from 0 to 15, or 20 to 25. The overall score or sub-scale scores can be used for analysis. Dupuy proposed that scores of 0–60 reflect 'severe distress', 61–72 'moderate distress', while 73 to 110 represent 'positive well-being'.

Validity

Fazio's (1977) study of 195 students found that the GWBS correlated moderately with interviewers' ratings of depression (0.47); and that the average correlation of the GWBS and six other depression scales was 0.69, and 0.64 with three anxiety scales. Fazio (1977) and Ware *et al.* (1979) also reported criterion correlations between the GWBS and interviewers' ratings generally ranging between 0.65 and 0.90.

Edwards *et al.* (1978) showed that psychiatric patients achieved different scores in comparison with national population norms provided by the HNS. The scale was also sensitive enough to detect the progress over three weeks of the 21 psychiatric day patients in their study. Kammann and Flett (1983) reported a correlation of 0.74 between the GWBS scale and their 96-item scale of general happiness and well-being (the Affectometer).

On the basis of the US HNS data, Dupuy (1978) and Wan and Livieratos (1977) reported factor analyses of the GWBS which showed three factors which explained 51 per cent of the variance: anxiety, tension and depression; health and energy; and positive well-being or life satisfaction.

Reliability

Extensive scaling and tests of reliability and validity were carried out on 1,209 respondents. A six-factor solution was produced confirming the six sub-scales. Internal consistency coefficients for the six sub-scales ranged between 0.72 and 0.88. Test-retest reliability produced good results (with the exception of a lowered test-retest coefficient of

0.50 when the interval was extended from one week to one month). Test-retest reliability co-efficients ranged from 0.50 to 0.86, with a median of 0.66.

These results were based on a wide range of studies from samples of students to the large sample of adults participating in the Rand Health Insurance Study. They have been reviewed by Dupuy (1984). Test-retest reliability coefficients of 0.68 and 0.85 for two sub-samples within the US HNS were reported by Monk (1981). It is difficult to know whether the lower correlations reflect the instability of the instrument or changes in individuals. The same data reported internal consistency coefficients of 0.93 on the basis of analyses of 6,913 people. Fazio (1977) reported internal consistency coefficients of 0.91 for males and 0.95 for females; and correlations among sub-scores ranging from 0.16 to 0.72. Ware et al.'s (1979) review reported three studies using the GWBS which found internal consistency coefficients of over 0.90. However, Edwards et al. (1978) reported a coefficient of 0.69.

This is a scale with good test results on the whole. One advantage of this scale is that it avoids reference to physical symptoms of emotional distress and so avoids problems of interpretation. Fluctuations in test-retest reliability may be problematic in assessing individuals. A major disadvantage is that most of the validation studies of it are unpublished, although these have been thoroughly reviewed by Brook et al. (1979a; 1979b).

SENSE OF COHERENCE SCALE (SOC)

A generic scale of coherence, which overlaps with life satisfaction, is included in this section: the Sense of Coherence Scale (Antonovsky and Sagy 1986; Antonovsky 1993). The author reviewed more specific scales of adjustment, coping and control in *Measuring Disease*. The Sense of Coherence Scale is global in content, and is increasingly popular in European studies of health outcome (to measure modifying factors).

The development of the concept and the scale was based on intensive interviews with 52 respondents who had suffered major life crises. The Sense of Coherence Scale was derived from a theoretical model designed to explain the maintenance or improvement of one's position on a health-ease/disease continuum (Antonovsky 1993). The sense of coherence was defined by Antonovsky (1987) as: 'a global orientation that expresses the extent to which one has a pervasive, enduring though dynamic feeling of confidence that (1) the stimuli deriving from one's internal and external environments in the course of living are structured, predictable, and explicable; (2) the resources are available to one to meet the demands posed by these stimuli; and (3) these demands are challenges, worthy of investment and engagement'. These three elements are called comprehensibility, manageability and meaningfulness. In effect, it is a global orientation to one's inner and outer environments, and can be used as an indicator of coping capacity in stressful life situations. Antonovsky argued that a strong sense of coherence is necessary for the successful management of tension due to stress, and the movement towards the healthy end of the ease–disease continuum (Antonovsky 1990).

Content

The scale is a 29-item 7-point numeric scale, comprising 11 items on comprehensibility, 10 on manageability and 8 on meaningfulness. A range of shorter versions have been described, but the 13-item version is the generally accepted short version, with acceptable levels of reliability and validity (Antonovsky 1987; Langius 1995). Examples from the 29-item version are:

Do you have the feeling that you don't really care about what goes on around you?

1	2	3	4	5	6	7

Very seldom   Very
or never   often

Has it happened that people whom you counted on disappointed you?

1	2	3	4	5	6	7

Never   Always
happened   happened

Life is:

1	2	3	4	5	6	7

Full of   Completely
interest   routine

Most of the things you do in the future will probably be:

| 1 | 2 | 3 | 4 | 5 | 6 | 7 |

Completely
fascinating

Deadly
boring

What best describes how you see life?

| 1 | 2 | 3 | 4 | 5 | 6 | 7 |

One can always find
a solution to painful
things in life

There is no solution
to painful things in
life

Doing the things you do every day is:

| 1 | 2 | 3 | 4 | 5 | 6 | 7 |

A source of deep
pleasure and
satisfaction

Deep source of pain
and boredom

You anticipate that your personal life in the future will be:

| 1 | 2 | 3 | 4 | 5 | 6 | 7 |

Totally without meaning
or purpose

Full of meaning
and purpose

Many people – even those with a strong character –
sometimes feel like sad sacks (losers) in certain situations.
How often have you felt this way in the past?

| 1 | 2 | 3 | 4 | 5 | 6 | 7 |

Very often

Very seldom
or never

Scoring

Each of the 29 items have a 7-point numeric scale,
which are simply summed to produce the scale's
score. Thus the 29 items are scored from 29 to 203,
the higher the score the stronger the sense of coherence. The scoring follows the same format for
the 13-item version. Langius *et al.* (1992) reported
testing the numeric semantic-differential format of
the scale with an alternative linear visual analogue
scale response method; no significant differences
were found between the two scaling formats.

Validity

Its validity and reliability have been tested in
studies in over 20 countries. It was judged to be
applicable cross-culturally (Antonovsky 1993),
although as it does use some culture specific col-
loquialisms, care in translation and testing for
meaning is required. Antonovsky (1993) presented
the evidence for the scale's validity from all published studies up to 1993, and reported significant
correlations between the Sense of Coherence Scale
and measures of health, illness, well-being, orientation to self and stress, indicating the scale's
criterion and construct (convergent) validity.

In addition, Björvell *et al.* (1994), in a study of
obese patients, reported a significant correlation of
-0.55 between the Sense of Coherence Scale and a
measure of motivation, indicating that the stronger
the self-rated sense of coherence, the greater the
perceived self-motivation.

In a study of 189 US veterans a factor analysis of
the scale revealed that all 29 items loaded on one true
factor at 0.40 or above (eigenvalue given: 12.45).

Reliability

The 29-item version of the scale was tested for
reliability in 26 studies reported by Antonovsky
(1993). The Cronbach alpha measure of internal
consistency was 0.82–0.95. The 13-item version
was used in 16 studies, and the Cronbach's alpha
was 0.74–0.91. Some of the studies reported the
test-retest correlations, which were stable at 0.54
over two years (Antonovsky 1993). Langius *et al.*
(1994) and Langius (1995), in studies of patients
with oral or pharyngeal cancer, reported the Cronbach's alpha to be 0.88–0.89.

SCALES OF SELF-ESTEEM

Among the most popular and commonly used
measures of self-esteem are: the Self-Esteem Scale
(Rosenberg 1965); the Tennessee Self-Concept
Scale (Fitts 1965); and the Self-Esteem Inventory
(Coopersmith 1967). Several other popular scales
have been reviewed by Crandall (1973), Robinson
and Shaver (1973), Wylie (1974) and by George and
Bearon (1980); the reader is referred to these
authors for a more detailed review. Most scales
appear to warrant further testing for validity, reliability and sensitivity, and they appear to suffer
from concentration on studies of students with
little information being provided on their applicability to other population groups.

THE SELF-ESTEEM SCALE

Rosenberg (1965) described self-esteem as self-acceptance or a basic feeling of self-worth. Rosenberg (1965) developed the Self-Esteem Scale, based on Guttman scaling, for a study of 5,024 students in public schools in New York. Little information exists about the development of the scale. Self-esteem scores were correlated with characteristics such as participation and leadership in school activities. The measure was intended to be brief, global and unidimensional. It has been widely used in varying settings. Evidence suggests it is suitable for use with older people. A study of around 5,000 retired teachers and telephone-company employees by Atchley (1976) reported that men had higher self-esteem than women. Kaplan and Porkorny (1969) in a study of 500 adults in Harris County, Texas, reported that age is unrelated to self-esteem. Ward (1977), on the basis of a study of 323 residents of Madison, Wisconsin, reported that predictors for women's self-esteem were current activities, age-related deprivations and health. Among the elderly (aged 60–92), attitudes towards old age are predictive of self-esteem, and for men income and education are predictive (Ward 1977).

Content

The scale consists of 10 items with responses reported along a four-point continuum from 'strongly agree' to 'strongly disagree'. Examples of items are:

I feel that I'm a person of worth, at least on an equal plane with others.
I feel that I have a number of good qualities.
All in all, I am inclined to feel that I am a failure.
I feel I do not have much to be proud of.
At times I think I am no good at all.
On the whole, I am satisfied with myself.
I take a positive attitude toward myself.

Strongly agree (1)/agree (2)/disagree (3)/strongly disagree (4)

Scoring

The measure was designed as a 10-item Guttman scale. The category responses were originally designed to be scored from 0 to 6 (strongly agree to strongly disagree). However, there is no agreement over the method of scoring, and some users score responses dichotomously as 'agree' or 'disagree', and other researchers use a simple summing scale.

Validity

Silber and Tippett (1965) assessed the convergent validity of the scale, and reported item correlations of 0.56 and 0.83. Rosenberg (1965) explicitly chose items for the scale which he felt had face validity. He reported that the scale had acceptable predictive validity in relation to depression levels among volunteers assessed by nurses. Robinson and Shaver (1973) reported that the scale correlated 0.59–0.60 with Coopersmith's Self-Esteem Inventory, depending on the scoring method.

Although there is some evidence to support the construct validity of the scale (Rosenberg 1965), there is little evidence of its sensitivity to change. Rosenberg (1965), in assessing its construct validity, reported that positive self-esteem was predictive of several social and psychological characteristics, such as reduced shyness, depression and more assertiveness and social activities.

Kaplan and Porkorny (1969) reported two uncorrelated factors which accounted for 45 per cent of the total variance. The items forming the first factor they called 'self-derogation', and they stated that the second factor reflected 'defense of individual worth'. Kohn (1969) reported similar results.

Reliability

Reliability (internal consistency and test-retest) has been shown to be good by Rosenberg (1965; 1986) who reported reproducibility coefficients of 0.85–0.92 and a scalability coefficient of 0.72; Ward (1977) reported a coefficient of alpha of 0.74 for internal consistency; Silber and Tippett (1965) reported a test-retest reliability coefficient of 0.85 from administrations of the scale to 28 students with a two-week interval.

In sum, the scale is attractive due to its brevity and simplicity but still requires further testing for validity, reliability and sensitivity to change. Also its method of scoring remains unresolved. It is highly recommended by George and Bearon (1980).

Little recent work has been carried out with the scale and Wylie (1974), in her extensive review of the scale, concluded that it is worthy of further research and development.

THE TENNESSEE SELF-CONCEPT SCALE

The Tennessee Self-Concept Scale is probably the most popular and most often used scale. It was developed for use in mental-health rehabilitation in 1956 and revised in 1965 (Fitts 1965). Fitts (1965; 1972) based the scale on Maslow's theory that individuals who are more self-actualizing are more able to realize their true potentialities and to function in a more creative and effective manner. Fitts saw self-concept related to performance. The person who has a clear, consistent, positive and realistic self-concept will behave in a healthy, confident, constructive and effective way. This is dependent on other things being equal, and this, of course, is not always the case.

The scale was developed from other scales and open-ended items, and from self-descriptions from samples of psychiatric patients and non-patients. These were placed on an internal–external scale. Ninety remaining statements were independently classified by seven clinical psychologists into 15 categories. There was perfect agreement on their negative and positive content. The scale was initially tested on 626 people, aged 12–68.

Administration takes approximately 20 minutes, and is based on self-completion.

Content

The scale consists of 100 self-descriptive items and is fairly complicated. Ninety items are categorized under the following labels: physical self, moral-ethical self, personal self, family self and social self. These labels are divided into statements about internal self-concept: self-identity, self-acceptance and behaviour. The scale is intended to summarize an individual's feeling of self-worth, and the degree to which the image is realistic or deviant. Ninety items tap both an internal and external dimension of self-concept. The remaining 10 items form a lie scale and measure defensive responses.

Depending on the intended use, two versions of the scale are available – one for counselling and one for clinical or research purposes.

Details of the scale, reviews of unpublished and published studies and population norms, are available in purchasable reports by Fitts (1965) and Roid and Fitts (1988). Its commercial nature prohibits the reproduction of more than a few items:

I have a healthy body.
I am satisfied with my moral behaviour.
I am a member of a happy family.
I am as sociable as I want to be.

Completely false (1)/mostly false (2)/partly false and partly true (3)/mostly true (4)/completely true (5)

Scoring

Scoring is complex. A set of scoring templates and a scoring matrix is required. A computerized scoring service is available from the publisher.

The response categories to 90 of the items lie along a five-point continuum, ranging from 'completely false' to 'completely true'. The total score is a positive self-esteem score. The 10 remaining items are the self-criticism (lie) scale, consisting of mildly negative statements.

The positive self-esteem score has a potential range of 90–450. Fitts (1965) reported a mean score, on the basis of his original sample of 628 adults, of 345.57.

Validity

Correlations demonstrating convergent validity, discriminant and predictive validity have been reported by Fitts (1965), Thompson (1972) and Roid and Fitts (1988), although much of the evidence to support the scale comes from relatively early or unpublished studies. Correlations with an anxiety scale of −0.70 suggest the convergent validity of the scale (Fitts 1965), this has been confirmed by Thompson (1972). Fitts (1965) also reports a correlation of 0.68 with a scale of positive affect.

Vincent (1968) undertook a factor analysis of the scale. Self-acceptance and personal self loaded with several similar measures.

Discriminant validity is partly suggested by a correlation of −0.21 with the F scale measure of authoritarianism; and predictive validity is suggested by its ability to distinguish between mental health and psychopathology (Fitts 1965). The scale has been widely used on samples of juveniles and psychiatric patients, as well as normal adults. Self-esteem has been found to be higher among older people than among adults generally (Grant 1966). While there are many variables that correlate significantly with the scale, there are also many that do not (Reed *et al.* 1980).

Wylie (1974) questions the discriminant validity on the scale on the grounds of lack of sufficient information reported by Fitts (1965) to suggest the validity of the scale. Moreover, Vacchiano and Strauss (1968) reported that their factor analysis of the scale revealed 20 factors. Other studies have been published which support the factor structure of the scale, although the factor structure remains unresolved (see McGuire and Tinsley 1981 and Roid and Fitts 1988).

Applications of the scale do not show a consistent pattern of results to be able to support the definition of self-concept as defined by Fitts (Walsh 1984). There is also little evidence of the scale's sensitivity to change.

Reliability

Test-retest reliability tests show high correlations of 0.92 for the positive self-esteem score and 0.75 for the self-criticism scale over a two-week period in a study of 60 students (Fitts 1965). Wylie (1974) again criticized Fitts (1965) for lack of sufficient information to make independent judgements about the reliability of the scale. This has been rectified in a subsequent manual by Roid and Fitts (1988). Estimates of internal consistency (alpha coefficients) for the scale range between 0.66 and 0.94 for the total scale score and sub-sets of the scale, with most being between 0.70 to 0.87 (Stanwyck and Garrison 1982; Tzeng *et al.* 1985; Roid and Fitts 1988). However, inter-item correlations appear to be relatively low for the various sub-sets of items (from 0.14 to 0.35) (Tzeng *et al.* 1985), although this is within the range expected for such scales (Roid and Fitts 1988).

In sum, it appears usable with older people, although the low self-criticism scores obtained by the elderly should make the user cautious (George and Bearon 1980). It is a popular scale but lengthy to administer.

COOPERSMITH SELF-ESTEEM INVENTORY

The Coopersmith Inventories were well researched (Coopersmith 1975; 1981a; 1981b), and are widely used in social science and by clinicians. Self-esteem is portrayed as a trait that is not evenly distributed in the population, but highly desirable to have.

The manual of the scale offers several sources of population norms (Coopersmith 1981a).

Coopersmith (1967) defined self-esteem as self-judgements of personal worth, a definition compatible with earlier definitions. The Self-Esteem Inventory measures attitudes towards the self, encompassing several domains: social, academic, family and personal experiences. The scale was devised by five psychologists for use with children who classified items according to high or low esteem to derive a 50-item scale. Items were reduced to 25, after an item analysis based on the responses of 121 children. The correlation of the longer with the shorter version was 0.95. The scale is self-administered and takes approximately 10 minutes.

The 50-item scale has an additional eight lie-scale items (Coopersmith 1967). A similar 25-item version also exists, and this can be used with adults (aged 16+). The version for adults has been published by Robinson and Shaver (1973).

Content

The items consist of short statements which the subject rates as either 'like me' or 'unlike me'. It is multi-dimensional, covering leadership-popularity, self-derogation, family-parents, and assertiveness-anxiety. Examples are:

I can make up my mind without too much trouble.
I'm a lot of fun to be with.
I'm popular with people my own age.
It's pretty tough to be me.
Things are all mixed up in my life.
I often feel upset about the work I do.
I'm not as nice looking as most people.
If I have something to say, I usually say it.
Things don't usually bother me.

Scoring

The scoring format remains untested. The item responses 'like me' or 'unlike me' are allocated a value and simply summed. A score is derived by multiplying X, the raw score, by 2 on the short scale and 4 on the long scale. A totally positive score is 100 and a totally negative score is 0.

Validity

Convergent-validity correlations between the scale and other self-esteem scales, based again on students, vary widely between 0.02 and 0.60 (Taylor and Reitz 1968; Ziller *et al*. 1969; Crandall 1973). More consistent correlations with the Rosenberg Self-Esteem Scale were reported by Robinson and Shaver (1973), again using students (total: 300): from 0.59 to 0.60. Hoffmeister (1976) compared two sub-scales of the Self-Esteem Questionnaire which he developed with Coopersmith's Self-Esteem Inventory and reported correlations of 0.40 and 0.61.

Discriminant validity correlations range between 0.44 and 0.75 when tested against a social desirability scale (Taylor and Reitz 1968), indicating that there is possible confounding with social desirability.

Correlations have been reported with scales measuring other concepts, which would be expected on theoretical grounds: Campbell (1967) reported a correlation of 0.31 with an achievement test; Boshier (1968) reported a correlation of 0.80 with the scale and liking one's first name; Wiest (1965) reported a correlation of 0.22 between the scale and the reporting of mutual liking between others and self. Not all correlations are in the direction expected. For example, Trowbridge (1970) reported a higher mean on the scale for children who were socioeconomically disadvantaged.

Robinson and Shaver (1973), on the basis of two samples of students (total: 500), carried out two factor analyses of the scale which indicated its multi-dimensional nature. Four factors emerged: self-derogation, leadership-popularity, family-parents and assertiveness-anxiety. The family-parents factor was reported to be the most stable and least ambiguous.

Kokenes (1974) estimated the validity of the sub-scales by factor analysis of the responses of 7,600 schoolchildren and reported that the four bipolar dimensions obtained were highly congruent with the test's sub-scales.

It is a stable measure over time and thus is not suitable for longitudinal use where changes require measurement (Coopersmith 1967).

Wylie (1974) questions Coopersmith's claims of validity for the scale, on the grounds of the large number of significance tests undertaken in its development and the non-reporting of the actual number of such tests. The number reaching statistical significance at the 0.5 level was unreported, thus making it impossible to estimate the number that could have occurred by chance alone.

Reliability

The scale was originally administered to 87 schoolchildren. Early testing for test-retest reliability reported high coefficients at 0.88 over five weeks and 0.70 over three years, based on the samples of pre-adolescent schoolchildren (Coopersmith 1967). Split-half reliability tests also show high correlations: 0.90 (Taylor and Reitz 1968). Spatz and Johnson (1973) administered the 50-item child version to 600 students and reported internal-consistency coefficients in excess of 0.80. However, internal consistency was reported to be low in another study of 453 college students (Crandall 1973), a probable consequence of its multi-dimensionality. In sum, the scale appears to have been well researched and is widely used. A major methodological limitation has been its restricted use with samples of students for the testing of the reliability and validity of the adult version (Adair 1984).

APPENDIX:
A SELECTION OF
USEFUL SCALE
DISTRIBUTORS AND
ADDRESSES

Abbreviated Mental Test Score (AMT) 7 item version Professor S. Ebrahim, Department of Public Health, Royal Free Hospital Medical School, Rowland Hill Street, London NW3 2PF, UK.

Arizona Social Support Interview Schedule (ASSIS) Department of Psychology, Arizona State University, Tempe AZ 85287, USA.

Arthritis Impact Measurement Scales Dr R.F. Meenan, Arthritis Center, Boston University Medical Center, Conte Building, 80 East Concord Street, Boston, MA 02118, USA.

Barthel Index (Granger's modified version and FIM+FAM replacement scale) Dr C.V. Granger, Center for Functional Assessment, Department of Rehabilitative Medicine, University of Buffalo, 232 Parker Hill, 3435 Main Street, Buffalo, NY 14214–3007, USA.

Beck Depression Inventory (BDI) (revised version) Psychological Corporation, 555 Academic Court, San Antonio, TX 78204–2498, USA.

Consulting Psychologists Press (scale distributors), 3803 East Bayshore Road, Box 10096, Palo Alto, CA 94303, USA.

Crichton Royal Behaviour Rating Scale Dr D.J. Jolley, South Manchester Old Age Psychiatry Service, Withington Hospital, Nell Lane, West Didsbury, Manchester M20 2LR, UK.

Dartmouth COOP Function Charts Dr Deborah Johnson, Dartmouth COOP Project, Dartmouth Medical School, Hinman Box 7265, Hanover, NH 03755–3862, USA; WONCA version: Northern Centre for Health Care Research, University of Groningen, Ant. Deusinglaan 4, 9713 AW Groningen, The Netherlands.

Family Relationship Index (FRI), Family Environ- ment Scale (FES) Consulting Psychologists Press, 3803 East Bayshore Road, Box 10096, Palo Alto, CA 94303, USA.

General Health Questionnaire (GHQ) NFER-NELSON, Darville House, 2 Oxford Road East, Windsor, Berks SL4 1DF, UK.

Geriatric Mental State (GMS) and CARE Professor J.R.M. Copeland, Department of Psychiatry, Royal Liverpool Hospital, Prescot Street, Liverpool L7 8XP, UK.

Hamilton Depression Scale Professor M. Hamilton, Department of Psychiatry, University of Leeds, Woodhouse Lane, Leeds, LS2 9JT, UK. Structured interview version: Dr M. Potts, Department of Social Work, California State University, 1250 Bellflower Blvd., Long Beach, CA 90840–0902, USA.

Health Outcomes Institute, 2001 Killebrew Drive, Suite 122, Bloomington, MN 55425, USA.

Health Status Questionnaire-12 Health Outcomes Institute, 2001 Killebrew Drive, Suite 122, Bloomington, MN 55425, USA.

Hospital Anxiety and Depression Scale (HAD) NFER-NELSON, Darville House, 2 Oxford Road East, Windsor, Berks SL4 1DF, UK.

Interview Schedule for Social Interaction Professor A.S. Henderson, NH & MRC Social Psychiatry Research Unit, Australian National University, Canberra ACT 0200, Australia.

McGill Pain Questionnaire (MPQ) Professor R. Melzack, Department of Psychology, Stewart Biological Sciences Building, McGill University, 1205 Docteur Penfield Avenue, Montreal, Quebec H3A 1B1, Canada.

McMaster Health Index Questionnaire (MHIQ) Dr L. Chambers, Department of Clinical

Epidemiology and Biostatistics, McMaster University Health Sciences Center, 1200 Main Street West, Hamilton, Ontario L8N 3Z5, Canada.

Montgomery-Asberg Depression Rating Scale Professor S.A. Montgomery, Department of Psychiatry, Paterson Centre for Mental Health, 20 South Wharf Road, London, W2 1PD.

Network Typology: The Network Assessment Instrument Professor G.C. Wenger, Centre for Social Policy Research and Development, University of Wales, Bangor, Gwynedd LL57 2DG, Wales. Training pack for practitioners from: Pavilion Publishers, 8 St George's Place, Brighton, East Sussex, BN1 4GB

NFER-Nelson (scale distributors – mainly psychological), Darville House, 2 Oxford Road East, Windsor, Berks SL4 1DF, UK.

Nottingham Health Profile (NHP) Galen Research, Southern Hey, 137 Barlow Moor Road, West Didsbury, Manchester M20 8PW, UK.

Older Americans' Resources and Services Schedule (OARS) Dr H.J. Cohen, Center for the Study of Aging and Human Development, Box 3003, Duke University Medical Center, Durham, NC 27710, USA.

Philadelphia Geriatric Center Morale Scale Dr M.P. Lawton, the Edward and Esther Polisher Research Institute, Philadelphia Geriatric Center, 5301 Old York Road, Philadelphia, PA 19141-2996, USA.

Psychological Corporation (scale distributors), 555 Academic Court, San Antonio, TX 78204-2498, USA.

Quality of Life Questionnaire Multi-Health Systems, Inc., 65 Overlea Blvd., Suite 210, Toronto, M4H 1P1, Canada.

Quality of Well-Being Scale (QWBS) Professor R.M. Kaplan, Division of Health Care Sciences, School of Medicine, University of California, 9500 Gilman Drive, La Jolla, CA 92093-0622, USA.

Rand Health Insurance/Medical Outcomes Study Batteries and Scales Rand Health Sciences Program, Distribution Services, 1700 Main Street, PO Box 2138, Santa Monica, CA 90407-2138, USA.

SEIQoL Professor C.A. O'Boyle, Department of Psychology, Medical School, Royal College of Surgeons in Ireland, Mercer Building, Mercer Street, Dublin 2, Ireland.

Short-Form-36 Technical queries to: The Health Institute, New England Medical Center Hospital, NEMCH Box 345, 750 Washington Street, Boston, MA 02111, USA; to obtain the questionnaires: Medi-

cal Outcomes Trust, PO Box 1917, Boston, MA 02205, USA (for other US versions of the SF-36, including that developed at Rand, see the author's *Measuring Disease*).

Short Form-36 (UK version) UK Clearing House for Information on the Assessment of Health Outcomes, Nuffield Institute for Health, University of Leeds, Fairburn House, 71-75 Clarendon Road, Leeds LS2 9PL, UK.

Short Form-12 Medical Outcomes Trust, PO Box 1917, Boston, MA 02205, USA (another version – the Health Status Questionnaire-12 – has been developed by the Health Outcomes Institute, 2001 Killebrew Drive, Suite 122, Bloomington, MN 55425, USA).

Sickness Impact Profile (SIP) Health Policy and Management, School of Hygiene and Public Health, The Johns Hopkins University, 624 North Broadway, Baltimore, MD, 21205-1901, USA.

Social Network Scale (SNS) Department of Psychology, University of Illinois at Chicago, P.O. Box 4348, Chicago, IL 60680, USA.

Social Support Questionnaire Professor I.G. Sarason, Department of Psychology, University of Washington, Mail Stop NI-25, Seattle, WA 98195, USA.

Social Support Scale Dr C.D. Sherbourne, Rand, 1700 Main Street, Santa Monica, CA 90407-2138, USA.

Stanford Arthritis Center Health Assessment Questionnaire (HAQ) Dr J.F. Fries, Department of Medicine, Room S-102B, Stanford University School of Medicine, Division of Immunology and Rheumatology, Stanford CA 94305, USA.

UK Clearing House for Information on the Assessment of Health Outcomes Nuffield Institute for Health, University of Leeds, Fairburn House, 71-75 Clarendon Road, Leeds LS2 9PL, UK.

Tennessee Self-Concept Scale Western Psychological Services, 12031 Wilshire Blvd., Los Angeles, CA 90025-1251, USA.

Western Psychological Services (scale distributors – psychology), 12031 Wilshire Blvd., Los Angeles, CA 90025-1251, USA.

WHOQOL The WHOQOL Group, Division of Mental Health, World Health Organization, 1211 Geneva 27, Switzerland.

Zung's Self Rating Depression Scale DISTA Products, Eli Lilly Corporate Center, Indianapolis, IN 46285, USA.

REFERENCES

Aaronson, N.K. (1993). The EORTC QLQ-C30: a quality of life instrument for use in international clinical trials in oncology (abstract). *Quality of Life Research*, 2: 51.

Aaronson, N.K., Acquadro, C., Alonso, J. *et al.* (1992). International quality of life assessment (IQOLA) project. *Quality of Life Research*, 1: 349–51.

Abelin, T., Brzezinski, Z.J. and Carstairs, V.D.L. (ed.) (1986). *Measurement in Health Promotion and Protection*. Copenhagen: World Health Organization, Regional Office for Europe, European Series no. 22.

Abramson, J.H., Terespolsky, L., Brook, J.G. *et al.* (1965). Cornell Medical Index as a health measure in epidemiological surveys. *British Journal of Preventive and Social Medicine*, 19: 103–10.

Adair, F.L. (1984). Coopersmith Self-Esteem Inventories, in D.J. Keyser and R.C. Sweetland (eds) *Test Critiques*, Vol. I. Kansas City, MI: Test Corporation of America.

Adams, B.N. (1967). Interaction theory and the social network. *Sociometry*, 30: 64–78.

Affleck, J.W., Aitken, R.C.B., Hunter, J. *et al.* (1988). Rehabilitation status: a measure of medico-social dysfunction. *Lancet*, i: 230–33.

Alonso, J., Anto, J.M., Gonzalez, M. *et al.* (1992) Measurement of a general health status of non-oxygen-dependent chronic obstructive pulmonary disease patients. *Medical Care*, 30: 125–35 (suppl. 5).

American Psychiatric Association (1987). *Diagnostic and Statistical Manual of Mental Disorders*, 3rd revised edn. Washington, DC: APA.

American Psychiatric Association (1994). *Diagnostic and Statistical Manual of Mental Disorders*, 4th edn. Washington, DC: APA.

American Psychological Association (1974). *Standards for Educational and Psychological Tests*. Washington, DC: APA.

Anderson, J., Sullivan, F. and Usherwood, T.P. (1990). The Medical Outcomes Study Instruments (MOSI) – use of a new health status measure in Britain. *Family Practice*, 7: 205–18.

Anderson, R. (1988). The quality of life of stroke patients and their carers, in R. Anderson and M. Bury (eds) *Living with Chronic Illness: The Experience of Patients and Their Families*. London: Unwin Hyman.

Anderson, R., Davies, J.K., McQueen, D.V. *et al.* (1989). *Health Behaviour Research and Health Promotion*. Oxford: Oxford University Press.

Anderson, R.T., Aaronson, N.K. and Wilkin, D. (1993). Critical review of the international assessments of health-related quality of life. *Quality of Life Research*, 2: 369–95.

Andersson, E. (1993). The Hospital Anxiety and Depression Scale: homogeneity of the subscales. *Journal of Social Behavior and Personality*, 21: 197–204.

Andrews, F.M. and Crandall, R. (1976). The validity of measures of self-reported well-being. *Social Indicators Research*, 3: 1–19.

Andrews, F.M. and McKennel, A.C. (1980). Measures of self-reported well-being: their affective, cognitive and other components. *Social Indicators Research*, 18: 127–55.

Andrews, F.M. and Robinson, J.P. (1991). Measures of subjective well-being, in J.P. Robinson, P.R. Shaver and L.S. Wrightsman (eds) *Measures of Personality and Social Psychological Attitudes*. London: Academic Press, Inc.

Andrews, F.M. and Withey, S.B. (1974). Developing measures of perceived life quality: results from several national surveys. *Social Indicators Research*, 1: 1–26.

Andrews, F.M. and Withey, S.B. (1976). *Social Indicators of Well-being: Americans' Perceptions of Life Quality*. New York: Plenum Press.

Antonovsky, A. (1987). *Unravelling the Mystery of Health: How People Manage Stress and Stay Well*. San Francisco: Jossey-Bass Publishers.

Antonovsky, A. (1990). A somewhat personal odyssey in studying the stress process. *Stress Medicine*, 6: 71–80.

Antonovsky, A. (1993). The structure and properties of the Sense of Coherence Scale. *Social Science and Medicine*, 36: 725–33.

Antonovsky, A. and Sagy, S. (1986). The development of a sense of coherence and its impact on responses to stress situations. *Journal of Social Psychology*, 126: 213–25.

Arfwidsson, L., Elia, G., D'Laurell, B. *et al.* (1974). Can self-rating replace doctors' rating in evaluating anti-depressive treatment? *Acta Psychiatrica Scandinavica*, 50: 16–22.

Argyle, M., Martin, M. and Crossland, J. (1989). Happiness as a function of personality and social encounters, in J.P. Forgas and J.M. Innes (eds) *Recent Advances in Social Psychology: An International Perspective*. North Holland: Elsevier Science Publishers.

Atchley, R.C. (1976). Selected social and psychological differences between men and women in later life. *Journal of Gerontology*, 31: 204–11.

Aylard, P.R., Gooding, J.H., McKenna, P.J. and Snaith, R.P. (1987). A validation study of three anxiety and depression self assessment scales. *Psychosomatic Research*, 31: 261–8.

Banks, M.H. (1983). Validation of the General Health Questionnaire in a young community sample. *Psychological Medicine*, 13: 349–53.

Bardelli, D. and Saracci, R. (1978). Measuring the quality of life in cancer clinical trials: a sample survey of published trials, in P. Armitage and D. Bardelli (eds) *Methods and Impact of Controlled Therapeutic Trials in Cancer*. Geneva: Union Internationale Contre le Cancer. Technical Report Series no. 36, 75–94.

Barrera, M. (1980). A method for the assessment of social support networks in community survey research. *Connections*, 3: 8–13.

Barrera, M. (1981). Social support in the adjustment of pregnant adolescent assessment issues, in B.H. Gottlieb (ed.) *Social Networks and Social Support*. Beverly Hills, CA: Sage Publications.

Barrera, M. and Ainlay, S. (1983). The structure of social support: a conceptual and empirical analysis. *Journal of Community Psychology*, 11: 133–43.

Barrera, M., Baca, L., Christiansen, J. *et al.* (1985). Informant corroboration of social support network data. *Connections*, 8: 9–13.

Bech, P. (1981). Rating scales for affective disorder: their validity and consistency. *Acta Psychiatrica Scandinavica*, suppl. 295: 1–101.

Bech, P., Gram, L.F., Dein, E. *et al.* (1975). Quantitative rating of depressive states. *Acta Psychiatrica Scandinavica*, 51: 161–70.

Beck, A.T. (1970). *Depression: Causes and Treatment*. Philadelphia, PA: University of Pennsylvania Press.

Beck, A.T. and Beck, R.W. (1972). Screening depressed patients in family practice: a rapid technic. *Postgraduate Medicine*, 52: 81–5.

Beck, A.T., Mendelson, M., Mock, J. *et al.* (1961). Inventory for measuring depression. *Archives of General Psychiatry*, 4: 561–71.

Beck, A.T., Rial, W.Y. and Rickels, K. (1974). Short form of depression inventory: cross validation. *Psychological Reports*, 34: 1184–6.

Beck, A.T., Steer, R.A. and Garbin, M.G. (1988). Psychometric properties of The Beck Depression Inventory: twenty-five years of evaluation. *Clinical Psychology Review*, 8: 77–100.

Becker, M. (1974). The health belief model and personal health behaviour. *Health Education Monographs*, 2: 326–73.

Bedford, A., Foulds, G.A. and Sheffield, B.F. (1976). A new personal disturbance scale (DSSI/SAD). *British Journal of Social and Clinical Psychology*, 15: 387–94.

Benjamin, S., Decalmer, P. and Haran, D. (1982). Community screening for mental illness: a validity study of the General Health Questionnaire. *British Journal of Psychiatry*, 140: 174–80.

Benner, P. (1985). Quality of life: a phenomenological perspective on explanation, prediction, and understanding in nursing science. *Advances in Nursing Science, Special Issue: Quality of Life*, 8: 1–14.

Berg, R.L., Hallauer, D.S. and Berk, S.N. (1976). Neglected aspects of the quality of life. *Health Services Research*, 11: 391–5.

Bergner, M. (1988). 'Development, testing and use of the Sickness Impact Profile', in S.R. Walker and R.M. Rosser (eds) *Quality of Life Assessment and Application*. Lancaster: MIT Press.

Bergner, M. (1993). 'Development, testing and use of the Sickness Impact Profile', in S.R. Walker and R.M. Rosser (eds) *Quality of Life Assessment: Key Issues in the 1990s* (2nd edn). Dordrecht: Kluwer Academic.

Bergner, M., Bobbitt, R.A., Carter, W.B. *et al.* (1981). The Sickness Impact Profile: development and final revision of a health status measure. *Medical Care*, 19: 787–805.

Bergner, M., Bobbitt, R.A., Kressel, S. *et al.* (1976a). The Sickness Impact Profile: conceptual formulation and methodology for the development of a health status measure. *International Journal of Health Services*, 6: 393–415.

Bergner, M., Bobbitt, R.A., Pollard, W.E. *et al.* (1976b). The Sickness Impact Profile: validation of a health status measure. *Medical Care*, 14: 57–67.

Berkanovic, E., Hurwicz, M.L. and Landsverk, J. (1988). Psychological distress and the decision to seek medical care. *Social Science and Medicine*, 27: 1215–21.

Berkman, L.F. and Syme, S.L. (1979). Social networks, host resistance and mortality: a nine-year follow-up study of Alameda County residents. *American Journal of Epidemiology*, 109: 186–204.

Berkman, P.L. (1971). Life stress and psychological well-being: a replication of Langner's analysis in the Midtown Manhattan study. *Journal of Health and Social Behaviour*, 12: 35–45.

Berwick, D.M., Budman, S., Damico-White, J. *et al.* (1987). Assessment of psychological morbidity in primary care: explorations with the General Health Questionnaire. *Journal of Chronic Diseases*, 40: 71S–79S.

Berwick, D.M., Murphy, J.M., Goldman, P.A. *et al.* (1991). Performance of five-item mental health screening test. *Medical Care*, 29: 169–76.

Berzon, R.A., Simeon, G.P., Simpson, R.L. *et al.* (1995). Quality of life bibliography and indexes: 1993 update. *Quality of Life Research*, 4: 53–74.

Bigelow, D.A., McFarland, B.H. and Olson, M.M. (1991). Quality of life of community mental health program clients: validating a measure. *Community Mental Health Journal*, 27: 43–55.

Biggs, J.T., Wylie, L.T. and Ziegler, V.E. (1978). Validity of the Zung self-rating depression scale. *British Journal of Psychiatry*, 132: 381–5.

Bild, B.K. and Havighurst, R.J. (1976). Life satisfaction. *Gerontologist*, 16: 70–5.

Billings, A.G. and Moos, R.H. (1981). The role of coping responses and social resources in attenuating the impact of stressful life events. *Journal of Behavioural Medicine*, 4: 139–57.

Billings, A.G. and Moos, R.H. (1982). Social support and functioning among community and clinical groups: a panel model. *Journal of Behavioural Medicine*, 5: 295–311.

Björvell, H., Aly, A., Langius, A. and Nördstrom, G. (1994). Indicators of changes in weight and eating behaviour in severely obese patients treated in a nursing behavioural program. *International Journal of Obesity*, 18: 521–5.

Black, S.E., Blessed, J.A., Edwardson, J.A. *et al.* (1990). Prevalence rates of dementia in an ageing population: are low rates due to the use of insensitive instruments? *Age and Ageing*, 19: 84–90.

Blazer, D.G. (1982). Social support and mortality in an elderly community population. *American Journal of Epidemiology*, 115: 684–94.

Blessed, G., Tomlinson, B.E. and Roth, M. (1968). The association between quantitative measures of dementia and of senile change in the cerebral grey matter of elderly subjects. *British Journal of Psychiatry*, 114: 797.

Blumenthal, M.D. (1975). Measuring depressive symptomatology in a general population. *Archives of General Psychiatry*, 32: 971–8.

Bombardier, C., Ware, J., Russell, J. *et al.* (1986). Auranofin therapy and quality of life in patients with rheumatoid arthritis. *American Journal of Medicine*, 81: 565–78.

Bond, J. and Carstairs, V. (1982). *Services for the Elderly*. Scottish Health Service Studies no. 42. Edinburgh: Scottish Home and Health Department.

Bond, J., Gregson, B., Atkinson, A. *et al.* (1989). *Evaluation of Continuing Care Accommodation for Elderly People*, vol. 2. *The Randomised Controlled Trial of the Experimental NHS Nursing Homes and Conventional Continuing Care Wards in NHS Hospitals*. Report no. 38. Newcastle upon Tyne: University of Newcastle upon Tyne Health Care Research Unit.

Borgatta, E.F. and Montgomery, R.J.V. (1987). *Critical Issues in Ageing Policy: Linking Research and Values*. Beverly Hills, CA: Sage Publications.

Boshier, R. (1968). Self esteem and first names in children. *Psychological Reports*, 22: 762.

Bowling, A. (1990). The prevalence of psychiatric morbidity among people aged 85 and over living at home. *Social Psychiatry and Psychiatric Epidemiology*, 25: 132–40.

Bowling, A. (1991). Social support and social networks: their relationship to the successful and unsuccessful survival of elderly people in the community. An analysis of concepts and a review of the evidence. *Family Practice*, 8: 68–83.

Bowling, A. (1994). Social networks and social support among older people and implications for emotional well-being and psychiatric morbidity. *International Review of Psychiatry*, 6: 41–58.

Bowling, A. (1995a). *Measuring disease: A review of disease-specific quality of life measurement scales*. Buckingham: Open University Press.

Bowling, A. (1995b). What things are important in people's lives? A survey of the public's judgements to inform scales of health related quality of life. *Social Science and Medicine*, Special Issue 'Quality of Life', 10: 1447–62.

Bowling, A. and Browne, P. (1991). Social support and emotional well-being among the oldest old living in London. *Journal of Gerontology*, 46: S20–32.

Bowling, A. and Cartwright, A. (1982). *Life after a Death: A Study of the Elderly Widowed*. London: Tavistock Press.

Bowling, A. and Charlton, J. (1987). Risk factors for mortality after bereavement: a logistic regression analysis. *Journal of the Royal College of General Practitioners*, 37: 551–4.

Bowling, A. and Farquhar, M. (1995). Changes in network composition among older people living in Inner

London and Essex. *Journal of Health and Place*, 3: 149–66.

Bowling, A. and Formby, J. (1990). *Evaluation of District Health Authority Funded Nursing Homes and Geriatric Wards in City and Hackney*. London, Department of Public Health, City and Hackney District Health Authority.

Bowling, A. and Salvage, A. (1986). Prevention of residential care among the elderly. *Community Care*, 13 March: 24–7.

Bowling, A., Farquhar, M. and Grundy, E. (1994a). Associations with changes in level of functional ability. *Ageing and Society*, 14: 53–73.

Bowling, A., Farquhar, M. and Grundy, E. (1994b). Changes in the ability to get outdoors among a community sample of people aged 85+ in 1987: results from a follow-up study in 1990. *International Journal of Health Sciences*, 5: 13–23.

Bowling, A., Leaver, J. and Hoeckel, T. (1988). *The Needs and Circumstances of People Aged 85+ Living at Home in City and Hackney*. London: Department of Public Health, City and Hackney Health Authority.

Bowling, A., Farquhar, M., Grundy, E. and Formby, J. (1992). Psychiatric morbidity among people aged 85+ in 1987. A follow-up study at two and a half years: associations with changes in psychiatric morbidity. *International Journal of Geriatric Psychiatry*, 7: 307–21.

Bowling, A., Farquhar, M., Grundy, E. and Formby, J. (1993). Changes in life satisfaction over a two and a half year period among very elderly people living in London. *Social Science and Medicine*, 36: 641–55.

Bowling, A., Edelmann, R., Leaver, J. *et al.* (1989). Loneliness, mobility, well-being and social support in a sample of over-65-year-olds. *Journal of Personality and Individual Differences*, 10: 1189–97.

Bradburn, N.M. (1969). *The Structure of Psychological Well-being*. Chicago: Aldine Publishing.

Bradburn, N.M. and Caplovitz, D. (1965). *Reports on Happiness: A Pilot Study of Behaviour Related to Mental Health*. Chicago: Aldine Publishing.

Bradlyn, A.S., Harris, C.V., Warner, J.E. *et al.* (1993). An investigation of the validity of the Quality of Well-Being Scale with pediatric oncology patients. *Health Psychology*, 12: 246–50.

Bradwell, A.R., Carmal, M.H. and Whitehead, T.P. (1974). Explaining the unexpected: abnormal results of biochemical profile investigations. *Lancet*, ii: 1071–4.

Brazier, J.E., Harper, R., Jones, N. *et al.* (1992). Validating the SF-36 health survey questionnaire: a new outcome measure for primary care. *British Medical Journal*, 305: 160–4.

Brazier, J.E., Jones, N. and Kind, P. (1993). Testing the validity of the EuroQol and comparing it with the SF-36 health survey questionnaire. *Quality of Life Research*, 2: 169–80.

Brodman, K., Erdman, A.J., Jr, Lorge, I. *et al.* (1953). The Cornell Medical Index–Health Questionnaire VI: the relation of patients' complaints to age, sex, race and education. *Journal of Gerontology*, 8: 339–42.

Brodman, K., Erdman, A.J., Jr, Lorge, I. *et al.* (1954). The Cornell Medical Index–Health Questionnaire VII: the prediction of psychosomatic and psychiatric disabilities in army training. *American Journal of Psychiatry*, 111: 37–40.

Brodman, K., Erdmann, A.J., Jr and Wolff, H.G. (1949). *Cornell Medical Index Health Questionnaire*. New York: Cornell University Medical College.

Brodman, K., Van Woerkom, A.J., Jr and Goldstein, L.S. (1959). Interpretation of symptoms with a data-processing machine. *Archives of Internal Medicine*, 103: 776–82.

Brook, R.H., Ware, J.E., Davies-Avery, A. *et al.* (1979a). Overview of adult health status measures fielded in Rand's health insurance study. *Medical Care*, 17 (supplement), 1–131.

Brook, R.H., Ware, J.E., Davies-Avery, A. *et al.* (1979b). *Conceptualization and Measurement of Health for Adults in the Health Insurance Study*, vol. VIII, *Overview*. Santa Monica, CA: Rand Corporation, R-1987/8-HEW.

Brorsson, B. and Asberg, K.H. (1984). Katz Index of Independence in ADL: reliability and validity in short-term care. *Scandinavian Journal of Rehabilitative Medicine*, 16: 125–32.

Brown, B., Bhrolchain, M. and Harris, T. (1975). Social class and psychiatric disturbance among women in an urban population. *Sociology*, 9: 225–54.

Brown, G.L. and Zung, W.W.K. (1972). Depression scales: self or physician rating? A validation of certain clinically observable phenomena. *Comprehensive Psychiatry*, 13: 361–7.

Brown, J.H., Lewis, M.D., Kazis, E. *et al.* (1984). The dimensions of health outcomes: a cross validated examination of health status measurement. *American Journal of Public Health*, 74: 159–61.

Bucquet, D., Condom, S. and Ritchie, K. (1990). The French version of the Nottingham Health Profile: a comparison of item weights with those of the source version. *Social Science and Medicine*, 30: 829–35.

Bullinger, M. (1995). German translation and psychometric testing of the SF-36 Health Survey: preliminary results from the IQOLA project. *Social Science and Medicine*, Special Issue 'Quality of Life' in Social Science and Medicine, 10: 1359–66.

Burnam, M.A., Wells, K.B., Leake, B. and Landsverk, J. (1988). Development of a brief screening instrument for detecting depressive disorders. *Medical Care*, 26: 775–89.

Bush, J.W. (1984). General health policy model: Quality of well-being (QWB) scale, in N.K. Wenger, M.E.

Mattson, C.D. Furberg *et al.* (eds) *Assessment of Quality of Life in Clinical Trials of Cardiovascular Therapies.* New York: Le Jacq.

Buxton, M. (1983). The economics of heart transplant programmes: measuring the benefits, in G. Teeling Smith (ed.) *Measuring the Social Benefits of Medicine.* London, Office of Health Economics.

Buxton, M., Acheson, R.M., Caine, N. *et al.* (1985). *Costs and benefits of the heart transplantation programmes at Harefield and Papworth Hospitals.* London: Her Majesty's Stationery Office.

Byrne, D.G. (1978). Cluster analysis applied to self reported depressive symptomatology. *Acta Psychiatrica Scandinavica,* 57: 1–10.

Caine, N., Harrison, S.C.W., Sharples, L.D. and Wallwork, J. (1991). Prospective study of quality of life before and after coronary artery bypass grafting. *British Medical Journal,* 302: 511–16.

Caine, N., Sharples, L.D., English, T.A.H. and Wallwork, J. (1990). Prospective study comparing quality of life before and after heart transplantation. *Transplantation Proceedings,* 22: 1437–9.

Cairl, R.E., Pfeiffer, E., Keller, D.M. *et al.* (1983). An evaluation of the reliability and validity of the functional assessment inventory. *Journal of the American Geriatric Society,* 31: 607–12.

Caldwell, J.R. (1985). Family Environment Scale, in D.J. Keyser and R.C. Sweetland (eds) *Test Critiques,* volume II. Kansas City, MI: Test Corporation of America.

Caldwell, R.A. and Reinhart, M.A. (1988). The relationship of personality to individual differences in the use of type and source of social support. *Journal of Social and Clinical Psychology,* 6: 140–6.

Campbell, A. (1976). Subjective measures of wellbeing. *American Psychologist,* 31: 117–24.

Campbell, A. (1981). *The sense of well-being in America.* New York: McGraw-Hill.

Campbell, A., Converse, P.E. and Rogers, W.L. (1976). *The Quality of American Life.* New York: Russell Sage Foundation.

Campbell, P.B. (1967). School and self concept. *Educational Leadership,* 24: 510–15.

Cantril, H. (1967). *The pattern of human concerns.* New Brunswick, NJ: Rutgers University Press.

Caplan, G. (1974). *Support Systems and Community Mental Health.* New York: Behavioral Publications.

Carp, F.M. (1977). What questions are we asking of whom?, in C.N. Nydegger (ed.) *Measuring Morale: A Guide to Effective Assessment.* Washington, DC: Gerontology Society.

Carr-Hill, R. (1989). Assumption of the QALY procedure. *Social Science and Medicine,* 29: 469–77.

Carr-Hill, R. and Morris, J. (1991). Current practice in

obtaining the 'Q' in QALYS – a cautionary note. *British Medical Journal,* 303: 699–701.

Carroll, B.J., Fielding, J.M. and Blash, T.G. (1973). Depression rating scales: a critical review. *Archives of General Psychiatry,* 28: 361–6.

Carroll, B.T., Kathol, R.G., Noyes, R. *et al.* (1993). Screening for depression and anxiety in cancer patients using the Hospital Anxiety and Depression Scale. *Journal of General Hospital Psychiatry,* 15: 69–74.

Carter, W., Bobbitt, R.A., Bergner, M. *et al.* (1976). Validation of an interval scaling: the Sickness Impact Profile. *Health Services Research,* 11: 516–28.

Cartwright, A. and Anderson, R. (1981). *General Practice Revisited: A Second Study of Patients and Their Doctors.* London: Tavistock Press.

Cassel, J. (1976). The contribution of the social environment to host resistance. *American Journal of Epidemiology,* 104: 107–23.

Cavanaugh, S. (1983). The prevalence of emotional and cognitive dysfunction in a general medical population: using the MMSE, GHQ and BDI. *General Hospital Psychiatry,* 5: 15–24.

Chambers, L.W. (1982). The McMaster Health Index Questionnaire (MHIQ): methodologic documentation and report of second generation of investigators. Hamilton, Ontario: McMaster University, Department of Clinical Epidemiology and Biostatistics.

Chambers, L.W. (1984). The McMaster Health Index Questionnaire, in N.K. Wenger, M.E. Mattson, C.D. Furberg *et al.* (eds) *Assessment of Quality of Life in Clinical Trials of Cardiovascular Therapies.* New York: Le Jacq.

Chambers, L.W., Haight, M., Norman, G. *et al.* (1987). Sensitivity to change and the effect of mode of administration on health status measurement. *Medical Care,* 25: 470–9.

Chambers, L.W., MacDonald, L.A., Tugwell, P. *et al.* (1982). The McMaster Health Index Questionnaire as a measure of quality of life for patients with rheumatoid disease. *Journal of Rheumatology,* 9: 780–4.

Chambers, L.W., Sackett, D.L., Goldsmith, C.H. *et al.* (1976). Development and application of an index of social function. *Health Services Research,* 11: 430–41.

Charlton, J.R.H., Patrick, D.L. and Peach, H. (1983). Use of multivariate measures of disability in health surveys. *Journal of Epidemiology and Community Health,* 37: 296–304.

Chaturvedi, S.K. (1990). Asian patients and the HAD scale. *British Journal of Psychiatry,* 156: 133.

Cherlin, A. and Reeder, L.G. (1975). The dimensions of psychological well being: a critical review. *Sociological Methods Research,* 4: 189–214.

Chiange, C.L. (1965). *An Index of Health: Mathematical Models.* Washington, DC: US Government Printing Office, PHS Publication no. 1000, Series 2, no. 5.

Cleary, P.D., Goldberg, D.M., Kessler, L.G. *et al.* (1982). Screening for mental disorder among primary care physicians: usefulness of the General Health Questionnaire. *Archives of General Psychiatry*, 39: 837–40.

Coates, A., Gebski, V., Stat, M. *et al.* (1987). Improving the quality of life during chemotherapy for advanced breast cancer. *New England Journal of Medicine*, 317: 1490–5.

Coates, A.K. and Wilkin, D. (1992). Comparing the Nottingham Health Profile with the Dartmouth COOP Charts, in J.H.G. Scholten (ed.) *Functional status assessment in family practice*. Lelystad: Meditekst.

Cobb, S. (1976). Social support as a moderator of life stress. *Psychosomatic Medicine*, 38: 300–14.

Cochrane, A.L. and Holland, W.W. (1971). Validation of screening procedures. *British Medical Bulletin*, 27: 3–8.

Cohen, C.I., Teresi, J. and Holmes, D. (1987). Social networks and mortality in an inner-city elderly population. *International Journal of Ageing and Human Development*, 24: 257–69.

Cohen, S., Mermelstein, R., Karmack, T. *et al.* (1985). Measuring the functional components of social support, in I.S. Saronson and B.R. Saronson (eds) *Social Support: Theory, Research and Applications*. Boston, MA: Martinus Nijhoff.

Collen, F.M., Wade, D.T. and Bradshaw, C.M. (1990). Mobility after stroke: reliability of measures of impairment and disability. *International Disability Studies*, 12: 6–9.

Collin, C., Wade, D.T., Davies, D. *et al.* (1988). The Barthel ADL Index: a reliability study. *International Disability Studies*, 10: 61–3.

Conner, K.A., Powers, E. and Bultena, G.L. (1979). Social interaction and life satisfaction: an empirical assessment of late life patterns. *Journal of Gerontology*, 34: 116–21.

Convery, F.R., Minteer, M.A., Amiel, D. and Connett, K.L. (1977). Polyarticular disability: a functional assessment. *Archives of Physical Medicine and Rehabilitation*, 58: 494–9.

Cooper, P.J. and Fairburn, C.G. (1986). The depressive symptoms of bulimia nervosa. *British Journal of Psychiatry*, 148: 268–74.

Coopersmith, S. (1967). *The Antecedents of Self-esteem*. San Francisco, CA: W.H. Freeman. Reprinted in 1981.

Coopersmith, S. (1975). *Developing motivation in young children*. San Francisco, CA: Albion Publishing.

Coopersmith, S. (1981a). *The Antecedents of Self-Esteem*. Palo Alto, CA: Consulting Psychologists Press.

Coopersmith, S. (1981b). *Self-esteem Inventories*. Palo Alto, CA: Consulting Psychologists Press.

Copeland, J.R.M. (1990). Suitable instruments for detecting dementia in community samples. *Age and Ageing*, 19: 81–3.

Copeland, J.R.M. and Gurland, B.J. (1978). Evaluation of diagnostic methods: an international comparison, in A.D. Isaacs and F. Post (eds) *Studies in Geriatric Psychiatry*. Chichester: John Wiley.

Copeland, J.R.M., Dewey, M.E., Wood, N. *et al.* (1987a). Range of mental illness among the elderly in the community: prevalence in Liverpool using the GMS-AGECAT package. *British Journal of Psychiatry*, 150: 815–23.

Copeland, J.R.M., Dewey, M.E. and Griffiths Jones, H.M. (1986). A computerized psychiatric diagnostic system and case nomenclature for elderly subjects: GMS and AGECAT. *Psychological Medicine*, 16: 89–99.

Copeland, J.R.M., Dewey, M.E., Henderson, A.S. *et al.* (1988). The Geriatric Mental State (GMS) used in the community: replication studies of the computerized diagnoses AGECAT. *Psychological Medicine*, 18: 219–23.

Copeland, J.R.M., Gurland, B.J., Dewey, M.E. *et al.* (1987b). The distribution of dementia, depression and neurosis in elderly men and women in an urban community: assessed using the GMS-AGECAT package. *International Journal of Geriatric Psychiatry*, 2: 177–84.

Copeland, J.R.M., Kelleher, M.J., Kellet, J.M. *et al.* (1976). A semi-structured clinical interview for the assessment of diagnosis and mental state in the elderly: The Geriatric Mental State: Schedule I. Development and reliability. *Psychological Medicine*, 6: 439–49.

Cornoni-Huntley, J.C., Foley, D.J., White, L.R. *et al.* (1985). Epidemiology of disability in the oldest old: methodologic issues and preliminary findings. *Milbank Memorial Fund Quarterly, Health and Society*, 63: 350–76.

Coulton, C.J., Hyduk, C.M. and Chow, J.C. (1989). An assessment of the Arthritis Impact Measurement Scales in 3 ethnic groups. *Journal of Rheumatology*, 16: 1110–15.

Crandall, R.C. (1973). The measurement of self esteem and related constructs, in J. Robinson and P. Shaver (eds) *Measures of Social Psychological Attitudes*. Ann Arbor, MI: Institute for Social Research.

Craven, P. and Wellman, B. (1974). The network city in M.P. Effrat (ed.) *The Community: Approaches and Applications*. New York: Free Press.

Crawford-Little, J. and McPhail, N.I. (1973). Measures of depressive mood at monthly intervals. *British Journal of Psychiatry*, 122: 447–52.

Cronbach, L.J. (1951). Coefficient alpha and the internal structure of tests. *Psychometrika*, 22: 293–6.

Cuffel, B.J. and Akamatsu, T.J. (1989). The structure of loneliness: a factor-analytic investigation. *Cognitive Therapy and Research*, 13: 459–74.

Davidson, I.A., Dewey, M. and Copeland, J.R.M. (1988). The relationship between mortality and mental disorder: evidence from the Liverpool longitudinal study. *International Journal of Geriatric Psychiatry*, 3: 95–8.

Davies, A.R. and Ware, J.E. (1981). *Measuring Health Perceptions in the Health Insurance Program*. Santa Monica, CA: Rand Corporation: R-2711-HHS.

Davies, A.R., Sherbourne, C.D., Peterson, J.R. and Ware, J.E. (1988). *Scoring Manual: Adult Health Status and Patient Satisfaction Measures Used in RAND's Health Insurance Experiment. Publication No. N-2190-HHS*. Santa Monica, CA: Rand Corporation.

Davies, B., Burrows, G. and Poynton, C.A. (1975). Comparative study of four depression rating scales. *Australian and New Zealand Journal of Psychiatry*, 9: 21–4.

de Bruin, A.F., Diederiks, J.P.M., de Witte, I.P. and Stevens, F.C.J. (1993). The first testing of the SIP-68, a short generic version of the Sickness Impact Profile. Paper presented to the Fifth European Health Services Research Conference, Maastricht, December.

de Bruin, A.F., de Witte, L.P. and Diederiks, J.P. (1992). Sickness Impact Profile: the state of the art of a generic functional status measure. *Social Science and Medicine*, 8: 1003–14.

Dean, K., Holst, E., Kreiner, S. et al. (1994). The measurement issues in research on social support and health. *Journal of Epidemiology and Community Health*, 48: 201–6.

Denniston, O.L. and Jette, A.M. (1980). A functional status assessment instrument: validation in an elderly population. *Health Services Research*, 15: 21–4.

Dewey, M.E. and Copeland, J.R.M. (1986). Computerized psychiatric diagnosis in the elderly: AGECAT. *Journal of Microcomputer Applications*, 9: 135–40.

Deyo, R.A., Inui, T.S., Leininger, J.D. et al. (1982). Physical and psychological functions in rheumatoid arthritis: clinical use of a self-administered instrument. *Archives of Internal Medicine*, 142: 879–82.

Deyo, R.A., Inui, T.S., Leininger, J.D. et al. (1983). Measuring functional outcomes in chronic disease: a comparison of traditional scales and a self-administered health status questionnaire in patients with rheumatoid arthritis. *Medical Care*, 21: 180–92.

Dobson, C., Powers, E.A., Keith, P.M. et al. (1979). Anomie, self-esteem, and life satisfaction: interrelationships among three scales of well-being. *Journal of Gerontology*, 34: 569–72.

Donald, C.A. and Ware, J.E. (1982). *The Quantification of Social Contacts and Resources*. Santa Monica, CA: Rand Corporation: R-2937-HHS.

Donald, C.A., Ware, J.E., Brook, R.H. et al. (1978). *Conceptualization and Measurement of Health for Adults in the Health Insurance Study, vol. IV, Social Health*. Santa Monica, CA: Rand Corporation R-1987/4-HEW.

Dorn, H.F. (1955). Some applications of biometry in the collection and evaluation of medical data. *Journal of Chronic Diseases*, 1: 638–64.

Dubuisson, D. and Melzack, R. (1976). Classification of clinical pain descriptions by multiple group discriminant analysis. *Experimental Neurology*, 51: 480–7.

Dunnell, K. and Cartwright, A. (1972). *Medicine Taker, Prescribers and Hoarders*. London: Routledge and Kegan Paul.

Dupuy, H.J. (1978). Self representations of general psychological well-being of American adults. Paper presented at American Public Health Association Meeting. Los Angeles, California, 17 October.

Dupuy, H.J. (1984). The psychological General Well-being Index, in N.K. Wenger, M.E. Mattson, C.D. Furberg et al. (eds) *Assessment of Quality of Life in Clinical Trials of Cardiovascular Therapies*. New York: Le Jacq.

Ebmeier, K.P., Beson, J.A.O., Eagles, J.N. et al. (1988). Continuing care of the demented elderly in Inverurie. *Health Bulletin*, 46: 32–41.

Edwards, D.W., Yarvis, R.M., Mueller, D.P. et al. (1978). Test-taking and the stability of adjustment scales: can we assess patient deterioration? *Evaluation Q*, 2: 275–91.

Edwards, J.N. and Klemmack, D.L. (1973). Correlates of life satisfaction: a re-examination. *Journal of Gerontology*, 28: 479–502.

Eskin, M. (1993). Swedish translations of the Suicide Probability Scale, Perceived Social Support from Family and Friends Scales, and the Scale for Interpersonal Behavior: a reliability analysis. *Scandinavian Journal of Psychology* 34: 276–81.

EuroQol Group (1990). EuroQol – a new facility for the measurement of health-related quality of life. *Health Policy*, 16: 199–208.

Evans, D. and Cope, W. (1994). *The Quality of Life Questionnaire – D. Complete Kit*. Northern Tonawanda, New York: Multi-Health Systems.

Evans, G., Hughes, B.C. and Wilkin, D. (1981). *The Management of Mental and Physical Impairment in Non-specialist Residential Homes for the Elderly*, Research Report no. 4. Manchester: Research Section, Psychiatric Unit, University Hospital of South Manchester.

Evans, R.W., Manninen, D.L., Overcast, T.D. et al. (1984). *The National Heart Transplantation Study: Final Report*. Seattle, WA: Battelle Human Affairs Research Centre.

Fallowfield, L.J., Baum, M. and Maguire, G.P. (1987). Do psychological studies upset patients? *Journal of the Royal Society of Medicine*, 80: 59.

Fanshel, S. and Bush, J.W. (1970). A health status index

and its applications to health services outcomes. *Operational Research*, 18: 1021–65.

Farquhar, M. (1995a). Definitions of quality of life: a taxonomy. *Journal of Advanced Nursing*, 22: 502–8.

Farquhar, M. (1995b). Elderly people's definitions of quality of life. Special Issue 'Quality of Life' in *Social Science and Medicine*, 10: 1439–46.

Fazio, A.F. (1977). *A Concurrent Validation Study of the NCHS General Well-Being Schedule*. Hyattsville, MA: US Department of Health, Education and Welfare, National Center for Health Statistics: Vital and Health Statistics Series 2, no. 73 DHEW Publication No. (HRA) 78–1347.

Fillenbaum, G.G. (1978). Multidimensional functional assessment: The OARS Methodology – A Manual, 2nd edn. Durham, NC: Center for the Study of Aging and Human Development, Duke University.

Fillenbaum, G.G. (1988). *Multidimensional functional assessment of older adults: the Duke Older Americans Resources and Services Procedures*. Hillsdale, NJ: Lawrence Erlbaum.

Fillenbaum, G.G. and Smyer, M.A. (1981). The development, validity and reliability of the OARS multidimensional functional assessment questionnaire: disability and pain scales. *Journal of Gerontology*, 36: 428–33.

Finch, J. (1989). *Family obligations and social change*. Cambridge: Policy Press.

Finlay-Jones, R.A. and Murphy, E. (1979). Severity of psychiatric disorder and the 30-item General Health Questionnaire. *British Journal of Psychiatry*, 134: 609–16.

Fiore, J., Coppel, D.B., Becker, J. *et al.* (1986). Social support as a multifaceted concept: examination of important dimensions for adjustment. *American Journal of Community Psychology*, 14: 93–111.

Fitts, W.H. (1965). *Tennessee Self-Concept Scale Manual*. Nashville, TN: Counselor Recordings and Tests.

Fitts, W.H. (1972). *The Self-Concept and Performance*, Research Monograph no. 5. Nashville, TN: Social and Rehabilitation Service.

Fitzpatrick, R., Newman, S., Lamb, R. and Shipley, M. (1988). Social relationships and psychological well-being in rheumatoid arthritis. *Social Science and Medicine*, 27: 399–403.

Fitzpatrick, R., Newman, S., Lamb, R. and Shipley, M. (1989). A comparison of measures of health status in rheumatoid arthritis. *British Journal of Rheumatology*, 28: 201–6.

Fitzpatrick, R., Ziebland, S., Jenkinson, C. and Mowat, A. (1992). A generic health status instrument in the assessment of rheumatoid arthritis. *British Journal of Rheumatology*, 31: 87–90.

Fletcher, A., McLoone, P. and Bulpitt, C. (1988). Quality of life on angina therapy: a randomized controlled trial of transdermal glyceryl trinitrate against placebo. *Lancet*, 2: 4–8.

Fortinsky, R.H., Granger, C.V. and Selzer, G.B. (1981). The use of functional assessment in understanding home care needs. *Medical Care*, 19: 489–97.

Francis, D. (1984). *Will You Still Need Me, Will You Still Feed Me, When I'm 84?* Bloomington, IN: Indiana University Press.

Freemantle, N., Long, A., Mason, J. *et al.* (1993). The treatment of depression in primary care. *Effective Health Care*, 5 (whole issue).

Fries, J.F. (1983). The assessment of disability: from first to future principles. Paper presented at conference Advances in Assessing Arthritis held at the London Hospital, March (mimeo).

Fries, J.F., Hess, E.V. and Klinenberg, J. (1974). A standard database for rheumatic disease. *Arthritis and Rheumatism*, 17: 327–36.

Fries, J.F., Spitz, P.W. and Young, D.Y. (1982). The dimensions of health outcomes: the Health Assessment Questionnaire, disability and pain scales. *Journal of Rheumatology*, 9: 789–93.

Fries, J.F., Spitz, P.W., Kraines, R.G. and Holman, H.R. (1980). Measurement of patient outcome in arthritis. *Arthritis and Rheumatism*, 23: 137–45.

Frisch, M.B., Cornell, J., Villanueva, M. and Retzlaff, P.J. (1992). Clinical validation of the Quality of Life Inventory, A measure of life satisfaction for use in treatment planning and outcome assessment. *Psychological Assessment*, 4: 92–101.

Gallagher, D., Nies, G. and Thompson, L.W. (1982). Reliability of the Beck Depression Inventory with older adults. *Journal of Consulting and Clinical Psychology*, 50: 152–3.

Garratt, A.M., Ruta, D.A., Abdalla, M.I. *et al.* (1993). The SF-36 health survey questionnaire: an outcome measure suitable for routine use within the NHS? *British Medical Journal*, 306: 1440–4.

Garratt, A.M., Ruta, D.A., Abdalla, M.I., Russell, I.T. (1994). SF-36 health survey questionnaire: II. Responsiveness to changes in health status in four common clinical conditions. *Quality in Health Care*, 3: 186–92.

Gatz, M., Pederson, N.L. and Harris, J. (1987). Measurement characteristics of the mental health scale from the OARS. *Journal of Gerontology*, 42: 332–5.

George, L.K. (1979). The happiness syndrome: methodological and substantive issues in the study of psychological well-being in adulthood. *Gerontologist*, 19: 210–16.

George, L.K. and Bearon, L.B. (1980). *Quality of Life in Older Persons: Meaning and Measurement*. New York: Human Sciences Press.

George, L.K., Blazer, D.G., Hughes, D.C. *et al.* (1989). Social support and the outcome of major depression. *British Journal of Psychiatry*, 154: 478–85.

Gibbons, R.D., Clark, D.C. and Kupfer, D.J. (1993). Exactly what does the Hamilton Depression Rating Scale measure? *Journal of Psychiatric Research*, 27: 259–73.

Gill, T.M. (1995). Quality of life assessment: values and pitfalls. *Journal of the Royal Society of Medicine*, 88: 680–2.

Gill, T.M. and Feinstein, A.R. (1994). A critical appraisal of the quality of quality-of-life measurements. *Journal of the American Medical Association*, 272: 619–26.

Gilson, B.S., Bergner, M., Bobbitt, R.A. *et al.* (1979). *The Sickness Impact Profile: Final Development and Testing: 1975–1978*. Seattle, WA: University of Washington Press.

Glass, T.A. and Maddox, G.L. (1992). The quality and quantity of social support: stroke recovery as psychosocial transition. *Social Science and Medicine*, 34: 1249–61.

Goldberg, D.P. (1978). *Manual of the General Health Questionnaire*. Windsor: NFER-NELSON.

Goldberg, D.P. (1985). Identifying psychiatric illness among general medical patients. *British Medical Journal*, 291: 161–3.

Goldberg, D.P. and Huxley, P. (1980). *Mental Illness in the Community: The Pathway to Psychiatric Care*. London: Tavistock.

Goldberg, D.P. and Williams, P. (1988). *A user's guide to the General Health Questionnaire*. Windsor: NFER-NELSON.

Goldberg, E.M. and Connelly, N. (1982). *The Effectiveness of Social Care for the Elderly*. London, Heinemann.

Goldstein, M.S., Siegel, J.M. and Boyer, R. (1984). Predicting changes in perceived health status. *American Journal of Public Health*, 74: 611–15.

Gompertz, P., Pound, P. and Ebrahim, S. (1993a). The reliability of stroke outcome measurement. *Clinical Rehabilitation*, 7: 290–6.

Gompertz, P., Pound, P. and Ebrahim, S. (1993b). *Kudo: A Kit for Describing the Outcome of Stroke*. London: Department of Public Health, Royal Free Hospital Medical School.

Goodchild, M.E. and Duncan Jones, P. (1985). Chronicity and the General Health Questionnaire. *British Journal of Psychiatry*, 146: 55–61.

Gough, I.R., Furnival, C.M., Schilder, L. *et al.* (1983). Assessment of the quality of life of patients with advanced cancer. *European Journal of Cancer and Clinical Oncology*, 19: 1161–5.

Graham, C., Bond, S.S., Gerkovich, M.M. *et al.* (1980). Use of the McGill pain questionnaire in the assessment of cancer pain: reliability and consistency. *Pain*, 6: 377.

Granger, C.V. (1982). Health accounting – functional assessment of the long term patient in F.J. Kottke, G.K. Stillwell and J.F. Lehmann (eds) *Krusen's Handbook of*

Physical Medicine and Rehabilitation, 3rd edn. Philadelphia, PA: W.B. Saunders.

Granger, C.V., Albrecht, G.L. and Hamilton, B.B. (1979). Outcome of comprehensive medical rehabilitation: measurement by PULSES profile and the Barthel Index. *Archives of Physical Medicine and Rehabilitation*, 60: 145–54.

Granger, C.V. and McNamara, M.A. (1984). Functional assessment utilization: the long-range evaluation system (LRES), in C.V. Granger and G.E. Gresham (eds) *Functional Assessment in Rehabilitation Medicine*. Baltimore, MD: Williams & Williams.

Grant, C.R.H. (1966). Age differences in self-concept from early adulthood through old age. Dissertation from the University of Nebraska.

Grasbeck, R. and Saris, N.E. (1969). Establishment and use of normal values. *Scandinavian Journal of Clinical and Laboratory Investigation*, Supplement no. 110: 62–3.

Greenblatt, H.N. (1975). *Measurement of Social Well-being in a General Population Survey*. Berkeley, CA: Human Population Laboratory, California State Department of Health.

Greenblatt, M.Y., Becerra, R.M. and Serafetinides, E.A. (1982). Social networks and mental health: an overview. *American Journal of Psychiatry*, 139: 977–84.

Greenwald, H.P. (1987). The specificity of quality of life measures among the seriously ill. *Medical Care*, 25: 642–51.

Gurin, G., Veroff, J. and Feld, S. (1960). *Americans View their Mental Health*. New York: Basic Books.

Gurland, B.J. (1980). The assessment of the mental health status of older adults, in J.E. Birren and R.B. Sloane (eds) *Handbook of Mental Health and Ageing*. Englewood Cliffs, NJ: Prentice-Hall.

Gurland, B.J., Copeland, J.R.M., Kelleher, M.J. *et al.* (1983). *The Mind and Mood of Ageing: The Mental Health Problems of the Community Elderly in New York and London*. London: Croom Helm.

Gurland, B.J., Golden, R.R., Teresi, J.A. and Challop, J. (1984). The SHORT-CARE: An efficient instrument for the assessment of depression, dementia and disability. *Journal of Gerontology*, 39: 166–9.

Gurtman, M.B. (1985). Self-rating Depression Scale in D.J. Keyser and R.C. Sweetland (eds) *Test Critiques*, vol. III. Kansas City, MO: Test Corporation of America.

Guttman, L. (1944). A basis for scaling qualitative data. *American Sociological Review*, 9: 139.

Guyatt, G.H., Nogradi, S., Halcrow, S. *et al.* (1989). Development and testing of a new measure of health status for clinical trials in heart failure. *Journal of General Internal Medicine*, 4: 101–7.

Haber, L.D. (1968). *Prevalence of Disability among Non-institutionalized Adults under Age 65: 1966 Survey of Disabled Adults*, Research and Statistics Note no. 4. US

Department of Health Education and Welfare, Office of Research and Statistics .

Hall, J., Hall, N., Fisher, E. *et al.* (1987). Measurement of outcomes of general practice: comparison of three health status measures. *Family Practice*, 4: 117–23.

Hall, R., Horrocks, J.C., Clamp, S.E. *et al.* (1976). Observer variation in assessment of results of surgery for peptic ulceration. *British Medical Journal*, i: 814–16.

Hamer, D., Sanjeev, D., Butterworth, E. and Barzak, P. (1991). Using the Hospital Anxiety and Depression Scale to screen for psychiatric disorders in people presenting with deliberate self-harm. *British Journal of Psychiatry*, 158: 782–4.

Hamilton, M. (1959). The assessment of anxiety states by rating. *British Journal of Medical Psychology*, 32: 50–5.

Hamilton, M. (1960). Rating scale for depression, *Journal of Neurology, Neurosurgery and Psychiatry*, 23: 56–62.

Hamilton, M. (1967). Development of a rating scale for primary depressive illness. *British Journal of Social and Clinical Psychology*, 6: 278–96.

Hamilton, M. (1976). Clinical evaluation of depression: clinical criteria and rating scales, including a Guttman Scale, in M. Gallant and G.M. Simpson (eds) *Depression: Behavioral, Biochemical Diagnostic and Treatment Concepts*. New York: Spectrum Publications.

Hammen, C.L. (1981). Assessment: a clinical and cognitive emphasis in L.P. Rehm (ed.) *Behaviour Therapy for Depression: Present Status and Future Directions*. New York: Academic Press.

Harman, H.H. (1976). *Modern Factor Analysis*. Chicago, IL: University of Chicago Press.

Harris, L. (1975). *The Myth and Reality of Ageing in America*. Washington, DC: National Council on the Ageing.

Hart, G.L. and Evans, R.W. (1987). The functional status of ESRD patients as measured by the Sickness Impact Profile. *Journal of Chronic Diseases*, 40: 117S–130S (Supplement).

Health Outcomes Institute (1990). Report on a Survey of Elderly Rural Residents: Health Status, Use of Health Care Services and Satisfaction with Quality of Care. Bloomington, IN: HOI.

Heasman, M.A. and Lipworth, L. (1966). *Accuracy of Certification of Cause of Death*. London: General Register Office. Studies on Medical and Population Subjects no. 20.

Henderson, A.S., Duncan Jones, P. and Finlay-Jones, R.A. (1983). The reliability of the Geriatric Mental State Examination. *Acta Psychiatrica Scandinavica*, 67: 281–9.

Henderson, S. (1981). Social relationships, adversity and neurosis: an analysis of prospective observations. *British Journal of Psychiatry*, 138: 391–8.

Henderson, S., Byrne, D.G. and Duncan Jones, P.

(1981a). *Neurosis and the Social Environment*. London: Academic Press.

Henderson, S., Duncan Jones, P., Byrne, D.G. and Scott, R. (1980). Measuring social relationships: the Interview Schedule for Social Interaction. *Psychological Medicine*, 10: 723–34.

Henderson, S., Lewis, I.C., Howell, R.H. *et al.* (1981b). Mental health and the use of alcohol, tobacco, analgesics and vitamins in a secondary school population. *Acta Psychiatrica Scandinavica*, 63: 186–9.

Herron, M.K., Michaux, W.W., Katz, M.M. *et al.* (1964). *Supplemental Instructions for the Administration of the Katz Adjustment Scales*. Baltimore, MD: Spring Grove State Hospital, Research Department.

Hill, S. and Harries, U. (1994). Assessing the outcome of health care for the older person in community settings: should we use the SF-36? *Outcomes Briefing*. UK Clearing House for Health Outcomes, 4: 26–7.

Hinterberger, W., Gadner, H., Hocker, P. *et al.* (1987). Survival and quality of life in 23 patients with severe aplastic anaemia treated with BMT. *Blut*, 54: 137–46.

Hirsch, B.J. (1980). Natural support systems and coping with major life changes. *American Journal of Community Psychology*, 8: 159–72.

Hirsch, B.J. (1981). Social networks and the coping process: creating personal communities, in B.H. Gottlieb (ed.) *Social Networks and Social Support*. Beverly Hills, CA: Sage Publications.

Hobbs, P., Ballinger, C.B., Greenwood, C. *et al.* (1984). Factor analysis and validation of the General Health Questionnaire in men: a general practice survey. *British Journal of Psychiatry*, 144: 270–5.

Hobbs, P., Ballinger, C.B. and Smith, A.H.W. (1983). Factor analysis and validation of the General Health Questionnaire in women: a general practice survey. *British Journal of Psychiatry*, 142: 257–64.

Hodkinson, H.M. (1972). Evaluation of a mental test score for the assessment of mental impairment in the elderly. *Age and Ageing*, 1: 233–8.

Hoffmeister, J.K. (1976). *Some Information Regarding the Characteristics of the Two Measures Developed from the Self-Esteem Questionnaire (SEQ-3)*. Boulder, CO: Test Analysis and Development Corporation.

Holahan, C.J. and Moos, R.H. (1981). Social support and psychological distress: a longitudinal analysis. *Journal of Abnormal Psychology*, 90: 365–70.

House, J.S. (1981). *Work, Stress and Social Support*. Reading, MA: Addison-Wesley.

House, J.S. and Kahn, R.L. (1985). Measures and concepts of social support, in S. Cohen and S.L. Syme (eds) *Social Support and Health*. Orlando, FL: Academic Press.

House, J.S., Robbins, C. and Metzner, H.L. (1982). The association of social relationships and activities with mortality: prospective evidence from the Tecumseh

Community Health Study. *American Journal of Epidemiology*, 116: 123–40.

Hoyt, D.R. and Creech, J.C. (1983). The life satisfaction index: a methodological and theoretical critique. *Journal of Gerontology*, 38: 111–16.

Hoyt, D.R., Kaiser, M., Peters, G. *et al.* (1980). Life satisfaction and activity theory: a multidimensional approach. *Journal of Gerontology*, 35: 935–41.

Hunt, S.M. (1984). Nottingham Health Profile, in N.K. Wenger, M.E. Mattson, C.D. Furberg *et al.* (eds) *Assessment of quality of life in clinical trials of cardiovascular therapies*. New York: Le Jacq.

Hunt, S.M. (1986). Measuring health in clinical care and clinical trials, in G. Teeling Smith (ed.) *Measuring health: a practical approach*. Chichester: John Wiley.

Hunt, S.M. (1988). Subjective health indicators and health promotion. *Health Promotion*, 3: 23–34.

Hunt, S.M. and McKenna, S.P. (1993). Measuring patients' views of their health. SF-36 misses the mark (letter). *British Medical Journal*, 307: 125.

Hunt, S.M., McEwan, J., McKenna, S.P. *et al.* (1984a). Subjective health assessments and the perceived outcome of minor surgery. *Journal of Psychosomatic Research*, 28: 105–14.

Hunt, S.M., McEwan, J. and McKenna, S.P. (1984b). Perceived health: age and sex comparisons in a community. *Journal of Epidemiology and Community Health*, 34: 281–6.

Hunt, S.M., McEwan, J. and McKenna, S.P. (1986). *Measuring Health Status*. London: Croom Helm.

Hunt, S.M., McKenna, S.P. and Williams, J. (1981). Reliability of a population survey tool for measuring perceived health problems: a study of patients with osteoarthritis. *Journal of Epidemiology and Community Health*, 35: 297–300.

Hunt, S.M., McKenna, S.P., McEwan, J. *et al.* (1980). A quantitative approach to perceived health status: a validation study. *Journal of Epidemiology and Community Health*, 34: 281–6.

Huppert, F.A. and Garcia, A.W. (1991). Qualitative differences in psychiatric symptoms between high risk groups assessed on a screening test (GHQ-30). *Social Psychiatry and Psychiatric Epidemiology*, 26: 252–8.

Hutchinson, T.A., Boyd, N.F. and Feinstein, A.R. (1979). Scientific problems in clinical scales as demonstrated in the Karnofsky index of performance status. *Journal of Chronic Diseases*, 32: 661–6.

Hyland, M.E. and Kenyon, P. (1992). A measure of positive health-related quality of life: the Satisfaction with Illness Scale. *Psychological Reports*, 71: 1137–8.

Inglehart, R. and Rabier, J.R. (1986). Aspirations adapt to situations – but why are the Belgians so much happier than the French? A cross-cultural analysis of the subjective quality of life, in F.M. Andrews (ed.) *Research on the quality of life*. Michigan: Survey Research Center, Institute for Social Research, University of Michigan.

Isaacs, B. and Walkey, P.A. (1964). Measurement of mental impairment in geriatric pratice. *Gerontology Clinics*, 6: 114–23.

Jachuck, S.J., Brierly, H., Jachuk, S. *et al.* (1982). The effect of hypotensive drugs on the quality of life. *Journal of the Royal College of General Practitioners*, 32: 103–5.

Jenkinson, C., Coulter, A. and Wright, L. (1993). Short Form-36 (SF-36) health survey questionnaire: Normative data for adults of working age. *British Medical Journal*, 306: 1437–40.

Jenkinson, C., Fitzpatrick, R. and Argyle, M. (1988). The Nottingham Health Profile: an analysis of its sensitivity in differentiating illness groups. *Social Science and Medicine*, 27: 1411–14.

Jette, A.M. (1980). The Functional Status Index: Reliability of a chronic disease evaluation instrument. *Archives of Physical Medicine and Rehabilitation*, 61: 395–401.

Jitapunkul, S., Pillay, I. and Ebrahim, S. (1991). The Abbreviated Mental Test: its use and validity. *Age and Ageing*, 20: 332–6.

Jones, D.A., Victor, C.R. and Vetter, N.J. (1985). The problem of loneliness in the elderly in the community: characteristics of those who are lonely and the factors related to the loneliness. *Journal of the Royal College of General Practitioners*, 35: 136–9.

Julious, S.A., George, S. and Campbell, J. (1995). Sample sizes for studies using the short form 36 (SF-36). *Journal of Epidemiology and Community Health*, 49: 642–4.

Kahn, R.L., Goldfarb, A.I., Pollack, M. *et al.* (1960a). The relationship of mental and physical status in institutionalized aged persons. *American Journal of Psychiatry*, 117: 120–4.

Kahn, R.L., Goldfarb, A.I., Pollack, M. *et al.* (1960b). Brief objective measures for the determination of mental status in the aged. *American Journal of Psychiatry*, 117: 326–8.

Kalra, L. and Crome, P. (1993). The role of prognostic scores in targeting stroke rehabilitation in elderly patients. *Journal of the American Geriatrics Society*, 41: 396–400.

Kalson, C. (1976). MASH – a program of social interaction between institutionalised aged and adult mentally retarded persons. *The Gerontologist*, 16: 340–8.

Kammann, R. and Flett, R. (1983). Affectometer 2: a scale to measure current level of general happiness. *Australian Journal of Psychology*, 35: 259–65.

Kaplan, B.H. (1975). An epilogue: toward further research on family and health, in B.H. Kaplan and J.C. Cassel (eds) *Family and Health: An Epidemiological Approach*. Chapel Hill, NC: University of North Carolina, Institute for Research and Social Science.

Kaplan, G.A. and Camacho, T. (1983). Perceived health and mortality: a nine-year follow-up of the Human Population Laboratory Cohort. *American Journal of Epidemiology*, 117: 292–8.

Kaplan, H.B. and Porkorny, A.D. (1969). Self derogation and psychosocial adjustment. *Journal of Nervous and Mental Disease*, 149: 421–34.

Kaplan, R. (1985). Social support and social health, in I. Saranson and B. Saranson (eds) *Social Support Theory, Research and Application*. The Hague: Nijhoff.

Kaplan, R.M. (1988). New health promotion indicators: the general health policy model. *Health Promotion*, 3: 35–48.

Kaplan, R.M. (1994). Using quality of life information to set priorities in health policy. *Social Indicators Research*, 33: 121–63.

Kaplan, R.M. and Bush, J.W. (1982). Health-related quality of life measurement for evaluation research analysis. *Health Psychology*, 1: 61–80.

Kaplan, R.M. and Ernst, J.A. (1983). Do category rating scales produce biased preference weights for a health index? *Medical Care*, 21: 193–207.

Kaplan, R.M., Bush, J.W. and Berry, C.C. (1976). Health status: types of validity and the Index of Wellbeing. *Health Services Research*, 11: 478–507.

Kaplan, R.M., Bush, J.W. and Berry, C.C. (1978). The reliability, stability and generalizability of a health status index. American Statistical Association, *Proceedings of the Social Statistics Section*, 704–9.

Kaplan, R.M., Bush, J.W. and Berry, C.C. (1979). Health Status Index: category rating versus magnitude estimation for measuring levels of well-being. *Medical Care*, 17: 501–23.

Kaplan, R.M., Anderson, J.P., Patterson, T.L. *et al.* (1995). Validity of the Quality of Well-Being Scale for persons with human immunodeficiency virus infection. *Psychosomatic Medicine*, 57: 138–47.

Kaplan, R.M., McCutchan, J.A., Navarro, A.M. *et al.* (1994). Quality adjusted survival analysis: a neglected application of the quality of well-being scale. *Psychology and Health*, 9: 131–41.

Karnofsky, D.A., Abelmann, W.H., Craver, L.F. *et al.* (1948). The use of nitrogen mustards in the palliative treatment of carcinoma. *Cancer*, I: 634–56.

Kasl, S.V. and Cooper, C.L. (1987). *Stress and Health Issues in Research Methodology*. Chichester: John Wiley.

Kaszniak, A.W. and Allender, J. (1985). Psychological assessment of depression in older adults, in G.M. Chaisson-Stewart (ed.) *Depression in the elderly: an interdisciplinary approach*. New York: John Wiley.

Katz, J.N., Larson, M.G., Phillips, C.B. *et al.* (1992). Comparative measurement sensitivity of short and longer health status instruments. *Medical Care*, 30: 917–25.

Katz, S. and Akpom, C.A. (1976). Index of ADL. *Medical Care*, 14: 116–18.

Katz, S., Akpom, C.A., Papsidero, J.A. *et al.* (1973). Measuring the health status of populations, in R.L. Berg (ed.) *Health Status of Populations*. Chicago, IL: Hospital Research and Educational Trust.

Katz, S., Downs, T.D., Cash, H.R. *et al.* (1970). Progress in the development of and index of ADL. *Gerontologist*, 10: 20–30.

Katz, S., Ford, A.B., Chinn, A.B. *et al.* (1966). Prognosis after strokes: long-term course of 159 patients with stroke. *Medicine*, 45: 236–46.

Katz, S., Ford, A.B., Moskowitz, R.W. *et al.* (1963). Studies of illness in the aged: the index of ADL – a standardized measure of biological and psychosocial function. *Journal of the American Medical Association*, 185: 914–19.

Katz, S., Vignos, P.J., Moskowitz, R.W. *et al.* (1968). Comprehensive outpatient care in rheumatoid arthritis: a controlled study. *Journal of the American Medicine Association*, 206: 1249.

Kaufman, A.V. (1990). Social network assessment: a critical component in case management for functionally impaired older persons. *International Journal of Ageing and Human Development*, 30: 63–75.

Kay, D.W.K., Beamish, R. and Roth, M. (1964). Old age mental disorders in Newcastle upon Tyne, Part I: a study of prevalence. *British Journal of Psychiatry*, 110: 146–58.

Kazis, L.E., Anderson, J.J. and Meenan, R.F. (1988). Health status information in clinical practice: the development and testing of patient profile reports. *Journal of Rheumatology*, 15: 338–44.

Kazis, L.E., Meenan, R.F. and Anderson, J.J. (1983). Pain in the rheumatic diseases: investigation of a key health status component. *Arthritis and Rheumatism*, 26: 1017–22.

Kearns, N.P., Cruickshank, C.A. and McGuigan, K.J. *et al.* (1982). A comparison of depression rating scales. *British Journal of Psychiatry*, 141: 45–9.

Kelley, T.L. (1927). *Interpretation of Educational Measurements*. Yonkers: World Books.

Kind, P. (undated). Scaling the Nottingham Health Profile. Mimeo. York: University of York, Centre for Health Economics.

Kind, P. and Carr-Hill, R. (1987). The Nottingham Health Profile: a useful tool for epidemiologists? *Social Science and Medicine*, 25: 905–10.

Kirwan, R.J. and Reeback, J.S. (1983). Using a modified Stanford Health Assessment Questionnaire to assess disability in UK patients with rheumatoid arthritis. *Annals of the Rheumatic Diseases*, 42: 219–20.

Knapp, M.R.J. (1976). Predicting the dimensions of life satisfaction. *Journal of Gerontology*, 31: 595–604.

Knesevich, J.W., Biggs, J.T., Clayton, P.J. and Ziegler,

V.E. (1977). Validity of the Hamilton rating scale for depression. *British Journal of Psychiatry*, 131:49–52.

Knight, R.G., Waal-Manning, H.J. and Spears, G.F. (1983). Some norms and reliability data for the State-Trait Anxiety Inventory and the Zung Self-Rating Depression Scale. *British Journal of Clinical Psychology*, 22: 245–9.

Kohn, M.L. (1969). *Class and Conformity: a Study in Values*. Homewood, IL: Dorsey.

Kokenes, B. (1974). Grade level differences in factors of self esteem. *Development Psychology*, 10: 954–8.

Korner, A., Nielsen, B.M., Eschen, F. *et al.* (1990). Quantifying depressive symptomatology: inter-rater and inter-item correlations. *Journal of Affective Disorders*, 20: 140–9.

Kozma, A. and Stones, M.J. (1987). Social desirability in measures of subjective well-being: a systematic evaluation. *Journal of Gerontology*, 42: 56–9.

Kovacs, M. and Beck, A.T. (1977). An empirical–clinical approach toward a definition of childhood depression, in J.G. Schulterbrandt and A. Raskin (eds) *Depression in Childhood: Diagnosis, Treatment and Conceptual Models*. New York: Raven Press.

Kurtin, P.S., Davies, A.R., Meyer, K.B. *et al.* (1992). Patient-based health status measurements in outpatient dialysis: Early experiences in developing an outcomes assessment program. *Medical Care*, 30: MS136–MS149 (suppl. 5).

Kushman, J. and Lane, S. (1980). A multivariate analysis of factors affecting perceived life satisfaction and psychological well-being among the elderly. *Social Science Quarterly*, 61: 264–77.

Kutner, B., Fansel, D., Togo, A.M. *et al.* (1956). *Five Hundred over 60*. New York: Russell Sage.

Kutner, N.G., Fair, P.L. and Kutner, M.H. (1985). Assessing depression and anxiety in chronic dialysis patients. *Journal of Psychosomatic Research*, 29: 23–31.

Lamb, K.L., Brodie, D.A. and Roberts, K. (1988). Physical fitness and health-related fitness as indicators of a positive health state. *Health Promotion*, 3: 171–82.

Landgraf, J.M. and Nelson, E.C. (1992). Summary of the WONCA/COOP international health assessment field trial. *Australian Family Physician*, 21: 255–69.

Landgraf, J.M., Nelson, E.C., Hays, R.D. *et al.* (1990). Assessing function: does it really make a difference? A preliminary evaluation of the acceptability and utility of the COOP function charts, in M. Lipkin (ed.) *Functional status measurement in primary care*. New York: Springer-Verlag.

Langius, A. (1995). Quality of life in a group of patients with oral and pharyngeal cancer. Sense of coherence, functional status and well-being. Stockholm, Department of Medicine, Centre of Caring Sciences North, Karolinska Institute.

Langius, A., Björvell, H. and Antonovsky, A. (1992). The sense of coherence concept and its relation to personality traits in Swedish samples. *Scandinavian Journal of Caring Science*, 6: 165–71.

Langius, A., Björvell, H. and Lind, M. (1994). Functional status and coping in patients with oral and pharyngeal cancer before and after surgery. *Head and Neck*, 16: 559–68.

Larson, R. (1978). Thirty years of research on the subjective well-being of older Americans. *Journal of Gerontology*, 33: 109–25.

Lawton, M.P. (1972). The dimensions of morale, in D. Kent, R. Kastenbaum and S. Sherwood (eds) *Research, Planning and Action for the Elderly*. New York: Behavioral Publications.

Lawton, M.P. (1975). The Philadelphia Geriatric Center Morale Scale: a revision. *Journal of Gerontology*, 30: 85–9.

Leff, J. (ed). (1993). The TAPS project: evaluating community placement of long stay psychiatric patients. *British Journal of Psychiatry*, 162: 1–56 (suppl. 19).

Leff, J. O'Driscoll, C., Dayson, D. *et al.* (1990). The TAPS project: V. The structure of social network data obtained from long-stay patients. *British Journal of Psychiatry*, 157: 848–52.

Lehman, A. (1983). The well-being of chronic mental patients. *Archives of General Psychiatry*, 40: 369–73.

Leighton, A.H. (1959). *My Name is Legion: Foundations for a Theory of Man in Relation to Culture*. New York: Basic Books.

Leighton Read, J., Quinn, R.J. and Hoefer, M.A. (1987). Measuring overall health: an evaluation of three important approaches. *Journal of Chronic Diseases*, 40: Supplement 1: 7S–21S.

Lerner, M. (1973). Conceptualization of health and well-being. *Health Services Research*, 8: 6–12.

Levine, M.N., Guyatt, G.H., Gent, M. *et al.* (1988). Quality of life in stage II breast cancer: An instrument for clinical trials. *Journal of Clinical Oncology*, 6: 1798–1810.

Lewis, G. and Wessely, S. (1990). Comparison of the General Health Questionnaire and the Hospital Anxiety and Depression Scale. *British Journal of Psychiatry*, 157: 860–4.

Liang, J. (1984). Dimensions of the life satisfaction Index A: a structural formation. *Journal of Gerontology*, 39: 613–22.

Liang, J. and Bollen, K.A. (1983). The structure of the Philadelphia Center Morale Scale: a reinterpretation. *Journal of Gerontology*, 30: 77–84.

Liang, M.H., Larson, M., Cullen, K. and Schwartz, J. (1995). Comparative measurement efficiency and sensitivity of five health status instruments for arthritis research. *Arthritis and Rheumatism*, 28: 524–47.

Liddle, J., Gilleard, C. and Neil, A. (1993). Elderly patients' and their relatives' views on CPR (letter). *Lancet*, 342: 1055.

Liem, G.R. and Liem, J.H. (1978). Social support and stress. Some general issues and their application to the problems of unemployment. Unpublished manuscript. Boston College and University of Massachusetts.

Likert, R. (1952). A technique for the development of attitude scales. *Educational and Psychological Measurement*, 12: 313–15.

Lin, N., Simeone, R., Ensel, W. *et al.* (1979). Social support, stressful life events and illness, a model and an empirical test. *Journal of Health and Social Behaviour*, 20: 108–19.

Linzer, M., Pontinen, M., Gold, D. *et al.* (1991). Impairment of physical and psychological function in recurrent syncope. *Journal of Clinical Epidemiology*, 44: 1037–43.

Little, A., Hemsley, D., Bergman, K. *et al.* (1987). Comparison of the sensitivity of three instruments for the detection of cognitive decline in the elderly living at home. *British Journal of Psychiatry*, 150: 808–14.

Lohmann, N. (1977). Correlations of life satisfaction, morale and adjustment measures. *Journal of Gerontology*, 32: 73–5.

Love, A., Loeboeuf, D.C. and Crisp, T.C. (1989). Chiropractic chronic low back pain sufferers and self-report assessment methods. Part 1. A reliability study of the Visual Analogue Scale, the pain drawing and the McGill pain Questionnaire. *Journal of Manipulative and Physiological Therapeutics*, 12: 21–25.

Lowe, D.J. (1975). *The Cornell Indices: A Bibliography of Health Questionnaires*. New York: Cornell University Medical College Library, Reference and Information Services.

Lowe, N.K., Walker, S.N. and McCallum, R.C. (1991) Confirming the theoretical structure of the McGill Pain Questionnaire in acute clinical pain. *Pain*, 46: 53–60.

Lowenthal, M.F. and Haven, C. (1968). Interaction and adaptation: intimacy as a critical variable. *American Sociological Review*, 33: 20–30.

McColl, E., Steen, I.N., Meadows, K.A. *et al.* (1995). Developing outcome measures for ambulatory care – an application to asthma and diabetes. Special Issue 'Quality of Life' in *Social Science and Medicine*, 10: 1339–48.

McCormick, I.A., Siegert, R.J. and Walkey, F.H. (1987). The dimensions of social support: a factorial confirmation. *American Journal of Community Psychology*, 15: 73–7.

McDowell, I. and Newell, C. (1987). *Measuring Health: A Guide to Rating Scales and Questionnaires*. New York: Oxford University Press.

McFarlane, A.H., Neale, K.A., Norman, G. *et al.* (1981). Methodological issues in developing a scale to measure social support. *Schizophrenia Bulletin*, 7: 90–100.

McGuire, B. and Tinsley, H.E.A. (1981). A contribution to the construct validity of the Tennessee Self-Concept Scale: a confirmatory factor analysis. *Applied Psychological Measurement*, 5: 449–57.

McHorney, C.A., Ware, J.E. and Raczek, A.E. (1993). The MOS 36-Item Short Form Health Survey (SF-36): II. Psychometric and clinical tests of validity in measuring physical and mental health constructs. *Medical Care*, 31: 247–63.

McHorney, C.A., Ware, J.E., Rogers, W. *et al.* (1992). The validity and relative precision of MOS short- and long-form health status scales and Dartmouth COOP Charts: results from the medical outcomes study. *Medical Care*, 30: MS253–MS265.

McKenna, S.P., Hunt, S.M. and McEwan, J. (1981). Weighting the seriousness of perceived health problems using Thurstone's method of paired comparisons. *International Journal of Epidemiology*, 10: 93–7.

McKenna, S.P., McEwan, J., Hunt, S.M. *et al.* (1984). Changes in the perceived health of patients recovering from fractures. *Public Health*, 98: 97–102.

McKennell, A.C. (1978). Cognitive and affect in perceptions of well-being. *Social Indicators Research*, 5: 389–426.

McMurdo, M.E.T. and Rennie, L. (1993). A controlled trail of exercise by residents of old people's homes. *Age and Ageing*, 22: 11–15.

McNab, A. and Phillip, A.S. (1980). Screening an elderly population for psychological well-being. *Health Bulletin*, 160–5.

McNaughton, M.J. and Wiklund, I. (1993). A critical review of dimension-specific measures of health-related quality of life in cross-cultural research. *Quality of Life Research*, 2: 397–432.

McNeil, B.J., Weichselbaum, R. and Pauker, S.G. (1978). Fallacy of the five year survival in lung cancer. *New England Journal of Medicine*, 299: 1397–401.

McNeil, B.J., Weichselbaum, R. and Pauker, S.G. (1981). Speech and Survival: tradeoffs between quality and quantity of life in laryngeal cancer. *New England Journal of Medicine*, 305: 982–7.

McPeek, B. and McPeek, A. (1984). Formen der Wiedergabe der Lebensqualitat in Klinischen Studien, in H. Rohde and H. Troidl (eds) *Das Magenkarzinom: Methodik Klinischer Studien und therapeutischer Ansatze*. New York: Georg Thieme Verlag.

McQuay, H.J. (1990). Assessment of pain, and effectiveness of treatment, in A. Hopkins and D. Costain (eds) *Measuring the Outcomes of Medical Care*. London: Royal College of Physicians.

McWhirter, B.T. (1990). Factor analysis of the Revised UCLA Loneliness Scale. *Current Psychology Research and Reviews*, 9: 56–68.

McWilliam, C., Copeland, J.R.M., Dewey, M.E. *et al.* (1988). The geriatric mental state examination as a case finding instrument in the community. *British Journal of Psychiatry*, 152: 205–8.

Maes, S., Vingerhoets, A. and Van Heck, G. (1987). The study of stress and disease: some developments and requirements. *Social Science and Medicine*, 25: 567–78.

Magne, I.U., Ojehagen, A. and Traskman, B.L. (1992). The social network of people who attempt suicide. *Acta Psychiatrica Scandinavica*, 86: 153–8.

Mahon, N.E. and Yarcheski, A. (1990). The dimensionality of the UCLA Loneliness Scale in early adolescents. *Research in Nursing and Health*, 13: 45–52.

Mahoney, F.I. and Barthel, D.W. (1965). Functional evaluation: the Barthel Index. *Maryland State Medical Journal*, 14: 61–5.

Mangione, C.M., Marcantonio, E.R., Goldman, L. *et al.* (1993). Influence of age on measurement of health status in patients undergoing elective surgery. *Journal of the American Geriatrics Society*, 41: 377–83.

Mari, J.D.J. and Williams, P. (1985). A comparison of the validity of two psychiatric screening questionnaires (GHQ-12 and SRQ-20) in Brazil, using relative operating characteristics (ROC) analysis. *Psychological Medicine*, 15: 651–9.

Martin, A.J. (1987). Patients and presentation: a profile from general practice. *Modern Medicine*, April: 14–18.

Mason, J.H., Anderson, J.J. and Meenan, R.F. (1988). A model for health status for rheumatoid arthritis: a factor analysis of the Arthritis Impact Measurement Scales. *Arthritis and Rheumatism*, 31: 714–20.

Mattison, P.G., Aitken, R.C.B. and Prescot, R.J. (1991). Rehabilitation status – the relationship between the Edinburgh Rehabilitation Status Scale (ERSS), Barthel Index and PULSES Profile. *International Disability Studies*, 13: 9–11.

Mauskopf, J., Austin, R., Dix. L. *et al.* (1994). The Nottingham Health Profile as a measure of quality of life in zoster patients: convergent and discriminant validity. *Quality of Life Research*, 3: 431–5.

Medical Outcomes Trust (1993). *How to score the SF-36 Health Survey*. Boston, MA: Medical Outcomes Trust.

Meenan, R.F. (1982). The AIMS approach to health status measurement: conceptual background and measurement properties. *Journal of Rheumatology*, 9: 785–8.

Meenan, R.F. (1985). New approaches to outcome assessment: the AIMS questionnaire for arthritis, in G.H. Stollerman (ed.), *Advances in Internal Medicine*, vol. 31. New York: Year Book Medical Publishers.

Meenan, R.F. and Mason, J.H. (1990). *AIMS2 users' guide*. Boston, MA: Boston University School of Medicine, Boston University Arthritis Center and Department of Public Health.

Meenan, R.F. and Mason, J.H. (1994). *AIMS2 users' guide* (revised). Boston, MA: Boston University School of Medicine, Boston University Arthritis Center and Department of Public Health.

Meenan, R.F., Gertman, P.M. and Mason, J.H. (1980). Measuring health status in arthritis: the arthritis impact measurement scales. *Arthritis and Rheumatism*, 23: 146–52.

Meenan, R.F., Anderson, J.J., Kazis, L.E. *et al.* (1984). Outcome assessment in clinical trials: evidence for the sensitivity of a health status measure. *Arthritis and Rheumatism*, 27: 1344–52.

Meenan, R.F., Gertman, P.M., Mason, J.H. *et al.* (1982). The arthritis impact measurement scales: further investigations of a health status measure. *Arthritis and Rheumatism*, 25: 1048–53.

Meenan, R.F., Mason, J.H., Anderson, J.J. *et al.* (1992). AIMS2. The content and properties of a revised and expanded Arthritis Impact Measurement Scales Health status Questionnaires. *Arthritis and Rheumatism*, 35: 1–10.

Mellor, K.S. and Edelmann, R.J. (1988). Mobility, social support, loneliness and well-being amongst two groups of older adults. *Journal of Personality and Individual Differences*, 9: 1–5.

Melzack, R. (1975). The McGill pain questionnaire: major properties and scoring methods. *Pain*, 1: 277–99.

Melzack, R. (1983). *Pain measurement and assessment*. New York: Raven Press.

Melzack, R. (1987). The short-form McGill Pain Questionnaire. *Pain*, 30: 191–7.

Melzack, R. and Katz, J. (1992). The McGill Pain Questionnaire: appraisal and current status, in D.C. Turk and R. Melzack (eds) *Handbook of pain assessment*. New York: The Guilford Press.

Melzack, R. and Torgerson, W.S. (1971). On the language of pain. *Anesthesiology*, 34: 50.

Melzack, R., Terrence, C., Fromm, G. and Amsel, R. (1986). Trigeminal neuralgia and atypical face pain: use of the McGill Pain Questionnaire for discrimination and diagnosis. *Pain*, 27: 297–302.

Mendola, W.F. and Pelligrini, R.V. (1979). Quality of life and coronary artery bypass surgery patients. *Social Science and Medicine*, 13A, 457–61.

Merrell, M. and Harris, L. (1975). *The Myth and Reality of Ageing in America*. Washington, DC: National Council on Ageing.

Merrell, M. and Reed, L.J. (1949). *The Epidemiology of Health, Social Medicine, its Deviations and Objectives*. New York: The Commonwealth Fund.

Messick, S. (1980). Test validity and the ethics of assessment. *American Psychologist*, 35: 1012–27.

Metcalfe, M. and Goldman, E. (1965). Validation of an inventory for measuring depression. *British Journal of Psychiatry*, 111: 240–2.

Meyboom-de Jong, B. and Smith, R.J.A. (1990). Studies with the Dartmouth COOP Charts in general practice: comparison with the Nottingham Health Profile and the General Health Questionnaire, in M. Lipkin (ed.) *Functional status measurement in primary care*. New York: Springer-Verlag.

Miller, I.W., Bishop, S., Norman, W.H. and Maddever, H. (1985). The modified Hamilton Rating Scale for Depression: Reliability and Validity. *Psychiatric Research*, 14: 131–42.

Milne, J.S., Maule, M.M., Cormack, S. et al. (1972). The design and testing of a questionnaire and examination to assess physical and mental health in older people using a staff nurse as the observer. *Journal of Chronic Diseases*, 25: 385–405.

Mitchell, J.C. (1969). The concept and use of social networks, in J.C. Mitchell (ed.) *Social Networks in Urban Situations: Analysis of Personal Relationships in Central African Towns*. Manchester: Manchester University Press.

Mitchell, R.E. and Trickett, E.J. (1980). Social networks as mediators of social support: an analysis of the effects and determinants of social networks. *Community Mental Health Journal*, 16: 27–44.

Monk, M. (1981). Blood pressure awareness and psychological well-being in the Health and Nutrition Examination Survey. *Clinical Investigative Medicine*, 4: 183–9.

Montgomery, S.A. and Asberg, M. (1979). A new depression scale designed to be sensitive to change. *British Journal of Psychiatry*, 134: 382–9.

Montgomery, S.A., Asberg, M., Traskman, L. and Montgomery, D. (1978). Cross cultural studies on the use of the CPRS in English and Swedish depressed patients. *Acta Psychiatrica Scandinavica*, 271: 3–37 (suppl.).

Moorey, S., Greer, S., Watson, M. et al. (1991). The factor structure and factor stability of the Hospital Anxiety and Depression Scale in patients with cancer. *British Journal of Psychiatry*, 158: 255–9.

Moos, R.H. and Moos, B.S. (1981). *Manual for Family Environment Scale*. Palo Alto, CA: Consulting Psychologists Press.

Moos, R.H. and Moos, B.S. (1994). *Family Environment Scale (FES) and Manual* 3rd edn. Palo Alto, CA: Consulting Psychologists Press.

Mor, V. (1987). Cancer patients' quality of life over the disease course: lessons from the real world. *Journal of Chronic Disease*, 40: 535–44.

Mor, V., Laliberte, L., Morris, J.N. et al. (1984). The Karnofsky performance status scale: an examination of its reliability and validity in a research setting. *Cancer*, 53: 2002–7.

Moreno, J.K., Fuhriman, A. and Selby, M.J. (1993). Measurement of hostility, anger, and depression in depressed and non-depressed subjects. *Journal of Personality Assessment*, 61: 511–23.

Morgan, K., Dallosso, H.M., Arie, T. et al. (1987). Mental health and psychological well-being among the old and the very old living at home. *British Journal of Psychiatry*, 150: 801–7.

Moriyama, I.M. (1968). Problems in the measurement of health status, in E.B. Sheldon and W.E. Moore (eds) *Indicators of Social Change*. New York: Russell Sage Foundation.

Morris, J. (1975). Changes in morale experienced by the elderly institutionalized applicants along the institutional path. *Gerontologist*, 15: 345–9.

Morris, J.C.D., Suissa, A., Sherwood, S. et al. (1986). Last days: a study of the quality of life of terminally ill cancer patients. *Journal of Chronic Disease*, 39: 47–62.

Morris, J.N. and Sherwood, S. (1975). A re-testing and modification of the Philadelphia Geriatric Center Morale Scale. *Journal of Gerontology*, 30: 77–84.

Morris, J.N. and Sherwood, S. (1987). Quality of life of cancer patients at different stages in the disease trajectory. *Journal of Chronic Disease*, 40: 545–53.

Morris, J.N., Wolf, R.S. and Klerman, L.V. (1975). Common themes among morale and depression scales. *Journal of Gerontology*, 30: 209–15.

Morris, L.W., Morris, R.G. and Britton, P.G. (1989). Social support networks and formal support as factors influencing the psychological adjustment of spouse caregivers of dementia sufferers. *International Journal of Geriatric Psychiatry*, 4: 47–51.

Morton-Williams, J. (1979). Alternative patterns of care for the elderly: Methodological report. *Social and Community Planning Research*. London.

Mowbray, R.M. (1972). The Hamilton Rating Scale for Depression: A factor analysis. *Psychological Medicine*, 2: 272.

Mulder, P.H. and Sluijs, E.M. (1993). Dependent elderly. Quality of life indicators. Bibliography no. 48. The Netherlands: Netherlands Institute of Primary Health Care (NIVEL).

Mulgrave, N.W. (1985). Clifton Assessment Procedures for the elderly, in D.J. Keyser and R.C. Sweetland (eds) *Test Critiques*, vol. II. Kansas City, MI: Test Corporation of America.

Mumford, D.B., Tareen, I.A., Bajwa, M.A. et al. (1991). The translation and evaluation of an Urdu version of the Hospital Anxiety and Depression Scale. *Acta Psychiatrica Scandinavica*, 83: 81–5.

National Center for Health Statistics (1964). *Health Survey Procedures: Concepts, Questionnaires, Develop-*

ment and Definitions in the Health Interview Survey, Publication No. 1000, Series 1, No. 2, Washington, Public Health Service, May.

National Heart and Lung Institute (1976). Report of a task group on cardiac rehabilitation, in *Proceedings of the Heart and Lung Institute Working Conference on Health Behaviour*. Bethesda, MD: US Department of Health, Education and Welfare.

Naughton, M.J. and Wiklund, I. (1993). A critical review of dimension-specific measures of health-related quality of life in cross-cultural research. *Quality of Life Research*, 2: 397–432.

Nayani, S. (1989). The evaluation of psychiatric illness in Asian patients by the HAD scale. *British Journal of Psychiatry*, 155: 545–7.

Nelson, E.C. and Berwick, D.M. (1989). The measurement of health status in clinical practice. *Medical Care*, 27 (Supplement to no. 3): S77–90.

Nelson, E.C., Conger, R., Douglas, D. et al. (1983). Functional health status levels of primary care patients. *Journal of the American Medical Association*, 249: 3331–8.

Nelson, E.C., Landgraf, J.M., Hays, R.D. et al. (1990a). The functional status of patients: how can it be measured in physicians offices? *Medical Care*, 28: 1111–26.

Nelson, E.C., Landgraf, R.D., Hays, J.W. et al. (1990b). The COOP Function Charts: a system to measure patient function in physician's office, in *WONCA Classification Committee: Functional status measurement in primary care*. New York: Springer-Verlag.

Nelson, E.J., Wasson, J., Kirk, A. et al. (1987). Assessment of function in routine clinical practice: description of the COOP Chart method and preliminary findings. *Journal of Chronic Diseases*, 40 (Supplement 1): 55S–63S.

Neugarten, B.L., Havighurst, R.J. and Tobin, S.S. (1961). The measurement of life satisfaction. *Journal of Gerontology*, 16: 134–43.

Noack, H. and McQueen, D. (1988). Towards health promotion indicators. *Health Promotion*, 3: 73–8.

Noelker, L. and Harel, Z. (1978). Predictors of well-being and survival among institutionalized aged. *Gerontologist*, 18: 562–7.

Nou, E. and Aberg, T. (1980). Quality of survival in patients with surgically treated bronchial carcinoma. *Thorax*, 35: 255–63.

Nunnally, J. (1978). *Psychometric Theory*, 2nd edn. New York: McGraw Hill.

O'Boyle, C.A., McGee, H., Hickey, A. et al. (1989). Reliability and validity of judgement analysis as a method for assessing quality of life. *British Journal of Clinical Pharmacology*, 27: 155.

O'Brien, B.J. (1988). Assessment of treatment in heart disease, in G. Teeling Smith (ed.) *Measuring Health: A Practical Approach*. Chichester: John Wiley.

O'Brien, B.J., Banner, N.R., Gibson, S. et al. (1988). The Nottingham Health Profile as a measure of quality of life following combined heart and lung transplantation. *Journal of Epidemiology and Community Health*, 42: 232–4.

Office of Population Censuses and Surveys (1987). *General Household Survey* (1985). London, HMSO.

Olsen, O. (1992). Impact of social network on cardiovascular mortality in middle-aged Danish men. *Journal of Epidemiology and Community Health*, 47: 176–80.

Olsson, G., Lubsen, J., Van Es, G.A. and Rehnqvist, N. (1986). Quality of life after myocardial infarction: effect of long-term metoprolol on mortality and morbidity. *British Medical Journal*, 292: 1491–3.

O'Reilly, P. (1988). Methodological issues in social support and social network research. *Social Science and Medicine*, 26: 863–73.

O'Riordan, T.G., Haynes, J.P. and O'Neil, D. (1990). The effect of mild to moderate dementia on the Geriatric Depression Scale and on the General Health Questionnaire. *Age and Ageing*, 19: 57–61.

Orth-Gomer, K., Britton, M. and Rehnqvist, N. (1979). Quality of care in an out-patient department: the patient's view. *Social Science and Medicine*, 13A: 347–57.

Orth-Gomer, K. and Johnson, J. (1987). Social network interaction and mortality. A six-year follow-up study of a random sample of the Swedish population. *Journal of Chronic Diseases*, 40: 949–57.

Orth-Gomer, K. and Unden, A.L. (1987). The measurement of social support in population surveys. *Social Science and Medicine*, 24: 83–94.

Ott, C.R., Sivarajan, E.S., Newton, K.M. et al. (1983). A controlled randomized study of early cardiac rehabilitation: the Sickness Impact Profile as an assessment tool. *Heart and Lung*, 12: 162–70.

Ottawa Charter for Health Promotion (1986). *Health Promotion*, 14: iii–v.

Oxman, T.E. and Berkman, L.F. (1990). Assessment of social relationships in elderly patients. *International Journal of Psychiatry in Medicine*, 20: 65–84.

O'Young, J. and McPeek, B. (1987). Quality of life variables in surgical trials. *Journal of Chronic Diseases*, 40: 513–22.

Parker, S.G., Du, X., Bardsley, M.J. et al. (1994). Measuring outcomes in care of the elderly. *Journal of the Royal College of Physicians of London*, 28: 428–33.

Paterson, M. (1988). Treatment in rheumatoid arthritis, in G. Teeling Smith (ed.) *Measuring Health: A Practical Approach*. Chichester, John Wiley.

Patterson, W. (1975). The quality of survival in response to treatment. *Journal of the American Medical Association*, 233: 280–1.

Patrick, D.L. (ed.) (1982). *Health and Care of the Physically Disabled in Lambeth*. Report of Phase II of the Longitudinal Disability Interview Survey. London: St Thomas's Hospital Medical School, Department of Community Medicine.

Patrick, D.L. and Erickson, P. (1993). *Health status and health policy. Quality of life in health care evaluation and resource allocation*. New York: Oxford University Press.

Patrick, D.L., Bush, J.W. and Chen, M.M. (1973a). Methods for measuring levels of well-being for a health status index. *Health Services Research*, 11: 516.

Patrick, D.L., Bush, J.W. and Chen, M.M. (1973b). Toward an operational definition of health. *Journal of Health and Social Behaviour*, 14: 6–23.

Pattie, A.H. and Gilleard, C.J. (1979). *Manual of the Clifton Assessment Procedures for the Elderly*. Sevenoaks: Hodder and Stoughton.

Paykel, E.S. (1985). Clinical interview for depression, development, reliability and validity. *Journal of Affective Disorders*, 9: 85–96.

Payne, R.L. and Graham-Jones, J. (1987). Measurement and methodological issues in social support, in S.V. Kasl and C.L. Cooper (eds) *Stress and Health: Issues in Research Methodology*. Chichester: John Wiley.

Perlman, D. and Peplau, L.A. (1981). Toward a social psychology of loneliness, in R. Gilmour and S. Duck (eds) *Personal relationships: 3. Personal relationships in disorder*. London: Academic Press.

Perlman, R.A. (1987). Development of a functional assessment questionnaire for geriatric patients: the comprehensive older persons' evaluation (COPE). *Journal of Chronic Diseases*, 40: 85S–94S, Supplement.

Perloff, J.M. and Persons, J.B. (1988). Biases resulting from the use of indexes: an application to attributional style and depression. *Psychological Bulletin*, 103: 95–104.

Permanyer-Miralda, G., Alonso, J., Anto, J.M. *et al.* (1991). Comparison of perceived health status and conventional functional evaluation in stable patients with coronary artery disease. *Journal of Clinical Epidemiology*, 44: 779–86.

Pfeiffer, E. (1975). A short portable mental status questionnaire for the assessment of organic brain deficit in elderly patients. *Journal of American Geriatrics Society*, 23: 433–41.

Pierce, G.R., Sarason, I.G. and Sarason, B.R. (1991). General and relationship-based perceptions of social support: are two constructs better than one? *Journal of Personality and Social Psychology*, 61: 1028–39.

Pollard, W.E., Bobbitt, R.A. and Bergner, M. (1978). Examination of variable errors of measurement in a survey-based social indicator. *Social Indicators Research*, 5: 279–301.

Pollard, W.E., Bobbitt, R.A., Bergner, M., *et al.* (1976). The Sickness Impact Profile: reliability of a health status measure. *Medical Care*, 14: 57–67.

Pomeroy, E., Cook, B. and Benjafield, J. (1992). Perceived social support in three residential contexts. *Canadian Journal of Community Mental Health*, 11: 101–7.

Potts, M.K., Daniels, M., Burnam, A. and Wells, K.B. (1990). A structured interview version of the Hamilton Depression Rating Scale: Evidence of reliability and versatility of administration. *Journal of Psychiatric Research*, 24: 335–50.

Pretorius, T.B. and Diedricks, M. (1993). A factorial investigation of the dimensions of social support. *South African Journal of Psychology*, 23: 32–5.

Priestman, T.J. and Baum, M. (1976). Evaluation of quality of life in patients receiving treatment for advanced breast cancer. *Lancet*, i: 899–901.

Prieto, E.J. and Geisinger, K.F. (1983). Factor analytic studies of the McGill Pain Questionnaire, in R. Melzack (ed.) *Pain Measurement and Assessment*. New York: Raven Press.

Procidano, M.E. and Heller, K. (1983). Measures of perceived social support from friends and from family: three validation studies. *American Journal of Community Psychology*, 11: 1–24.

Qureshi, K.N. and Hodkinson, H.M. (1974). Evaluation of a 10 question mental test in the institutionalized elderly. *Age and Ageing*, 3: 152–7.

Radloff, L.S. (1977). Sex differences in depression: the effects of occupation and marital status. *Sex Roles*, 1: 249–65.

Radosevich, D.M. and Husnik, M.J. (1995). An abbreviated health status questionnaire: the HSQ-12. Update. Bloomington, IN: Newsletter of the Health Outcomes Institute, 2: 1–4.

Radosevich, D.M. and Pruitt, M.J.H. (1995). HSQ-12 Cooperative validation project: phase 1 reliability, validity and comparability. Update. Bloomington, IN: Newsletter of the Health Outcomes Institute, 2: 3.

Ramey, D.R., Fries, J.F. and Singh, G. (1996). The Health Assessment Questionnaire 1995 – Status and review, in B. Spilker (ed.) *Pharmacoeconomics and quality of life in clinical trials*, 2nd edn. Philadelphia: Lippincott-Raven.

Ramey, D.R., Raynauld, J.P. and Fries, J.F. (1992). The Health Assessment Questionnaire 1992. *Arthritis Care and Research*, 5: 119–29.

Ranhoff, A.H. and Laake, K. (1993). The Barthel ADL Index: scoring by the physician from patient interview is not reliable. *Age and Ageing*, 22: 171–4.

Read, L.J., Quinn, R.J. and Hoefer, M.A. (1987). Measuring overall health: an evaluation of three important approaches. *Journal of Chronic Diseases*, 40: 7S–21S.

Reading, A.E. (1979). The internal structure of the McGill Pain Questionnaire in dysmenorrhoea patients. *Pain*, 7: 353–8.·

Reading, A.E., Everitt, B.S. and Sledmere, C.M. (1982). The McGill Pain Questionnaire: a replication of its construction. *British Journal of Clinical Psychology*, 21: 339–49.

Reed, P.F., Fitts, W.H. and Boehm, L. (1980). *Tennessee Self Concept Scale: Bibliography of Research Studies*. Nashville, TN: Councillor Recordings and Tests.

Rehm, L.P. (1981). *Behaviour Therapy for Depression*. New York: Academic Press.

Renne, K.S. (1974). Measurement of social health in a general population survey. *Social Sciences Research*, 3: 25–44.

Revicki, D.A. and Kaplan, R.M. (1993). Relationship between psychometric and utility-based approaches to the measurement of health related quality of life. *Quality of Life Research*, 2: 477–87.

Reynolds, W.M. and Gould, J.W. (1981). A psychometric investigation of the standard and short form Beck Depression Inventory. *Journal of Consulting and Clinical Psychology*, 49: 306–7.

Riggio, R.E., Watring, K.P. and Throckmorton, B. (1993). Social skills, social support, and psychosocial adjustment. *Journal of Personality and Individual Differences*, 15: 275–80.

Robins, L.N., Helzer, J.E., Croughan, J.L. and Ratcliff, K. (1981). The NIMH diagnostic interview schedule: Its history, characteristics and validity, in J.K. Wing, P. Bebbington and L.N. Robins (eds) *What is a case? The Problem of definition in Psychiatric Community Surveys*. London: Grant MacIntyre.

Robinson, J.P. and Shaver, P.R. (1973). *Measures of Social Psychological Attitudes*. Ann Arbor, MI. Survey Research Centre, Institute for Social Research.

Robinson, R.A. (1968). The organisation of a diagnostic and treatment unit for the aged, in U.K. Giegy *Psychiatric Disorders in the Aged*. Manchester: World Psychiatric Association.

Rodgers, H., Curless, R. and James, O.F.W. (1993). Standardized functional assessment scales for elderly patients. *Age and Ageing*, 22: 161–3.

Roid, G.H. and Fitts, W.H. (1988). *Tennessee Self-Concept Scale (TSCS)*. Los Angeles, CA: Western Psychological Services.

Rosenberg, M. (1965). *Society and the Adolescent Self Image*. Princeton, NJ: Princeton University Press.

Rosenberg, M. (1986). *Conceiving the self*. 2nd edn. Malabar, FL: Krieger.

Rosenberg, R. (1995). Health-related quality of life between naturalism and hermeneutics. Special Issue 'Quality of Life' in *Social Science and Medicine*, 10: 1411–15.

Rosser, R.M. and Watts, V.C. (1971). The sanative outputs of hospitals. Dallas, 39th conference of the Operational Research Society of America.

Rosser, R.M. and Watts, V.C. (1972). The measurement of hospital output. *International Journal of Epidemiology*, 1: 361–8.

Roth, M., Tym, E., Mountjoy, C.Q. *et al.* (1986). CAMDEX: a standardized instrument for the diagnosis of mental disorder in the elderly with special reference to the early detection of dementia. *British Journal of Psychiatry*, 149: 698–709.

Russell, D. (1982). The measurement of loneliness, in L.A. Peplau and D. Perlman (eds) *Loneliness: A Sourcebook of Current Theory, Research and Therapy*. New York: John Wiley.

Russell, D., Peplau, L.A. and Cutrona, C.E. (1980). The revised UCLA Loneliness Scale: concurrent and discriminant validity evidence. *Journal of Personality and Social Psychology*, 39: 472–80.

Russell, D., Peplau, L.A. and Ferguson, M.L. (1978). Developing a measure of loneliness. *Journal of Personality Assessment*, 42: 290–4.

Ruta, D.A., Abdalla, M.I., Garratt, A.M. *et al.* (1994a). SF 36 health survey questionnaire: I. Reliability in two patient based studies. *Quality in Health Care*, 3: 180–5.

Ruta, D.A., Garratt, A.M., Leng, M. *et al.* (1994b). A new approach to the measurement of quality of life. The Patient-generated Index. *Medical Care*, 32: 1109–26.

Sackett, D.L., Spitzer, W.O., Gent, M. *et al.* (1974). The Burlington Randomized Trial of the nurse practitioner: health outcomes of patients. *Annals of Internal Medicine*, 80: 137–42.

Sainsbury, S. (1973). *Measuring Disability*. London: Bell.

Sandler, I.N. and Barrera, M. (1984). Towards a multimethod approach to assessing the effects of social support. *American Journal of Community Psychology*, 12: 37–52.

Sarason, B.R., Sarason, I.G., Hacker, T.A. and Basham, R.B. (1985). Concomitants of social support: social skills, physical attractiveness, and gender. *Journal of Personality and Social Psychology*, 49: 469–80.

Sarason, B.R., Shearin, E.N., Pierce, G.R. and Sarason, I.G. (1987a). Interrelationships of social support measures: theoretical and practical implications. *Journal of Personality and Social Psychology*, 52: 813–32.

Sarason, I.G., Sarason, B.R. and Pierce, G.R. (1994). Social support: global and relationship-based levels of analysis. *Journal of Social and Personal Relationships*, 11: 295–312.

Sarason, I.G., Levine, H.M., Basham, R.B. and Sarason, B.R. (1983). Assessing social support: the social support questionnaire. *Journal of Personality and Social Psychology*, 44: 127–39.

Sarason, I.G., Sarason, B.R., Shearin, E.N. and Pierce, G.R. (1987b). A brief measure of social support. Practical and theoretical implications. *Journal of Social and Personal Relationships*, 4: 497–510.

Saronson, S.B., Carroll, C., Maton, K. *et al.* (1977). *Human Services and Resource Networks*. San Francisco, Jossey-Bass.

Sauer, W.J. and Warland, R. (1982). Morale and life satisfaction, in D.J. Mangen and W.A. Peterson (eds) *Research instruments in social gerontology, vol. 1. Clinical and social psychology*. Minneapolis, MN: University of Minnesota Press.

Saunders, P.A., Copeland, J.R., Dewey, M.E. *et al.* (1989). Alcohol use and abuse in the elderly: findings from the Liverpool longitudinal study of continuing health in the community. *International Journal of Geriatric Psychiatry*, 4: 103–8.

Sayer, N.A., Sackheim, H.A., Moeller, J.R. *et al.* (1993). The relations between observer-rating and self-report of depressive symptomatology. *Journal of Psychological Assessment*, 5: 350–60.

Schaafsma, J. and Osoba, D. (1994). The Karnofsky performance status scale re-examined: a cross-validation with the EORTC-C30. *Quality of Life Research*, 3: 413–24.

Schag, C.A.C., Heinrich, R.L. and Ganz, P.A. (1984). Karnofsky Performance Status revisited: reliability, validity and guidelines. *Journal of Clinical Oncology*, 2: 187–93.

Schneiderman, L.J., Kaplan, R.M., Pearlman, R.A. *et al.* (1993). Do physicians' own preferences for life sustaining treatment influence their perceptions of patients' preferences? *Journal of Clinical Ethics*, 4: 28–33.

Scholten, J.H.G. and van Weel, C. (1992). Manual for the use of the Dartmouth COOP Functional Health Assessment Charts/WONCA in measuring functional status in family practice (Part I), in J.H. Scholten and C. van Weel (eds) *Functional status assessment in family practice*. Lelystad: Meditekst.

Schuling, J., Greidanus, J., Meyboom-de Jong, B. (1993). Measuring functional status of stroke patients with the Sickness Impact Profile. *Disability and Rehabilitation*, 15: 19–23.

Schuling, J. and Meyboom-de Jong, B. (1992). Change in clinical status in patients with stroke, in J.H. Scholten and C. van Weel (eds) *Functional status assessment in family practice*. Lelystad: Meditekst.

Schwab, J.J., Brolow, M.R. and Holser, C.E. (1967). A comparison of two rating scales for depression. *Journal of Clinical Psychology*, 23: 94–6.

Schwartz, A.N. (1975). An observation of self-esteem as the linchpin of quality of life for the aged. An essay. *Gerontologist*, 15: 470–2.

Scott, P.J., Ansell, B.M. and Huskisson, E.C. (1977). The measurement of pain in juvenile chronic polyarthritis. *Annals of the Rheumatic Diseases*, 36: 186–7.

Scottish Health Education Group (1984). *European Monographs in Health Education Research*, no. 6. Edinburgh, Scottish Health Education Group.

Seedhouse, D. (1986). *Health: the Foundations of Achievement*. Chichester: John Wiley.

Seeman, T.E. and Berkman, L.F. (1988). Structural characteristics of social networks and their relationship with social support in the elderly: who provides support? *Social Science and Medicine*, 26: 737–49.

Seeman, T.E., Kaplan, G.A., Knudsen, L. *et al.* (1987). Social network ties and mortality among the elderly in the Alameda County study. *American Journal of Epidemiology*, 126: 714–23.

Shah, S., Frank, V. and Cooper, V. (1989). Improving the sensitivity of the Barthel Index for stroke rehabilitation. *Journal of Clinical Epidemiology*, 42: 703–9.

Shanas, E., Townsend, P. and Wedderburn, D. *et al.* (1968). *Old People in Three Industrial Societies*. London: Routledge and Kegan Paul.

Sherbourne, C.D. and Hays, R.D. (1990). Marital status, social support and health transitions in chronic disease patients. *Journal of Health and Social Behaviour*, 31: 328–43.

Sherbourne, C.D., Meredith, L.S., Rogers, W. and Ware, J.E. (1992). Social support and stressful life events: Age differences in their effects on health related quality of life among the chronically ill. *Quality of Life Research*, 1: 235–46.

Sherbourne, C.D. and Stewart, A.L. (1991). The MOS Social Support Survey. *Social Science and Medicine*, 32: 705–14.

Sherwood, S.J., Morris, J., Mor, V. and Gutkin, C. (1977). Compendium of Measures for Describing and Assessing Long Term Care Populations. Boston, MA: Hebrew Rehabilitation Center for the Aged.

Shin, D.C. and Johnson, D.M. (1978). Avowed happiness as an overall assessment of the quality of life. *Social Indicators Research*, 5: 475–92.

Silber, E. and Tippett, J. (1965). Self esteem: clinical assessment and measurement validation. *Psychological Reports*, 16: 1017–71.

Sims, A.C.P. and Salmons, P.H. (1975). Severity of symptoms of psychiatric out-patients: use of the General Health Questionnaire in hospital and general practice patients. *Psychological Medicine*, 5: 62–6.

Singer, E., Garfinkel, R., Cohen, S.M. *et al.* (1976). Mortality and mental health: evidence from the midtown Manhattan re-study. *Social Science and Medicine*, 10: 517–21.

Skinner, D.E. and Yett, D.E. (1972). Debility index for long-term care patients, in R.L. Berg (ed.) *Health Status Indexes*. Chicago, IL: Hospital Research and Education Trust.

Slevin, M.L. (1984). Quality of life in cancer patients. *Clinics in Oncology*, 371–90.

Slevin, M.L., Plant, H., Lynch, D. *et al*. (1988). Who should measure quality of life, the doctor or the patient? *British Journal of Cancer*, 57: 109–12.

Smith, A. (1987). Qualms about Qalys. *Lancet*, 1: 1134–6.

Smith, A.H.W., Ballinger, B.R. and Presley, A.S. (1981). The reliability and validity of two assessment scales for the elderly mentally handicapped. *British Journal of Psychiatry*, 138: 15–16.

Smith, T.W. (1979). Happiness: time trends, seasonal variations, inter-survey differences and other mysteries. *Social Psychology Quarterly*, 42: 18–30.

Snaith, R.P. (1987). The concepts of mild depression. *British Journal of Psychiatry*, 150: 387–93.

Snaith, R.P. and Taylor, C.M. (1985). Rating scales for depression and anxiety: a current perspective. *British Journal of Clinical Pharmacology*, 19: 17S–20S (suppl.).

Sokolovsky, J. (1986). Network methodologies in the study of ageing, in J. Keith (ed.) *New Methods for Old Age Research*. Westport, CT: Greenwood Press, Bergin and Garvey.

Spatz, K. and Johnson, F. (1973). Internal consistency of the Coopersmith Self Esteem Inventory. *Educational and Psychological Measurements*, 33: 875–6.

Spector, W.D., Katz, S., Murphy, J.B. *et al*. (1987). The hierarchical relationship between activities of daily living and instrumental activities of daily living. *Journal of Chronic Diseases*, 40: 481–9.

Spilker, B., Simpson, R. and Tilson, H. (1992a). Quality of life bibliography and indexes: 1991 update. *Journal of Clinical Research Pharmacoepidemiology*, 6: 205–66.

Spilker, B., Molinek, F.R., Johnson, K.A. *et al*. (1990). Quality of life bibliography and indexes. *Medical Care*, 28 (supplement 12): DS1–DS77.

Spilker, B., White, W.S.A., Simpson, R.L. and Tilson, H.H. (1992b). Quality of life bibliography and indexes: 1990 update. *Journal of Clinical Research Pharmacoepidemiology*, 6: 87–156.

Spitzer, R.L., Burdock, E.I. and Hardesty, A.S. (1964). *Mental Status Schedule*. New York: Department of Psychiatry, College of Physicians and Surgeons, Columbia University and Biometrics Research Section, New York State Department of Mental Hygiene.

Spitzer, R.L., Endicott, J. and Robins, E. (1978). Research Diagnostic Criteria: rationale and reliability. *Archives of General Psychiatry*, 35: 773–82.

Spitzer, R.L., Endicott, J., Fliess, J.L. *et al*. (1970). Psychiatric status schedule: a technique for evaluating psychopathology and impairment in role functioning. *Archives of General Psychiatry*, 23: 41–55.

Spitzer, W.O., Dobson, A.J., Hall, J. *et al*. (1981). Measuring quality of life of cancer patients: a concise QL-index for use by physicians. *Journal of Chronic Diseases*, 34: 585–97.

Springfield, V.A. (1976). *Perceived Health and Patient Role*

Propensity. Washington, DC: Department of Commerce, National Technical Information Service.

Stansfeld, S.A. and Marmot, M.G. (1992). Social class and minor psychiatric disorder in British civil servants: a validated screening survey using the GHQ. *Psychological Medicine*, 22: 739–49.

Stanwyck, D.J. and Garrison, W.M. (1982). Detecting on faking on the Tennessee Self-Concept Scale. *Journal of Personality Assessment*, 46: 426–31.

Steer, R.A., Beck, A.T. and Garrison, B. (1986). Applications of the Beck Depression Inventory, in N. Sartorius and T.A. Ban (eds) *Assessment of Depression*. Berlin: Springer-Verlag.

Stehouwer, R.S. (1985). Beck Depression Inventory, in D.J. Keyser and R.C. Sweetland (eds) *Test Critiques*, vol. II. Kansas City, MI: Test Corporation of America.

Stewart, A.L. and Ware, J.E. (1992). *Measuring functioning and well-being: The medical outcomes study approach*. Durham, NC: Duke University Press.

Stewart, A.L., Hays, R.D. and Ware, J.E. (1988). The MOS Short-form General Health Survey. Reliability and validity in a patient population. *Medical Care*, 26: 724–35.

Stewart, A.L., Ware, J.E. and Brook, R.H. (1981). Advances in the measurement of functional status: construction of aggregate indexes. *Medical Care*, 19: 473–88.

Stewart, A.L., Greenfield, S., Hays, R.D. *et al*. (1989). Functional status and well-being of patients with chronic conditions: results from the medical outcomes study. *Journal of the American Medical Association*, 262: 907–13.

Stewart, A.L., Ware, J.E., Brook, R.H. *et al*. (1978). *Conceptualization and Measurement of Health for Adults in the Health Insurance Study*: vol. II: *Physical Health in Terms of Functioning*. Santa Monica, CA: Rand Corporation: R-1987/2-HEW.

Stineman, M.G., Escarce, J.J., Goin, J.E. *et al*. (1994). A case mix classification system for medical rehabilitation. *Medical Care*, 32: 366–79.

Stock, W.A. and Okun, M.A. (1982). The construct validity of life satisfaction among the elderly. *Journal of Gerontology*, 37: 625–7.

Stokes, J.P. (1983). Predicting satisfaction with social support from social network structure. *American Journal of Community Psychology*, 11: 141–52.

Stokes, J.P. (1985). The relation of social network and individual difference variables to loneliness. *Journal of Personality and Social Psychology*, 48: 981–90.

Stokes, J.P. and Wilson, D.G. (1984). The Inventory of Socially Supportive Behaviours: dimensionality, prediction and gender differences. *American Journal of Community Psychology*, 12: 53–70.

Stones, M.L. and Kozma, A. (1980). Issues relating to

the usage of conceptualizations of mental constructs employed by gerontologists. *International Journal of Ageing and Human Development*, 11: 269–81.

Streiner, D.L. and Norman, G.R. (1989). *Health Measurement Scales: A Practical Guide to their Development and Use*. Oxford: Oxford University Press.

Stueve, A. and Lein, L. (1979). Problems in network analysis: the case of the missing person. Paper presented at 32nd annual general meeting of the Gerontological Society of America.

Stull, D.E. (1987). Conceptualization and measurement of well-being: implications for policy evaluation, in E.F. Borgatta and R.J.V. Montgomery (eds) *Critical Issues in Ageing Policy*. Beverly Hills, Sage Publications.

Sullivan, C.F., Copeland, J.R.M., Dewey, M.E. *et al.* (1988). Benzodiazepine usage amongst the elderly: findings of the Liverpool community survey. *International Journal of Geriatric Psychiatry*, 3: 289–92.

Sullivan, M., Ahlmen, M. and Bjelle, A. (1990). 'Health status assessment in rheumatoid arthritis:' 1. Further work on the validity of the Sickness Impact Profile. *Journal of Rheumatology*, 17: 439–47.

Sullivan, M., Karlsson, J. and Ware, J.R. (1995). The Swedish SF-36 Health Survey – I. Evaluation of data quality, scaling assumptions, reliability and construct validity across general populations in Sweden. Special Issue 'Quality of Life' in *Social Science and Medicine*, 10: 1349–58.

Tamaklo, W., Schubert, D.S., Mentari, A. *et al.* (1992). Assessing depression in the medical patient using the MADRS, a sensitive screening scale. *Journal of Integrative Psychiatry*, 8: 264–70.

Tardy, C.H. (1985). Social support measurement. *American Journal of Community Psychiatry*, 13: 187–202.

Tarnopolsky, A., Hand, D.J., McLean, E.K. *et al.* (1979). Validity and uses of a screening questionnaire (GHQ) in the community. *British Journal of Psychiatry*, 134: 508–15.

Taylor, J. and Reitz, W. (1968). *The Three Faces of Self-esteem*. London: University of Western Ontario, Department of Psychology. Research Bulletin no. 80.

Teeling Smith, G. (1988). *Measuring Health: A Practical Approach*. Chichester: John Wiley.

Tennant, C. (1977). The General Health Questionnaire: a valid index of psychological impairment in Australian populations. *Medical Journal of Australia*, 2: 392–4.

Thoits, P.A. (1982). Conceptual, methodological and theoretical problems in studying social support as a buffer against life stress. *Journal of Health and Social Behaviour*, 23: 145–59.

Thomas, M.R. and Lyttle, D. (1980). Patient expectations about success of treatment and reported relief from low back pain. *Journal of Psychosomatic Research*, 24: 297–301.

Thompson, C. (1984). *The Reliability of a Schedule for Assessing Dependency in the Elderly in Residential Care*. Manchester: University of Manchester. Working papers in applied social research, no. 2.

Thompson, P. (1989). Affective disorders, in P. Thompson (ed.) *The Instruments of Psychiatric Research*. Chichester: John Wiley.

Thompson, P. and Blessed, G. (1987). Correlation between the 37-item Mental Test Score and abbreviated 10-item Mental Test Score by psychogeriatric day patients. *British Journal of Psychiatry*, 151: 206–9.

Thompson, W. (1972). *Correlates of the Self Concept*. Nashville, TN: Counselor Recordings and Tests.

Thuriaux, M.C. (1988). Health promotion and indicators for health for all in the European Region. *Health Promotion*, 3: 89–99.

Toevs, C.D., Kaplan, R.M. and Atkins, C.J. (1984). The costs and effects of behavioral programs in chronic obstructive pulmonary disease. *Medical Care*, 22: 1088–1100.

Tollefson, G.D. and Holman, S.L. (1993). Analysis of the Hamilton Depression Rating Scale factors from a double-bind, placebo-controlled trial of fluoxetine in geriatric major depression. *International Journal of Clinical Psychopharmacology*, 8: 253–9.

Tolsdorf, C.C. (1976). Social networks, support and coping: an exploratory study. *Family Process*, 15: 407–17.

Toner, J., Gurland, B. and Teresi, J. (1988). Comparison of self-administered and rater-administered methods of assessing levels of severity of depression in elderly patients. *Journal of Gerontology*, 43: 136–40.

Torrance, G.W. (1986). Measurement of health state utilities for economic appraisal. *Journal of Health Economics*, 5: 1–30.

Torrance, G.W. (1987). Utility approach to measuring health related quality of life. *Journal of Chronic Diseases*, 40: 593–600.

Torrance, G.W., Boyle, M.H. and Horwood, S.P. (1982). Application of multiattribute utility theory to measure social preferences for health states. *Operations Research*, 30: 1043–69.

Torrance, G.W., Thomas, W.H. and Sackett, D.L. (1972). A utility maximisation model for the evaluation of health care programs. *Health Services Research*, 7: 118–33.

Townsend, P. (1962). *The Last Refuge*. London: Routledge and Kegan Paul.

Townsend, P. (1979). *Poverty in the United Kingdom*. Harmondsworth: Pelican.

Trowbridge, N. (1970). Effects of socio-economic class on self-concept of children. *Psychology in the Schools*, 7: 304–6.

Twining, T.C. and Allen, D.G. (1981). Disability factors among residents in old people's homes.

Journal of Epidemiology and Community Health, 36: 303–5.

Tyrer, P., Seivewright, N., Murphy, S. *et al.* (1988). The Nottingham study of neurotic disorder: comparison of drug and psychological treatments. *Lancet*, 2: 235–40.

Tzeng, O.C., Maxey, W.A., Fortier, R. and Landis, D. (1985). Construct evaluation of the Tennessee Self Concept Scale. *Educational and Psychological Measurement*, 45: 63–78.

Unden, A.L. and Orth-Gomer, K. (1989). Development of a social support instrument for use in population surveys. *Social Science and Medicine*, 29: 1387–92.

Usui, W.M., Keil, T.J. and Durig, K.R. (1985). Socioeconomic comparisons and life satisfaction of elderly adults. *Journal of Gerontology*, 40: 110–14.

Vacchiano, R.B. and Strauss, P.S. (1968). The construct validity of the Tennessee Self Concept Scale. *Journal of Clinical Psychology*, 24: 323–6.

Valdenegro, J. and Barrera, M. (1983). Social support as a moderator of life stress: a longitudinal study using a multi-method analysis. Paper presented at the meeting of the Western Psychological Association, San Francisco, California.

van Agt, H.M.E., Esssink-Bot, M.L., van der Meer, J.B.W. and Bonsel, G.J. (1993). The NHP (Dutch version) in general and specified populations. Paper presented to the Fifth European Health Services Research Conference, Maastricht, December.

van de Lisdonk, E.H. and van Weel, C. (1992). Cataract and functional status, in J.H. Scholten and C. van Weel (eds) *Functional Status Assessment in Family Practice*. Lelystad: Meditekst.

van Weel, C., König-Zahn, C., Touw-Otten, F.W.M.M. *et al.* (1995). *COOP/WONCA Charts. A Manual*. The Netherlands: World Organization of Family Doctors, European Research Group on Health Outcomes, Northern Centre for Health Care Research: University of Groningen.

van Weel, C. and Scholten, J.H.G. (1992). Report of an international workshop of the WONCA Research and Classification committee, in J.H. Scholten and C. van Weel (eds) *Functional status assessment in family practice*. Lelystad: Meditekst.

Vardon, V.M. and Blessed, G. (1986). Confusion ratings and abbreviated mental test performance: a comparison. *Age and Ageing*, 15: 139–44.

Vaux, A. and Wood, J. (1985) Social support resources, behaviors and appraisals: a path analysis. Paper presented at the meeting of the Midwestern Psychological Association, Chicago.

Vaux, A., Burda, P. and Stewart, D. (1986a). Orientation toward utilizing support resources. *Journal of Community Psychology*, 14: 159–70.

Vaux, A., Phillips, J., Holly, L. *et al.* (1986b). The social support appraisals (SS-A) scale: studies of reliability and validity. *American Journal of Community Psychology*, 14: 195–219.

Vaux, A., Riedel, S. and Stewart, D. (1987). Modes of social support: the social support behaviours (SS-B) scale. *American Journal of Community Psychology*, 15: 209–337.

Vetter, N. and Ford, D. (1989). Anxiety and depression scores in elderly fallers. *International Journal of Geriatric Psychiatry*, 4: 159–63.

Vetter, N., Jones, D.A. and Victor, C.R. (1982). The importance of mental disabilities for the use of services by the elderly. *Journal of Psychosomatic Research*, 26: 607–12.

Vetter, N., Smith, A., Sastry, D. and Tinker, G. (1989). *Day hospital – pilot study report*. Research Team for the Care of Elderly People, Department of Geriatrics, St David's Hospital, Cardiff, S. Wales.

Vieweg, B.W. and Hedlund, J.L. (1983). The General Health Questionnaire: a comprehensive review. *Journal of Operational Psychiatry*, 14: 74–81.

Vincent, J. (1968). An explanatory factor analysis relating to the construct validity of self concept labels. *Educational and Psychological Measurement*, 28: 915–21.

Wade, D.T. (1992). *Measurement in Neurological Rehabilitation*. Oxford: Oxford University Press.

Wade, D.T. and Collin, C. (1988). The Barthel ADL Index: a standard measure of physical disability. *International Disability Studies*, 10: 64–7.

Wade, D.T. and Langton-Hewer, R. (1987). Functional abilities after stroke: Measurement, natural history and prognosis. *Journal of Neurology, Neurosurgery and Psychiatry*, 50: 177–82.

Wade, D.T., Legh-Smith, G.L. and Langton-Hewer, R. (1985). Social activities after stroke: Measurement and natural history using the Frenchay Activities Index. *International Rehabilitation Medicine*, 7: 176–81.

Wade, D.T., Collen, F.M., Robb, G.F. and Warlow, C.P. (1992). Physiotherapy intervention late after stroke and mobility. *British Medical Journal*, 304: 609–13.

Walker, K., Macbride, A. and Vachon, M.L.S. (1977). Social support networks and the crisis of bereavement. *Social Science and Medicine*, 11: 34–41.

Walkey, F.H., Seigert, R.J., McCormick, I.A. and Taylor, A.J. (1987). Multiple replication of the factor structure of the inventory of socially supportive behaviors. *Journal of Community Psychology*, 15: 513–19.

Wallace, J.L. and Vaux, A. (1993). Social network orientation: the role of adult attachment style. *Journal of Social and Clinical Psychology*, 12: 354–65.

Wallston, K.A., Brown, G.K., Stein, M.J. and Dobbins, C.J. (1989). Comparing the long and short versions of the Arthritis Impact Measurement Scales. *Journal of Rheumatology*, 16: 1105–9.

Wallwork, J. and Caine, N. (1985). A comparison of the quality of life of cardiac transplant patients and coronary artery bypass graft patients before and after surgery. *Quality of Life and Cardiovascular Care*, 1: 317–31.

Walsh, J.A. (1984). Tennessee Self Concept Scale, in D.J. Keyser and R.C. Sweetland (eds) *Test Critiques*, vol. 1. Kansas City, MI: Test Corporation of America.

Wan, T.T.H. and Livieratos, B. (1977). A validation of the General Well-being Index: a two-stage multivariate approach. Paper presented at American Public Health Association meeting, Washington, DC.

Ward, R.A. (1977). The impact of subjective age and stigma on older persons. *Journal of Gerontology*, 32: 227–32.

Ward, R.A., Sherman, S.R. and LaGory, M. (1984). Subjective network assessments and subjective well-being. *Journal of Gerontology*, 39: 93–101.

Ware, J.E. (1984). Methodological considerations in the selection of health status assessment procedures, in N.K. Wenger, M.E. Mattson, C.D. Furberg *et al.* (eds) *Assessment of Quality of Life in Clinical Trials of Cardiovascular Therapies*. New York: Le Jacq.

Ware, J.E. (1986). The assessment of health status, in L.H. Aiken and D. Mechanic (eds) *Applications of Social Science to Clinical Medicine and Health Policy*. New Brunswick, NJ: Rutgers University Press.

Ware, J.E. (1993). Measuring patients' views: the optimum outcome measure. *British Medical Journal*, 306: 1429–30.

Ware, J.E. and Karmos, A.H. (1976). *Development and Validation of Scales to Measure Perceived Health and Patient Role Propensity*, vol. 2 of a final report. Carbondale, IL: Southern Illinois University School of Medicine, publication no. PB 288–331.

Ware, J.E. and Young, J. (1979). Issues in the conceptualization and measurement of value placed on health, in S.J. Mushkin and D.W. Dunlop (eds) *Health: what is it worth?* New York: Pergamon Press.

Ware, J.E., Kosinski, M. and Keller, S.D. (1995). *How to score the SF-12 Physical and Mental Health Summary Scales*. Boston, MA: The Health Institute, New England Medical Center, 2nd edn.

Ware, J.E., Kosinski, M. and Keller, S.D. (1996a). *SF-12. An even shorter health survey*. Boston, MA: Medical Outcomes Trust Bulletin, 4: 2.

Ware, J.E., Kosinski, M. and Keller, S.D. (1996b). A 12-item short-form health survey. Construction of scales and preliminary tests of reliability and validity. *Medical Care*, 34: 220–33.

Ware, J.E., Sherbourne, C.D. and Davies, A.R. (1992). Developing and testing the MOS 20-item Short Form Health Survey: A general population application, in A.L. Stewart and J.E. Ware (eds) *Measuring Functioning and Well-being: The Medical Outcomes Study Approach*. Durham, NC: Duke University Press.

Ware, J.E., Snow, K.K., Kosinski, M. and Gandek, B. (1993). *SF-36 Health Survey: Manual and Interpretation Guide*. Boston, MA: The Health Institute, New England Medical Center.

Ware, J.E., Brook, R.H., Davies-Avery, A. *et al.* (1980). *Conceptualization and Measurement of Health for Adults in the Health Insurance Study*, vol. 6, *Analysis of Relationships among Health Status Measures*. Santa Monica, CA: Rand Corporation: R1987/6-HEW.

Ware, J.E., Johnson, S.A., Davies-Avery, A. *et al.* (1979). *Conceptualization and Measurement of Health for Adults in the Health Insurance Study*, vol. III, *Mental Health*. Santa Monica, CA: Rand Corporation: R-1987/3-HEW.

Warr, P. (1978). A study of psychological well-being. *British Journal of Psychology*, 69: 111–21.

Watchel, T., Piette, J., Mor, V. *et al.* (1992). Quality of life in persons with human immunodeficiency virus infection: Measurement by the medical outcomes study instrument. *Annals of Internal Medicine*, 116: 129–37.

Watson, E. and Evans, S. (1986). An example of cross-cultural measurement of psychological symptoms in post-partum mothers. *Social Science and Medicine*, 23: 869–74.

Webb, E.J., Campbell, D.T., Schwartz, R.D. *et al.* (1966). *Unobtrusive Measures: Non-reactive Research in the Social Sciences*. Chicago, IL: Rand McNally College Publishing.

Weckowicz, T., Muir, W. and Cropley, A. (1967). A factor analysis of the Beck Inventory of Depression. *Journal of Consulting Psychology*, 31: 23–8.

Weinberger, M., Tierney, W.M., Booher, P. and Hiner, S.L. (1990). Social support, stress and functional status in patients with osteoarthritis. *Social Science and Medicine*, 30: 503–8.

Weiss, R.S. (1969). The fund of sociability. *Transactions*, 6: 36.

Weiss, R.S. (1973). *Loneliness: The Experience of Emotional and Social Isolation*. Cambridge, MA: MIT Press.

Wells, E. and Marwell, G. (1976). *Self Esteem*. Beverly Hills, CA: Sage Publications.

Wells, K.B., Hays, R.D., Burnam, M.A., *et al.* (1989a). Detection of depressive disorder for patients receiving pre-paid or fee for service care: results from the medical outcomes study. *Journal of the American Medical Association*, 262: 3298–3302.

Wells, K.B., Stewart, A., Hays, R.D. *et al.* (1989b). The functioning and well-being of depressed patients: results from the medical outcomes study. *Journal of the American Medical Association*, 262: 914–19.

Wenger, G.C. (1989). Support networks in old age –

constructing a typology, in M. Jefferys (ed.) *As Britain Ages*. London: Routledge.

Wenger, G.C. (1992). *Help in old age – facing up to change*. Liverpool: Liverpool University Press.

Wenger, G.C. (1994). *Support networks of older people: A guide for practitioners*. Bangor: Centre for Social Policy Research and Development, University of Wales.

Wenger, G.C. (1995). *Practitioner assessment of network type (PANT). Training and resource pack*. Brighton: Pavilion Press.

Wenger, G.C. and Shahtahmasebi, S. (1991). Survivors: support network variation and sources of help in rural communities. *Journal of Cross-Cultural Gerontology*, 6: 41–82.

Wenger, N.K., Mattson, M.E., Furberg, C.D. *et al.* (eds) (1984). *Assessment of Quality of Life in Clinical Trials of Cardiovascular Therapies*. New York, Le Jacq.

Wentowski, G. (1982). Reciprocity and the coping strategies of older people: cultural dimensions of network building. *Gerontologist*, 21: 600–9.

Wiest, W.M. (1965). A qualitative extension of Heider's theory of cognitive balance applied to interpersonal perception and self esteem. *Psychological Monographs: General and Applied*, 79: 1–20.

Wilkin, D. (1987). Conceptual problems in dependency research. *Social Science and Medicine*, 24: 867–73.

Wilkin, D. and Jolley, D.J. (1979). *Behavioural Problems among Old People in Geriatric Wards, Psychogeriatric Wards and Residential Homes, 1976–78*. Research Report no. 1, Research Section, Psychiatric Unit, University Hospital of South Manchester.

Wilkin, D. and Thompson, C. (1989). *User's Guide to Dependency Measures for Elderly People*. Sheffield Social Services Monographs: Research in Practice. University of Sheffield, Joint Unit for Social Services Research.

Wilkin, D., Hallam, L. and Doggett, M. (1992). *Measures of need and outcome for primary care*. New York: Oxford Medical Publications.

Wilkin, D., Mashiah, T. and Jolley, D.J. (1978). Changes in behavioural characteristics of elderly populations of local authority homes and long stay hospital wards, 1976–77. *British Medical Journal*, 2: 1274–6.

Wilkinson, M.J.B. and Barczak, P. (1988). Psychiatric screening in general practice: Comparisons of the General Health Questionnaire and the Hospital Anxiety and Depression Scale. *Journal of the Royal College of General Practitioners*, 38: 311–13.

Willcocks, D., Peace, S. and Kellaher, L. (1987). *Private Lives in Public Places*. London: Tavistock Press.

Williams, A. (1985). The value of QALYS. *Health and Social Services Journal*, 95: 3–5.

Williams, J.G., Barlow, D.H. and Agras, W.S. (1972). Behavioural measurement of severe depression. *Archives of General Psychiatry*, 27: 330–3.

Williams, J.M.G. (1984). *The Psychology of Depression*. Beckenham: Croom Helm.

Williams, P. (1987). Depressive thinking in general practice patients, in P. Freeling, L.J. Downey and J.C. Malkin (eds) *The Presentation of Depression: Current Approaches*. Royal College of General Practitioners, Occasional Paper, 36: 17–20.

Williams, R.G.A., Johnston, M., Willis, M. *et al.* (1976). Disability: a model and measurement technique. *British Journal of Preventive and Social Medicine*, 30: 71–8.

Williams, S.J. and Bury, M.J. (1989). Impairment, disability and handicap in chronic respiratory illness. *Social Science and Medicine*, 29: 609–16.

Wilson, L.A. and Brass, W. (1973). Brief assessment of the mental state in geriatric domiciliary practice: the usefulness of the mental status questionnaire. *Age and Ageing*, 2: 92–101.

Wilson, L.A., Roy, S.K. and Bursill, A.E. (1973). The reliability of the mental status questionnaire in geriatric practice. (Unpublished, cited in Wilson and Brass.)

Wilson Barnett, J. (1981). Assessment of recovery: with special reference to a study with post-operative cardiac patients. *Journal of Advanced Nursing*, 6: 435–45.

Wing, J.K. (1991). Measuring and classifying clinical disorders: learning from the PSE, in P.E. Bebbington (ed.) *Social psychiatry: theory, methodology and practice*. London: Transaction Publishers.

Wing, J.K., Cooper, J.E. and Sartorius, N. (1974). *The Measurement and Classification of Psychiatric Symptoms: An Instruction Manual for the PSE and catego program*. Cambridge, Cambridge University Press.

WHOQOL Group (1993). *Measuring quality of life: the development of the World Health Organization Quality of Life Instrument (WHOQOL)*. Geneva: World Health Organization.

WHOQOL Group (1995). The World Health Organization quality of life assessment (WHOQOL): position paper from the World Health Organization. Special Issue 'Quality of Life' in *Social Science and Medicine*, 10: 1403–9.

Wood, V., Wylie, M.L. and Scheafor, B. (1969). An analysis of a short self-report measure of life satisfaction: correlation with rater judgements. *Journal of Gerontology*, 24: 465–9.

World Health Organization (1958). *The First Ten Years. The Health Organization*. Geneva: World Health Organization.

World Health Organization (1979). *Handbook for Reporting Results of Cancer Treatments*. WHO Offset Publication No. 48. Geneva: World Health Organization.

World Health Organization (1980). *International Classification of Impairments, Disabilities and Handicaps*. Geneva: World Health Organization.

World Health Organization (1982). *Basic Documents* (32nd edition). Geneva: World Health Organization.

World Health Organization (1985). *Targets for Health for All by the Year 2000*. Copenhagen: World Health Organization. Regional Office for Europe.

World Health Organization (1992). *International Classification of Diseases* (10th edn). Vols. I–III. Geneva: World Health Organization.

World Health Organization (1994). *Quality of life assessment. An annotated bibliography*. Geneva: Division of Mental Health, World Health Organization.

Wylie, C.M. and White, B.K. (1964). A measure of disability. *Archives of Environmental Health*, 8: 834–9.

Wylie, M.L. (1970). Life satisfaction as a program impact criterion. *Journal of Gerontology*, 25: 36–40.

Wylie, R.C. (1974). *The Self Concept*. Lincoln, NE, University of Nebraska Press.

Yates, J.W., Chalmer, B. and McKegney, F.P. (1980). Evaluation of patients with advanced cancer using the Karnofsky Performance Status. *Cancer*, 45: 2220–4.

Zigmond, A.S. and Snaith, R.P. (1983). The Hospital Anxiety and Depression Scale. *Acta Psychiatrica Scandinavica*, 67: 361–70.

Ziller, R., Hagey, J., Smith, M.D. *et al.* (1969). Self-esteem: a social construct. *Journal of Consulting and Clinical Psychology*, 33: 84–95.

Ziller, R.C. (1974). Self-other orientations and quality of life. *Social Indicators Research*, 1: 301–27.

Zubrod, C.G., Schneiderman, M., Frei, E. *et al.* (1960). Appraisal of methods for the study of chemotherapy of cancer in man: Comparative therapeutic trial of nitrogen mustard and triethylene thiophosphoramide. *Journal of Chronic Diseases*, 11: 7–33.

Zung, W.W.K. (1965). A self-rating depression scale. *Archives of General Psychiatry*, 12: 63–70.

Zung, W.W.K. (1967). Depression in the normal aged. *Psychosomatics*, 8: 287–92.

Zung, W.W.K. (1972). The Depression Status Inventory: An adjunct to the self-rating depression scale. *Journal of Clinical Psychology*, 28: 539–43.

Zung, W.W.K. (1986). Zung Self-Rating Depression Scale and Depression Status Inventory, in N. Sartorius and T.A. Ban (eds) *Assessment of Depression*. Heidelberg: Springer-Verlag.

Zung, W.W.K., Richards, C.B. and Short, M.J. (1965). Self rating depression scale in an out-patient clinic: further validation of the ZDS. *Archives of General Psychiatry*, 13: 508–15.

INDEX

MEASURING DISEASE

Ann Bowling

This book is intended to supplement the author's previous work *Measuring Health: A Review of Quality of Life Measurement Scales*. In assessing the outcomes of disease and treatments, measurement scales must be relevant to their specific effects. Generic health related quality of life, or health status, scales will need to be supplemented with, or replaced by, disease specific items and scales.

Some specialities, particularly in psychiatry and cancer, have made considerable progress in the development of disease specific scales of quality of life. Others still use batteries of single domain and generic measures in the assessment of quality of life. There is now considerable interest in measures which go beyond one dimensional assessments, and which are also highly sensitive to specific disease and treatment effects.

This book reviews disease specific measures of quality of life and, where appropriate, pertinent symptom and single domain scales which are still sometimes used to supplement them. It is intended as a source book for health services researchers, health care professionals, and others who are involved in the measurement of outcome of therapies in relation to broader health status and quality of life.

Contents
Preface – Health-related quality of life: a discussion of the concept, its use and measurement – Cancers – Psychiatric conditions and psychological morbidity – Respiratory conditions – Neurological conditions – Rheumatological conditions – Cardiovascular diseases – Other disease- and condition-specific scales – Comments on measurement issues and sources of information – Appendix: a selection of useful scale distributors and addresses – References – Index.

400pp   0 335 19225 4 (paperback)